Cla Insel.

DIAGNOSTIC METHODS IN VETERINARY MEDICINE

By the same Author

INTRODUCTION TO VETERINARY
THERAPEUTICS

FIRST PUBLISHED 1952

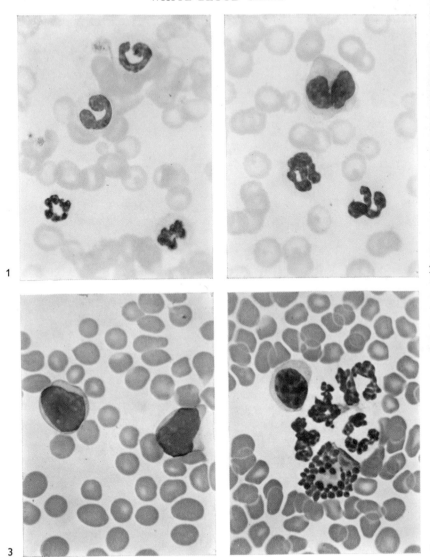

1. DOG : Neutrophils, Non-lobulated, Lobulated.
2. DOG : Monocyte, Lobulated neutrophils.
3. COW : Lymphocytes.
4. HORSE : Lymphocyte, Lobulated, Neutrophils and Eosinophil.

Leishman. Approx. × 1000.

DIAGNOSTIC METHODS IN VETERINARY MEDICINE

BY

GEO. F. BODDIE, B.Sc. (Edin.), M.R.C.V.S., F.R.S.E.

WILLIAM DICK PROFESSOR OF VETERINARY MEDICINE, EDINBURGH UNIVERSITY
(ROYAL DICK SCHOOL OF VETERINARY STUDIES)

WITH A CHAPTER ON
DIAGNOSIS OF POULTRY DISEASES
BY J. G. CAMPBELL, D.Sc., Ph.D., F.R.C.V.S.
POULTRY RESEARCH CENTRE, KING'S
BUILDINGS, EDINBURGH

FIFTH EDITION

OLIVER AND BOYD
EDINBURGH AND LONDON
1962

OLIVER AND BOYD LTD.
Tweeddale Court
Edinburgh

39A Welbeck Street
London, W. 1

FIRST EDITION . . . 1944
SECOND EDITION . . 1946
THIRD EDITION . . 1950
REPRINTED . . . 1953
FOURTH EDITION . . 1956
FIFTH EDITION . . 1962

PRINTED AND PUBLISHED IN GREAT BRITAIN BY
OLIVER AND BOYD LTD., EDINBURGH

PREFACE TO FIFTH EDITION

IN preparing the fifth edition of this work, the text has been extensively revised. This has entailed a large number of changes throughout the book. Major changes have been made in the section dealing with the digestive system in cattle.

That part of the book dealing with clinical laboratory methods has been re-cast. In the course of this re-arrangement the chapter on the techniques used in clinical chemistry has been revised and somewhat extended, while that on clinical hæmatology has been curtailed to a description of techniques. These chapters are followed by a new chapter on the application and interpretation of clinical laboratory methods as an aid to diagnosis.

A colour frontispiece showing the various forms of white blood cell serves to illustrate the re-cast chapter on clinical hæmatology.

Dr. J. G. Campbell has revised the chapter on the diagnosis of poultry diseases.

I am indebted to Mr. E. A. McPherson for his help in revising the chapter dealing with allergic reactions and to Mr. H. S. McTaggart for his help in revising the chapter on clinical helminthology.

I wish to thank Mr. R. Brown, my chief technician, and Mr. R. Hood, Head of the Photography Department in the Royal (Dick) School of Veterinary Studies for the production of the colour photo-micrographs used in making the frontispiece.

G. F. B.

EDINBURGH
August 1961

CONTENTS

ILLUSTRATIONS

CHAPTER I

INTRODUCTION

General Discussion
Development of Symptoms and Signs
    Disease—Lesion—Functional Disturbance—Symptoms—Signs
Methods of Examination
    Inspection—Palpation—Percussion—Auscultation. Smell. Other
    diagnostic procedures

GENERAL DISCUSSION

THE wide scope of veterinary science, including as it does all the domestic animals, presents the veterinary clinician with a great diversity of problems in diagnosis. While diagnostic methods may be equally applicable to the various animal species that the veterinarian is called upon to examine, the anatomical, physiological and pathological differences between them modify the results obtained by the application of these diagnostic methods to animals of different species.

As the economic and national importance of veterinary science depends principally on the service rendered to the community by securing and maintaining the health of farm animals, attention to the needs of smaller pet animals must occupy a subsidiary, though not unimportant, position. But it is well to bear in mind that the preservation of the health of pet animals is essential to the safety of the community that houses them ; further, the good health of these animals may be a useful factor in maintaining the morale and happiness of the populace.

The basis of the study of clinical methods must be a sound knowledge of anatomy, physiology and pathology, as well as an intimate acquaintance with the appearance and behaviour of the animal in normal health. Some of this knowledge can be acquired in the class room, dissecting room and laboratory, but at least part of it can only be secured by actually working with the various species of animals ; it follows that a period of some months spent living and working on a farm must form an essential part of the preliminary education of the veterinary student.

Only when he has become familiar with the normal animals that are to be his patients, should the student turn his attention to the abnormal. In the lecture room and laboratory he learns of the causes of disease and the changes that take place in the tissue as a result of disease processes. In clinical science there is to be found the means of co-relating these processes with the deviations from normal health that permit the existence and character of abnormalities to be recognised and identified in the

A

living animal. In many instances it is a matter of importance that what appear to be relatively minor deviations from the normal are promptly and correctly interpreted. This can only be done if the individual clinician is intimately familiar with his patients in good health as well as in ill health.

DIAGNOSIS may be defined as the art of recognising a disease and of distinguishing it from other diseases. The first essential step in dealing with any disease must be the establishment of a diagnosis, for the nature of treatment, control measures and prophylaxis all depend on the diagnosis.

To-day preventive medicine is an extremely important part of the activities of veterinary science. There is every reason to believe that there will be a great extension of the section of veterinary science devoted to the maintenance of animal health. This service to the community entails the control of epidemics and the prevention of their development by means of the provision of immunity where possible, and by means of hygienic and veterinary police measures. In some instances the cause of disease is found to be a dietetic deficiency, correction of this will remedy the condition. Methods applicable to one disease may not be effective in dealing with another, so each disease or outbreak of disease necessitates the selection of methods that have been found to be most suitable to treat, control, or prevent that disease. This selection can only take place after an accurate diagnosis has been formed. The diagnosis in most cases is made in the first instance on one individual animal, thereafter its existence in other animals in the herd or flock may be confirmed. Obviously diagnosis in cases of this kind is the determining factor in deciding the procedure to be adopted, and so the development of preventive medicine has emphasised more than ever the importance of diagnosis, and it might even be contended that accuracy in diagnosis is of greater economic importance in the control and prevention of epidemics than in the treatment of individual cases.

Diagnosis in any animal—including man—may be difficult, but there are certain inherent difficulties in veterinary diagnosis that are either absent or not frequently so pronounced in the case of human patients. The veterinarian's patients do not co-operate with the clinician in his endeavour to determine the site and nature of disease, in consequence the clinician is entirely dependent on his own powers of observation ; further, on account of fear or pain caused by the examination, the patient may actually obstruct the examination. The circumstances in which the animal is placed may not be conducive to a satisfactory examination : the byre or stable may be dark, the animal may be loose in a field, and, before an examination can be made, it is necessary to catch it and secure it, thereby greatly exciting and disturbing it. Most of these difficulties can be overcome or greatly reduced by the exercise of patience and perseverance. Quietness, and as far as possible, gentleness in handling the animal will be found of material assistance in securing a thorough and satisfactory examination of the patient.

The clinical examination of the patient may in many cases reveal the nature of the malady from which the animal is suffering, but in other cases it is necessary to employ one or more of the various aids to diagnosis that are available. It is usually found that the nature of the aid to be employed will be indicated by the findings of the clinical examination ; some of these aids may be applied by the practitioner himself, but others require the facilities provided in a laboratory. The veterinarian very frequently requires to make use of allergic reactions, such as tuberculin and mallein tests : these tests are employed not only as an aid to diagnosis in an individual clinical case, but as they can be employed to detect non-clinical cases are also an essential part of any scheme for the eradication of tuberculosis and glanders. The eradication of glanders from Great Britain was made possible by the mallein test used as a means of detection of animals infected with that disease. It was by means of the mallein test that glanders was kept under control in the British Army in the war of 1914-1918, and by means of the tuberculin test that bovine tuberculosis has been eliminated from several countries in various parts of the world.

The identification of the causal organism may in some cases be the only means of establishing a diagnosis ; thus the diagnosis of anthrax in cattle is dependent on the demonstration of *Bacillus anthracis* in the blood ; the presence of tuberculosis of the udder can only be determined with complete certainty by the demonstration of *Mycobacterium tuberculosis* in milk withdrawn from the affected quarter or quarters. While the veterinary practitioner may himself carry out a microscopic examination for tubercle bacillus, he will often find it necessary to submit material to a biological test, and for this purpose material is forwarded to a bacteriological laboratory and is there injected into guinea-pigs. In order to differentiate the various forms of bovine mastitis a bacteriological examination of the secretion from the affected quarter of the udder is required.

The physical and chemical analysis of a specimen of urine is not only of value in the diagnosis of disease of the urinary system, but frequently provides valuable information regarding the functional activity of other tissues. Thus the diagnosis of diabetes mellitus in the dog is dependent on the findings of a urine analysis. Diseased states of the liver may produce changes in the blood and urine.

Helminth infestations, especially in cattle, sheep and horses, may necessitate the examination of fæces and the estimation of the number of eggs present in a given weight of fæces. The diagnosis of parasitic skin diseases is dependent upon the demonstration of the causal parasite. For this purpose skin scrapings are prepared and examined microscopically.

It may be necessary to submit blood to a bacteriological laboratory for agglutination tests before a suspected diagnosis can be confirmed ; this is the method employed in the diagnosis of bovine contagious abortion and in the detection of hens that are carriers of the causal organism of bacillary white diarrhœa in chickens. Complement fixation tests are for instance used in the diagnosis of Johne's Disease.

Radiological examination of veterinary patients for purely medical reasons are largely confined to the smaller animals and are only regularly conducted in the dog and cat.

Biochemical examination of the blood, with a view to determining the amount of certain constituents present in comparison with normal, may be required to establish with certainty a diagnosis that is otherwise doubtful. Thus an accurate estimate of the hæmoglobin content of the blood may prove of value in the diagnosis of anæmia. On the other hand, in a disease such as hypo-magnesiæmia of cattle, it is necessary to form a diagnosis on the clinical signs, and carry out treatment at once, for to be successful treatment must be prompt in application. But with a view to confirming the existence of the hypo-magnesiæmia, samples of blood must be taken and forwarded to a biochemical laboratory, these samples being taken not only from the animal or animals that are obviously ill but also from other animals at risk, i.e. animals of the same sex and age exposed to the same environment as those that are ill. If the presence of a hypo-magnesiæmia is confirmed appropriate steps, such as feeding a mineral supplement rich in magnesium, may then be taken to prevent the occurrence of further cases. The accurate diagnosis of trace element deficiencies in ruminants can only be achieved by the demonstration that the quantity of the element in soil and herbage is below the normal figure. On the other hand it is often useful to apply what has come to be known as " test therapy." That is to say specific treatment for the suspected condition is applied and if recovery takes place some confirmation of the suspected diagnosis is obtained. A satisfactory response to " test therapy " in an individual animal is not necessarily conclusive but effective response to the group application of " test therapy " obviously carries more conviction.

Red blood cell counts, hæmoglobin estimations and hæmatocrit readings provide the information that may be required in the investigation of cases of anæmia. Differential white cell counts are helpful in the diagnosis of occult infected processes and in the diagnosis of some diseases such as leukæmia and lymphosarcoma, and for a differentiation between myeloid and lymphatic leukæmia.

Finally, it may be that an irrefutable diagnosis cannot be established in a particular case until a post-mortem examination has been made. Even when that post-mortem examination has been made it may be necessary for chemical analysis of tissues and bowel contents to be conducted ; and it may also be necessary for material to be examined by a pathologist and bacteriologist before the final diagnosis can be reached. Thus in lead poisoning, as neither the symptoms nor clinical signs nor the post-mortem findings are conclusive, a chemical analysis is required to complete the diagnosis. The distinction between a chronic inflammatory growth and a tumour may only be achieved by the microscopic examination of sections of the tissue. Reference has already been made to the value of bacteriological examinations in diagnosis.

Among domestic animals it may be necessary to make a post-mortem examination before the diagnosis of an enzootic disease can be confirmed. The existence of swine fever may be suspected on account of the history of the case, the symptoms and clinical signs, but a post-mortem examination, to demonstrate the characteristic lesions of the disease, is essential to diagnosis. In helminth infestations in sheep, such as liver fluke in ewes, a post-mortem examination may prove the simplest and most accurate method of diagnosis of the disease affecting the flock as a whole.

With such a diversity of aids to diagnosis available to the practitioner, their effective utilisation can only be obtained if the clinical examination is conducted in a methodical manner. It is obviously unlikely to lead to accuracy in diagnosis if the assistance of first one of these aids and then another is sought, until finally a tentative diagnosis is reached by the method of trial or error. It is therefore of the utmost importance that the criteria for the application of laboratory tests and diagnosis should be thoroughly understood. It is equally important that the interpretation to be placed on the results of the various tests should be clearly appreciated. Careful and methodical examination, coupled with a knowledge of the information to be obtained from the individual diagnostic aids will lead to their profitable utilisation. It must be borne in mind that these aids to diagnosis are not short-cuts providing an easy way to diagnosis. The basis of all diagnosis is still to be found in the clinical examination of the patient.

DEVELOPMENT OF SYMPTOMS AND SIGNS

DISEASE has been defined as an injurious deviation from the normal. This deviation may consist of an organic change in the tissue of an organ, or the deviation may consist of a functional disturbance with no obvious organic change. Lobular pneumonia obviously involves an organic change of the lung tissue, whereas cardiac arrhythmia may appear to be a functional disturbance of the heart because the organic change causing it cannot be demonstrated by an ordinary clinical examination but it may be demonstrated by an electrocardiograph; nevertheless in both instances the deviation from the normal is injurious to the patient.

LESION.—Pathological change in an organ or in part of the tissue of that organ leads to the production of a *lesion*. Lesions on the surface of the body may be seen and handled as, for example, the oedematous swelling of the limb of a horse suffering from acute sporadic lymphangitis. On the other hand, the lesion may be situated in a tissue within the body in such a position that it can neither be seen nor palpated in the living animal, for example, the lesion of chronic interstitial nephritis in the dog. Macroscopic lesions can be seen by the naked eye, but frequently important lesions are only microscopic in character ; even in macroscopic lesions it may be necessary to study the tissue microscopically to appreciate the nature and character of the lesion. The disease process leading to the production of these lesions may be the result of either inflammation or neoplasm (tumour). If the process be inflammatory in character it may be suppurative or non-suppurative ; if the process is one of tumour growth the tumour may be benign or malignant in character.

The presence in any organ or tissue of a lesion inevitably interferes with its normal function. In some organs the presence of even a very small lesion has serious effects on the animal, but in other organs the lesion may attain considerable dimensions before sufficiently interfering with the function of the organ concerned to cause effects that will be noticeable to the observer ; thus extensive damage to the liver may occur before the animal is noticed to be in any way ill ; chronic inter-stitial nephritis is usually present in a dog for some considerable time before its presence is clinically manifest.

FUNCTIONAL DISTURBANCE.—The disturbance of function, that results from the presence in an organ of a lesion, leads to the appearance of symptoms and clinical signs by means of which it is possible to recognise and identify disease. Similarly, functional disturbances that occur in organs within the body, without any gross lesions in the tissue of the organ concerned, give rise to symptoms and clinical signs by which their presence is revealed.

A SYMPTOM is any evidence that indicates the presence of disease. There is some difference of opinion in regard to the classification of symptoms and their differentiation from clinical signs.

Under one system symptoms are classified as subjective symptoms and objective symptoms. Subjective symptoms are those that are perceptible to the patient only ; therefore, no subjective symptoms are available to the veterinary clinician. Objective symptoms are those that are obvious to the senses of the observer. Under this system the symptomatology of a disease is divided into (1) THE SYMPTOMS, being those objective symptoms that are seen by the lay observer, and (2) THE CLINICAL SIGNS, being those objective signs that are appreciated only by the veterinary clinician.

Under the other system all symptoms are regarded as being sub-jective and therefore none fall to be considered in veterinary medicine, all evidence of disease being classified under the heading of CLINICAL SIGNS or more briefly SIGNS. This system has the merits of brevity and clarity.

Under the first system evidence of disease is considered under the two headings exemplified below but under the second system the evidence is considered under the one heading of clinical signs.   In order to avoid any confusion as between symptoms and signs all recognisable manifestations of disease may be dealt with under a common and simple heading CLINICAL FINDINGS.

(1) *Symptoms.*—When an animal becomes ill it attracts attention to itself by alterations in its behaviour that vary in character in the different species of animals, and also according to the nature of the illness from which the animal is suffering.   A horse affected with colic shows evidence of the pain it is suffering by pawing at the ground with the fore feet, lying down, rolling and groaning ; it may also break out in a sweat. A cow suffering from a comparable digestive disturbance tends to present a dull, stupid appearance, the only active action drawing attention to itself being a grunt or groan.   A cow suffering from foot and mouth disease may be noticed lame and long strings of ropy saliva are hanging from the mouth, which is being constantly opened and shut with a characteristic smacking sound.   A pig with foot and mouth disease will be noticed to be acutely lame, but evidence of mouth lesions is seldom seen.   As has been said, when on the surface of the body the lesion may be examined directly and its nature determined.   But attention may be drawn to the presence of the lesion by an alteration in the function, or the product of the function of the organ involved, thus alteration in the appearance of a cow's milk draws attention to the presence of mastitis in that udder, and examination of the udder will reveal the character and extent of the lesion in the udder.   These deviations from the normal may be discerned by any observer and constitute the symptoms of the disease.

(2) *Clinical Signs.*—When the veterinarian carries out a clinical examination of his patient after observing the symptoms, he endeavours to determine the presence of further evidence that will indicate to him the nature of the disease process.   If, however, the lesion is situated within the body it may be impossible directly to examine it, but a knowledge of the symptoms and clinical signs that arise from the presence of a lesion in the organ, make it possible to recognise the presence of that lesion.   Thus the symptoms in pneumonia include coughing, respiratory distress, loss of appetite and rigors.   Clinical examination of the animal reveals acceleration of pulse, elevation of temperature, the respiratory movement fast and shallow.   Physical examination of the chest reveals abnormalities characteristic of pneumonia.   The evidence obtained by the general examination and physical examination of the chest constitutes the clinical signs of this disease.   The rational understanding of the significance of clinical signs must be based on a sound knowledge of clinical pathology.

METHODS OF EXAMINATION

The clinical examination of patients necessitates the utilisation of various methods of examination. As interrogation of the patient is not possible in the domestic animals, the veterinarian is entirely dependent on his ability to ascertain by clinical examination the details of each case. It should be realised that each method of examination provides certain possibilities and also possesses certain limitations. These methods are applicable to both the preliminary general examination of the patient and the detailed examination of the individual body systems that will become necessary following on the information obtained by the preliminary general examination. In all these methods continued practice will greatly increase the amount and value of the information to be obtained by them in the examination of the patient. The student must assiduously practise the methods for himself as no demonstration can take the place of his individual efforts to master them.

These methods are as follows :

I. INSPECTION.—Inspection entails, in the first place, a visual examination of the whole animal, this being described as a general inspection. Subsequently this visual examination is extended to include a detailed inspection of individual tissues and organs.

II. PALPATION.—The act of handling the tissues. Palpation consists of the application of firm but gentle pressure with the fingers ; one or both hands may be employed. By palpation information may be obtained regarding the presence or absence of pain in particular tissues. If pain is present it may be possible, by palpation, to determine a point where there is the maximum intensity of pain. By palpation it may be possible to demonstrate abnormalities in shape, size, or consistency of organs or tissues.

III. PERCUSSION.—The act of striking a short sharp blow on a part of the body, with the object of provoking an audible response that will provide information regarding the condition of the parts of the body beneath the point being struck. When the part is struck directly with the finger tips, the procedure is termed *Immediate Percussion*. When the fingers of one hand are laid flat on the part concerned and the blow is struck on these fingers with the other hand, the procedure is termed *Mediate Percussion*. The fingers lying on the part must be maintained in the same relative position to the part, otherwise the character of the sound will be altered. Percussion may be carried out with vigour when it is known as *Strong Percussion* ; it may be carried out gently when it is known as *Weak Percussion*.

In place of the fingers percussion may be performed with two instruments known as a *plexor* and *pleximeter*. The plexor is a form of hammer used to strike the pleximeter, which is a circular disc with a small rim round the edge, this being laid flat on the part with the hollow side next to the skin. There is considerable difference of opinion among veterinary clinicians as to the advantage to be gained in the examination of the domestic animals by the use of the plexor and pleximeter instead of the fingers.

It should be realised that the thick coat and the heavy chest or abdominal wall in some of the domestic animals may mitigate against percussion providing the measure of information that might be desired.

IV. AUSCULTATION.—The act of listening to the sounds produced by functional activity in various parts of the body. Auscultation may be carried out by direct application of the ear to the part. There are obvious objections to this method; the friction between the clinician's own tissues and the animal's coat may create abnormal sounds interfering with the examination. The animal's coat may be soiled with dirt or skin secretions, it may be wet with rain or sweat, or the skin may be infested with parasites, such as lice or mange mites or ringworm. It is, therefore, preferable to use a *stethoscope*. After the technique of using the stethoscope has been mastered, it will be found that much more accurate results are obtained by its use than by the naked ear.

The most satisfactory and most suitable form of stethoscope for veterinary practice is the binaural type. The chest piece should be fitted with a rubber cover so that the hard ebonite portion does not come directly into contact with the hairs of the animal's coat, as the friction so created produces sounds that simulate some of the adventitious sounds that develop in the lungs in pneumonia. For similar reasons friction between the rubber tubing and the operator's clothes must be avoided. As there is little benefit in elaborate stethoscopes with complex fittings the student is advised to purchase a simple but reasonably robust instrument. The single wooden stethoscope is of very little value in veterinary practice, as the friction sounds caused by the contact between it and the animal's coat are exaggerated by the instrument; it is also an added disadvantage that only one ear is utilised.

The *phonendoscope* is an instrument used for auscultation that differs from a stethoscope in that the chest piece contains a diaphragm which is placed in contact with the patient's skin. The advantages of greater sensitivity produced by this diaphragm are to some extent counteracted by the friction sounds produced between the diaphragm and the hairs of the coat. The phonendoscope is, however, a very useful instrument in the detection and localisation of abnormal heart sounds.

V. USE OF SENSE OF SMELL.—The methods already described require the use of the senses of sight, touch and hearing. The sense of smell is frequently of value to the veterinary surgeon in that certain diseases are associated with the development of characteristic odours. The recognition of these odours may be of some assistance in diagnosis.

VI. OTHER DIAGNOSTIC PROCEDURES.—The site of the disease process may preclude a direct approach by means of any of the methods of examination just described. In order to overcome this, special diagnostic procedures are adopted. These include the passage of sounds and catheters, exploratory puncture, rectal examination, the use of the œsophagoscope and ophthalmoscope and radiological examination. In addition to these special diagnostic procedures laboratory aids to diagnosis are employed. These include chemical, hæmatological, bacteriological and parasitological examinations.

CHAPTER II

PRELIMINARY GENERAL EXAMINATION

THE clinical examination entails first a preliminary general examination of the patient and then a detailed examination of the individual systems and regions of the body. The preliminary general examination is designed so that the general condition of the animal may be determined and an indication obtained as to the systems and regions of the body that are principally involved in the disease process. In the domestic animals the absence of subjective symptoms makes the preliminary general examination of outstanding importance as it is by this means that the veterinary clinician is able to obtain a correctly proportioned view of the case as a whole as well as arriving at a conclusion of the site or sites of the disease. It is a fundamental truth that no disease is so local in character that only one organ or tissue is involved. Though the lesion may appear discrete and entirely localised, secondary effects will inevitably occur in both neighbouring and remote tissues. The extent of these secondary effects must be determined if an accurate diagnosis is to be accomplished, and this can be secured if the preliminary general examination is conducted thoroughly and methodically.

The owner's complaint, details of the patient, and the history of the case may be obtained before proceeding to make any examination of the animal, but it is often convenient to conduct the necessary enquiries whilst making a general inspection of the patient.

OWNER'S COMPLAINT

Frequently the owner's complaint is readily vouchsafed or may have been included in the message asking professional attendance. If it is not thus forthcoming it may be obtained by a suitable query. It is wise to avoid a direct question such as, " What is wrong with the animal ? " if for no other reason than that it may provoke the retort that the owner would have had no need to call in professional assistance had he known what was wrong.

Sometimes the owner's complaint takes the form of a statement of his opinion as to the nature of the illness. This may or may not be correct, and obviously should not be accepted as of any significance beyond indicating the possible general nature of the case. It is well to remember that such opinions on the part of the owner are sometimes very wide of the mark, and would be most misleading if too much attention were paid to them.

History

The history is usually obtained by discreet questioning from the owner of the animal or the person in attendance on it. Care must be taken to avoid asking leading questions that may encourage the person giving the history to make statements that have no real foundation on fact. In many instances a satisfactory history containing all the relevant details is readily obtained from the owner or animal attendant. It is well for the student to bear in mind that many stockmen are very careful and accurate observers, and frequently the history obtained from such a person is of great assistance in diagnosis. It may be that the history contains much irrelevant detail : this is particularly so when dealing with a verbose individual. It will be necessary to sift such a history and separate the relevant from the irrelevant; but care must be exercised in checking verbosity on the part of the individual giving the history, in case, as a result of such action, important details are withheld.

In the majority of cases the history given is reasonably accurate, but, on occasion, it may be coloured by the person's own idea of the case. When this has been done it usually becomes obvious in the course of discussion that such preconceived ideas exist, and their possible influence on the history can be realised. It is exceptional to find that a deliberately untrue history has been given, but this may be done to cover the effects of incompetence, negligence, or fraudulent action. Frequently the fact that the history is untrue is revealed by contradictory statements contained in it. Or it may be revealed during the clinical examination of the patient that the history is not consistent with the clinical findings. Probably the most common inaccuracy encountered in case histories is the claim that the illness is of recent origin when it is obvious that the diseased state must have been present for a very considerable time. It should, however, be remembered that many diseased states in the domestic animals are for a long time only obvious to a skilled observer.

The inarticulate person presents a difficulty when endeavouring to obtain the history. It is frequently profitable to indulge in a little general conversation before bringing the discussion round to the case in point, and if this is done gradually a satisfactory history may be obtained.

Misconceptions due to ignorance on the part of the individual from whom the history is sought may lead to statements that, if accepted, would be grossly misleading. Fortunately such statements are often so glaringly impossible that their true character is readily appreciated. The history in any case may refer only to a single animal, but frequently in veterinary medicine the history must extend to the other animals of the stud, herd or flock.

The history of a case is divisible into two main parts, (1) the past history and (2) the immediate history.

Past History.—In respect of an individual animal information is sought as to previous illness, previous pregnancies and any complications arising from such pregnancies. Such information may be of assistance in diagnosis in that it may indicate the presence of acquired weaknesses that render the animal more susceptible to disease affecting the tissues previously involved.

In regard to the herd history various points may suggest possible sources of infection or causes of illness. The term epidemiology covers the history in so far as it relates to contagious or infectious diseases. The introduction into the herd of new animals, especially if they have passed through markets, may well prove to be the source of an outbreak of infectious disease. The presence of epidemics in the neighbourhood or in the case of disease such as foot and mouth disease, even in a relatively remote neighbourhood, is of importance in that it raises the possibility of such a disease being present in the animal or animals that are to be examined. The history of the herd may indicate that some condition is present that is proving deleterious to the animals in the herd. A history of unexplained sudden deaths in cattle may suggest the existence of anthrax in the herd ; deaths among sows, or the failure of a number of breeding sows to produce and rear their litters may be due to the presence of chronic swine fever in the piggery.

An outbreak of disease may be found to affect several species, thus foot and mouth disease affects cattle, sheep and pigs, but not horses, or it may be found that the disease is confined to one species of animal, for instance, contagious pustular dermatitis of sheep (orf). It may be that a particular age group of animals only is affected, as is the case in outbreaks of piglet influenza and necrotic enteritis, both of these diseases affecting young pigs only. Lamb dysentery affects lambs in the first fortnight of their life, pulpy kidney affects lambs in the period from six to sixteen weeks of age, and braxy occurs in young sheep in their first autumn and winter. One group of animals only may have been exposed to infection, in consequence disease is limited to that group. In some diseases certain signs tend to be predominant in one species, whereas in other species these signs are less marked ; in foot and mouth disease salivation is profuse in cattle but not so profuse in sheep and absent in pigs ; lameness is always very noticeable in sheep and pigs suffering from foot and mouth disease.

The character of the feeding may be sufficient to cause a number of cases of digestive disturbance : the knowledge that the previous harvest was a bad one may be a useful pointer to the quality of the home-grown foodstuffs. Changes of foodstuffs, especially if sudden, may lead to what appears to be, and indeed almost amounts to, an outbreak of epidemic illness. It is important to realise that a change in foodstuff or an increase in food intake may activate what is sometimes termed the " trigger mechanism." Thus an outbreak of pulpy kidney in lambs or entero-toxæmia in older sheep caused by *Clostridium welchii* (Type D) often follows the sudden increase in food intake. Even a complete change of pasture may be sufficient to cause serious mischief ; cases of grass tetany in cattle may appear suddenly after a change of pasture. The knowledge that an antibiotic supplement has been fed to pigs may be relevant in the investigation of an outbreak of diarrhœa in the piggery.

When acquiring the past history it is necessary to obtain information concerning the geographical incidence of disease. Thus louping ill, affecting principally sheep and cattle, is confined to clearly delineated areas.

Seasonal incidence also has a bearing on the probable nature of the disease being investigated. Grass sickness of horses is mostly encountered during the height of summer, parasitic bronchitis of cattle is a disease of summer and autumn, while louping ill occurs following the period of seasonal activity of the ticks that transmit the causal virus. Climatic conditions may influence the incidence of helminth disease in grazing animals. This is exemplified by the increased prevalence of liver fluke infestation in cattle and sheep during the autumn and winter following a wet summer.

Immediate History.—The immediate history deals with the present case and should be as complete as is possible.

First, it is necessary to ascertain when the present illness developed, and thereby it is possible to assess the length of this illness. It is important that at this stage the clinician is informed as to whether one or more animals are involved.

It is desirable to enquire what symptoms the animal showed at the time the illness commenced and what other symptoms have subsequently been noticed. It will frequently be found that the person giving the history may omit symptoms that are of significance to the diagnostician. If it appears that any of these symptoms might have been present a direct question dealing with them may be addressed to the person in charge of the animal. Enquiries of this nature may deal with such symptoms as coughing, straining, frequent attempts at micturition, attacks of frenzy. Special attention must be paid to the previous existence of symptoms no longer in evidence.

The circumstances under which the illness developed may indicate certain possibilities ; thus in equine myohæmoglobinuria it is often found that the horse has been idle for a few days, but during that period received a full diet; when taken out it was in great spirits, but after going a short distance became acutely lame and began to sweat. In cases of colic in horses it is desirable to ascertain if any relation appears to exist between the onset of symptoms and the last meal or the period of work. The history may suggest a possible, or even probable, cause of the illness, but care is necessary in seeking information from the owner as to his opinion of such a cause lest a fictitious story be evolved.

It is important to ascertain whether the normal functional activities of life are being maintained or whether these are abnormal in any way, information being required in regard to appetite, thirst, defæcation, urination, rumination and lactation. In this connection, if not already dealt with under past history, enquiry should be made concerning the nature and quality of the foodstuffs being given to the animal.

Finally, it is necessary to try to find out what steps have been taken to deal with the condition. Previous cases may have been disposed of privily or publicly. The animal may have received some treatment, and some at least of the symptoms now exhibited may be due to the treatment and not to the original disease. Violent purgation may arise from an excessive dose of an active cathartic or from irritation of the bowel by a drastic remedy for worms. All too frequently the information obtained on this point is unreliable, as there may be a desire to hide the fact that an attempt has been made to treat the animal empirically.

DESCRIPTION OF ANIMAL

In the majority of cases encountered in practice, it is sufficient to obtain the description of the animal under the following headings :

Species and Breed.

Sex and Age.

Such a description supplies sufficient detail to enable the patient to be recognised at subsequent visits, and it fulfils a useful part in assisting diagnosis by narrowing the field of maladies to which that patient is susceptible ; but whenever there is any likelihood of it being necessary to grant a certificate, or when there is a possibility of litigation, the description of the animal requires to contain sufficient details to enable the animal to be accurately identified at a later date.

In the case of a horse this entails details of the height, colour, markings and distinguishing marks, such as brands on the hip, numbers tattooed on the upper gums. In pedigree cattle numbers are tattooed on the ears, and these numbers should be used in describing the animal in any document. A herd number is tattooed on one ear, and on the other ear a letter indicating the year of the animal's birth, followed by the animal's own pedigree number. A similar system may be employed for pedigree pigs.

The salient points that require to be considered under each of four headings may now be considered.

SPECIES.—The susceptibility of the individual species varies not only in regard to infectious and contagious diseases but also in regard to sporadic and functional diseases. Thus the horse tribe is susceptible to glanders, but cattle are immune. Cattle are susceptible to rinderpest but horses are not. On the other hand, all animals are susceptible to anthrax and rabies, though the incidence varies in the different species. In sheep *Cl. welchii* infections of different types occur in all ages of sheep.

Cardiac disease of cattle is encountered as cardiac palpitation, traumatic pericarditis and tuberculous pericarditis. Functional irregularity and cardiac dilatation represent the form of circulatory disturbance most common in the horse. In the dog, chronic valvular disease of the heart is present in a considerable proportion of adult and older dogs. Verrucose endocarditis due to chronic swine erysipelas, is the only important type of cardiac disturbance to which pigs are susceptible.

BREED.—In cattle the breed usually determines the purpose for which the animals are kept. Dairy cattle are particularly susceptible to diseases such as milk fever and acetonæmia (post-parturient dyspepsia) both of these diseases being relatively rare in the beef breeds. Both types of cattle are susceptible to grass tetany.

The breed determines the nature of the work a horse is likely to perform, and this may influence the development of various forms of disease. The breed also influences the susceptibility to certain types of disease, thus heavy-legged coarse-skinned horses are the subjects affected with symbiotic mange and seborrhœa, diseases not seen in light, thin-legged horses. Sporadic lymphangitis is practically unknown among arabs and ponies, but frequently seen in other breeds. All breeds of horses are equally susceptible to colic.

SEX.—It must be obvious that there are certain diseases to which only the members of one sex are susceptible. In the female it is necessary to take into consideration the connection of pregnancy with various diseases. Many febrile diseases in the female are due to disease of the uterus or udder. In cows an examination of the udder should always be made in cases of fever. In the male it is desirable to determine whether the animal is castrated or not. Strangulated hernia is not uncommon in stallions.

AGE.—Young animals are more susceptible to certain infectious diseases than adults. Intussusception is more common in foals than in adult horses. Septicæmia due to umbilical infection occurs only in very young animals. Rickets is a disease of young animals occurring prior to the union of the epiphyses. Lamb dysentery occurs in lambs under a fortnight old; pulpy kidney develops in forward lambs. Symptoms of helminthiasis are seldom seen in lambs less than one month old.

Old animals are particularly prone to circulatory disease, and in the dog chronic renal disease is usually seen in adult and elderly dogs.

GENERAL INSPECTION

A preliminary general examination of the patient commences with a general inspection of the patient, when any symptoms will be noted. The accurate observation of symptoms at this stage is of the utmost importance if an accurate picture of the case as a whole is to be obtained. It is frequently profitable before moving the animal at all to inspect it with a view to the observation of details that may not be noticeable after the animal has been disturbed by removing it from the stall, or by catching it if free in a box, courtyard, pen or field. This general inspection should be carried out at a distance of a few feet from the animal, and the animal should be viewed from all convenient angles, as any abnormality on one side may not be seen if the animal is viewed only from the opposite side. It is desirable that in conducting the general inspection a method be adopted and followed in all cases, though the exact order is a matter of personal preference.

APPEARANCE.—Any abnormality of conformation or stature must receive careful attention. Thus the deformity of the limbs caused by rickets in either a dog or pig will be appreciated when making a general inspection of the animal. Chronic swine fever in young pigs retards growth so that the animal has a stunted appearance, but the head is large in proportion to the rest of the body.

BEHAVIOUR.—The behaviour of the animal often provides a useful indication of the nature of the disease from which the animal is suffering. In the horse acute digestive disturbances give rise to the syndrome characteristic of colic, this being manifested by restlessness amounting in some cases to violence. In cattle acute digestive disturbances are characterised by dullness, and only in exceptional cases does the animal show signs of colic similar to the horse.

The animal may be dull, as is a horse suffering from sub-acute impaction of the colon, or it may be comatose, as is a cow suffering from milk fever ; on the other hand, the animal may be excited, as are some cows when suffering from lead poisoning. Muscular spasms may be noticed : these occur in cases of tetanus in all animals, and in chorea in the dog. General convulsions may be evident and develop in such diseases at the later stages of grass tetany in the cow and post-distemper encephalitis in the dog. The frenzy of a rabid dog is an outstanding example of grossly abnormal behaviour.

EXPRESSION.—Particular attention is paid to the facial appearance.

B

Wasting diseases lead to a particular type of woebegone, haggard expression that is rather characteristic; the "rocking horse" nostril appearance of a case of acute tetanus in the horse is easily recognised; and there is a peculiar, anxious expression on the face of a dog suffering from rabies.

The general appearance of the eye will be noticed at this stage, but a more detailed inspection is usually made later when a closer inspection of the animal is being made.

BODILY CONDITION.—The bodily condition is noticed. It is easy to distinguish between a fat animal and one that is emaciated, but the circumstances of the animal must be taken into account; an Ayrshire dairy cow is normally thin compared with a beef Shorthorn cow. In animals with a heavy coat or fleece emaciation may not be appreciated by visual inspection and so its existence may only be realised when the body surfaces are palpated. Actual emaciation usually indicates the presence of a chronic wasting disease, but it must be borne in mind that under certain conditions the domestic animals may lose bodily condition extremely rapidly. A cow with a painful suppurating hind foot, though in good bodily condition when the disease developed, may in a few days become very thin.

Among the more common causes of emaciation in cattle due to chronic disease may be mentioned tuberculosis, Johne's disease and so-called pine due to mineral deficiencies. In addition, the effect of parasitic helminths must be kept in mind. In the horse, besides many chronic diseases, parasitism, defective teeth and malnutrition cause grave loss of bodily condition. Horses can lose bodily condition very rapidly: a horse suffering from grass sickness in its chronic form, even though in good plump condition at the commencement of the illness, will in ten days or less become pitifully emaciated with every rib showing and the abdomen empty and completely tucked up. In sheep, chronic disease, mineral deficiency, parasitism and malnutrition all cause emaciation. In pigs, anæmia, helminthiasis and the chronic form of diseases such as swine fever and piglet influenza are common causes of emaciation.

SKIN AND COAT.—The state of the skin and coat will depend on whether the animal is housed, and also whether it has been groomed. Animals running out in winter have longer, rougher coats than those housed in warm buildings, but unless the coat is wet it is usually smooth and soft, though lacking the sleekness of the well-groomed house-fed animal. In cattle "lick marks" are often noticed on the coat; they are usually taken as an indication that the animal is in good health.

In febrile conditions the hairs of the coat tend to become erect, and in consequence the coat has a harsh staring appearance. In wasting diseases the coat has lost its lustre, has a dull lifeless appearance and can easily be pulled out. The presence of ectoparasites, such as lice, leads to itchiness, and by scratching and rubbing the hairs are broken and bald patches appear. Careful observation of an animal heavily infested with lice will often show fine twitching of the subcutaneous muscle. This may be particularly noticeable if the surface of the skin is being warmed by the rays of the sun or the heat from a fire.

Many skin diseases lead to the loss of hair and appearance of bald patches on the skin; among such conditions are mange, sheep scab, ringworm and eczema. The skin of a dog suffering from diabetes mellitus is particularly susceptible to the effects of minor injuries, and has little resistance to infection.

Discoloration of the skin can only readily be observed in pigs. In these animals it occurs as diffuse blotching in swine fever, as clearly defined areas in swine erysipelas and as cyanosis in any disease causing asphyxia.

Loss of hair may occur in certain metabolic disturbances. Pregnant and lactating bitches often lose a good deal of the hair of their coats and in consequence have a very shabby appearance. Similarly, sheep in spring, especially pregnant ewes, may lose some of the fleece. In sheep the specific disease known as scrapie leads to such intense pruritus that large parts of the fleece may be torn away. Wasting diseases of sheep such as Johne's disease and chronic progressive pneumonia frequently lead to considerable loss of wool.

In copper deficiency in black cattle the coat loses its normal colour and assumes a russet brown hue.

RESPIRATION.—The respiratory movements are now observed, disturbances in rate, depth and the character of the movement being noticed. Though it will probably not be possible to form an opinion as to the cause of the disturbance of respiration by these observations, a knowledge of their presence is essential to diagnosis.

The respiratory rate varies in the normal animal in proportion to its size and age. In very small animals and in very young animals the respiratory rate is fast. The respiratory rate is accelerated in the increased metabolism associated with fever. Diseases of the respiratory system that interfere with respiratory function cause marked changes in the respiratory rate.

The depth of the respiratory movement is determined by noting the excursion made by the ribs and abdominal muscles.

Certain respiratory movements are very characteristic, for instance, the double expiratory movement or "lift" of the horse suffering from chronic alveolar emphysema or broken wind, and the abdominal type of breathing associated with the early painful stages of pleurisy, in which the pleuritic line or ridge along the lower third of the chest wall may be discerned by inspection.

Acutely painful conditions in parts of the body remote from the respiratory system frequently cause profound alterations in the character of the respiratory movements. Thus in the early very painful stages of acute lymphangitis in the horse the respirations are so greatly accelerated that the condition superficially resembles acute congestion of the lungs. In acute abdominal catastrophes, such as volvulus, the respirations become short and shallow as well as extremely fast.

When inspecting the respiratory movements the presence and nature of any nasal discharge are also observed. During this part of the examination special attention is paid to the existence of a cough.

ABDOMEN.—Attention should be directed to the state of the abdomen ; this may be empty, replete or distended. Thus the presence of tympany of the rumen in bovines will be observed, or the acute distension of the abdomen of a horse suffering from tympanitic colic, or the pendulous abdomen of a dog affected with ascites.

In connection with the abdomen and alimentary system the clinician will ascertain whether his patient is feeding or not, and it may be of some significance if one animal in a group is not feeding when all the others are doing so. Similarly, in ruminants attention may be directed at this stage to whether rumination is being performed.

POSTURE.—The posture of the animal may supply much useful assistance in differential diagnosis. If the animal is recumbent it normally adopts a characteristic posture varying according to its species. But if found in an abnormal position this should be noticed. For example, a cow with milk fever may sit up on her sternum, but the neck is flexed and the head lies limply on her flank ; later she becomes more comatose, and if left alone will slide down on her side, where she lies with her legs stuck out stiffly and, owing to interference with the normal eructation of gas from the rumen, becomes tympanitic. If a recumbent animal is made to rise or attempts to rise, it will become evident whether it possesses normal control of its limbs or if it is suffering from partial or complete paraplegia.

The effect of some diseases is to make an animal adopt a characteristic posture. A horse suffering from tetanus may stand in a stiff manner with its four legs abducted from the body in such a way that the simile of a four-legged byre stool has been used to describe the appearance. The posture of a case of acute laminitis is due to the horse endeavouring to carry as much weight as possible on the hind feet to relieve the pressure on the acutely painful fore feet, so that the hind feet are carried forward under the body, and the fore feet are advanced in front of the body. In a case of acute lymphangitis the affected leg is held so that the toe just touches the ground, and while the limb may be used to assist balance, little or no weight is carried on it ; consequently the horse leans over to the unaffected side. A cow suffering from traumatic pericarditis stands with her elbows abducted so that she may relieve the pressure on the anterior part of the chest. In order to relieve the respiratory embarrassment that arises from the pressure of fluid on the lungs in tuberculous pleurisy, a dog will often sit erect for long periods. Horses with colic causing an increase in the intra-abdominal pressure frequently adopt the posture of urination.

Both horses and cattle affected with pneumonia remain standing, and only lie down when completely exhausted.

GAIT.—The gait of an animal when it is made to move may furnish the clinician with evidence that is vital to the completion of the diagnosis. The diagnosis of " shivering " in the horse is almost entirely dependent on the recognition of abnormalities in the gait, and in the performance of special movements, such as backing. The existence of tetanus may be suspected if a horse is noticed moving stiffly and no other adequate explanation of the stiffness can be found.

The stumbling gait encountered in the later stages of grass tetany in a cow may result in the cow falling forward in such a way as practically to turn a somersault. Cattle affected with pericarditis turn stiffly, holding the whole body rigidly. The disease of sheep known as louping ill produces in some cases a characteristic alteration in the gait, so that the sheep appears to progress forward by a succession of jumps. Sheep and cattle suffering from sturdy, caused by the presence within the cranium of the cystic stage of *Tænia multiceps*, may move in circles with the head turned towards the affected side. Sheep affected with scrapie adopt an unusually erect posture giving an exaggerated appearance of alertness.

The gait of a pig suffering from foot and mouth disease draws attention to the acute pain that it is suffering in all four feet.

ABNORMAL ACTIONS.—The clinician must be on the look-out for any abnormal actions on the part of the animal. Reference has already been made to the symptoms of colic in the horse, these attracting attention in virtue of their abnormality.

Tenesmus or straining may originate in the alimentary canal, in the urinary tract or in the genital tract. It is sometimes possible to determine by observation which system is involved, but in other cases it is necessary to carry out a clinical examination of the patient before doing so. Horses suffering from colic are often seen to posture and strain as though attempting to urinate. This may lead to the false impression that an obstruction is present in the urinary tract ; further examination will indicate that the case is one of colic.

Male dogs may posture in a similar manner to a bitch when attempting to urinate if the urethra is obstructed with a calculus ; a similar posture is sometimes adopted by a male dog suffering from cystitis. Frequent attempts to urinate may indicate obstruction of the urethra causing retention of the urine with acute distension of the bladder, or may indicate that, owing to irritation of the mucous membrane of the bladder and urethra, there is a continuous stimulation of the micturition reflex. Increased frequency of urination may result from polyuria that is itself a symptom of such diseases as diabetes insipidus in the horse or chronic interstitial nephritis in dogs. In diabetes mellitus in dogs the increased molecular concentration of the urine causes so great an augmentation of the volume of the urine that increased frequency is inevitable.

Abnormal actions due to nervous affections are best observed before the animal has been disturbed by a more detailed clinical examination. The animal may be hypersensitive as in tetany or strychnine poisoning when an exaggerated muscular response is given to afferent stimuli ; this response may be so pronounced as to amount to a convulsive seizure. Retraction of the angles of the mouth, giving a sardonic grin, is observed in diseases associated with local muscular spasm and is sometimes very noticeable in cases of tetanus.

Salivation, grinding of the teeth and unusual actions with the mouth will all attract attention to the existence of some abnormality in the mouth. Thus both cattle and sheep affected with foot and mouth disease salivate ; in this disease cattle working their mouths produce a sucking, smacking sound, and sheep an abrupt snapping noise.

Evidence of depraved appetite may be observed during the general inspection of the animal, when it is seen to pick up filth. In some cases attention is focussed on the depraved appetite by the history.

Yawning may be evidence of nausea associated with shock or hæmorrhage ; it is sometimes seen in cases of persistent indigestion. Lameness will have been observed when inspecting the animal's gait. Lameness is a leading sign in the differential diagnosis of diseases such as black quarter in cattle and sporadic lymphangitis in horses.

The movements of an animal that is choked will attract attention to the possible cause of the trouble. Coughing, though an abnormal act, has already received mention in the preliminary inspection of the respiratory system.

GENERAL CLINICAL EXAMINATION

Having completed the general inspection of the patient the practitioner now proceeds to make a general clinical examination. While, of course, he may wish to make a more detailed examination of some abnormality that has attracted his attention when making a general inspection, this should not deter him from carrying out the systematic examination now to be described. Particular attention should be paid to the response of the animal to the near approach of the clinician. Thus the animal may be in a hypersensitive state, or it may be in a dull, stupid condition. Allowance must be made for the reflex effects on pulse and respiration of the approach of a stranger in highly strung animals.

Visible Mucous Membranes

Inspection of the conjunctiva, the nasal mucous membrane and the mucous membrane of the mouth may provide much useful information. It is essential that this inspection be carried out in a good light, if need be the animal must be moved to the door or window, so that sufficient light be made available. Artificial light, but especially the yellow light of an oil lamp, may mask the slight yellow discoloration of the mucous membrane in a mild case of jaundice.

CONJUNCTIVA. The conjunctiva is examined by depressing and slightly everting the lower eyelid. The conjunctiva of both eyes must be examined, so that abnormalities due to local disease are appreciated as such and are not confused with general clinical signs. The appearance of the normal conjunctiva varies in the different domestic animals. In the horse the colour is pale roseate ; in cattle and sheep the conjunctival mucosa is paler than in the horse ; in the pig it is of a reddish tinge ; in the dog the conjunctiva much resembles that of the horse in colour ; in the cat the colour is pale. The student is advised to make himself familiar with the normal appearance of the conjunctiva of the different domestic animals. When inspecting the conjunctiva it is convenient to examine the eye as far as is necessary at this stage. Details are given later in this section.

Various changes in the conjunctival mucous membrane may be observed. The mucous membrane is pale and watery in appearance in case of anæmia, whether resulting from wasting diseases or due to defective blood formation. A pale blanched membrane is seen in shock and hæmorrhage. Intense injection of the conjunctiva may be associated with acute inflammatory conditions such as enteritis, encephalitis and acute pulmonary congestion. Cyanosis (bluish-grey discoloration) is observed whenever there is defective oxygenation of the blood, which may be due to a number of causes ; these chiefly involve either the lungs or the circulatory system. Staining of the mucous membrane with bile pigment, jaundice, is of a yellow colour varying from a slight orange tint to such an intense yellow that the mucosa almost appears to have a greenish tint. A bright pink œdematous condition of the conjunctiva is seldom seen in the domestic animals, except in the effusive form of equine influenza, known colloquially as " pink eye." Petechial hæmorrhages on the conjunctiva are found principally in association with diseases, such as purpura hæmorrhagica and glanders of the horse, or hæmorrhagic septicæmia of cattle.

The presence of any conjunctival discharge should be noted and its character observed. The discharge may be serous, mucoid, muco-purulent, or purulent in character. Such discharges are frequently of diagnostic significance, being associated with various specific diseases of the domestic animals, e.g., strangles of young horses, malignant catarrh of cattle, swine fever and canine distemper.

NASAL MUCOSA.—The nasal mucosa in the lower part of the nasal passages can be thoroughly inspected in horses ; the extent of inspection possible in cattle is limited, and comparatively little can be seen in the pig, dog and cat. Where possible, changes such as pallor, injection, discoloration, petechiation, or ulceration should be noticed. These changes are of comparable significance to those involving the conjunctiva. Ulceration of the nasal mucosa is an important and characteristic clinical sign of glanders in the horse.

The presence of nasal discharge is particularly significant, and both nostrils should be examined for its presence. A slight serous discharge from the nostrils may be the first obvious sign of the onset of one of the catarrhal fevers that affect domestic animals. Nasal discharges may have characters similar to those arising from the conjunctiva, but in addition foetid, hæmorrhagic and rusty nasal discharges are observed. A foetid nasal discharge may arise from diseased bone, diseased teeth, or empyema of the sinuses. When ulceration of the nasal mucosa has occurred the discharge is frequently hæmorrhagic. In purpura hæmorrhagica of the horse the nasal discharge is pale pink in colour and serous in character. In intense congestion of the lungs the nasal discharge may have a reddish-brown tinge due to the presence of blood-stained exudate. A rusty-coloured foetid discharge is observed in pulmonary gangrene.

MOUTH.—Examination of the mouth includes inspection of the mucous membrane and other tissues of the mouth, palpation of the tongue when necessary and the detection of abnormalities such as trismus.

Excessive salivation, if not already noticed during the general inspection of the animal, will now be appreciated. The inspection of the mouth should be directed towards elucidating the cause of excessive salivation. This may arise from local irritation such as ulceration, vesication, diseased conditions of the tongue, cheeks or jaws, or direct trauma in the mouth. Excessive salivation is an important symptom of foot and mouth disease in cattle.

Ulceration may arise from injuries due to defective teeth ; in the dog it occurs in toxæmia associated with acute nephritis, leptospiral infections, and acute vitamin deficiencies. It is also seen following the rupture of vesicles in foot and mouth disease. Ulceration of the buccal mucous membranes is seen in cattle in the condition known as mucosal disease. The ulcers are very superficial and heal rapidly. They are most easily seen on the mucosa below the dental pad and below the incisor teeth. Ulceration is present in well-established cases of actinobacillosis of cattle (wooden tongue), whether involving the tongue or soft structures of the mouth, such as the gums or cheeks. Ulceration occurs on the buccal mucous membrane in cases of actinomycosis involving the jaw.

Vesication, as has been already stated, may be a clinical sign of foot and mouth disease ; it may also be caused by irritation of the mouth with drugs or irritant poisonous plants or blister gases. Foreign bodies fixed in the mouth, whether they are sharp and penetrating the soft tissues, or merely jammed between the teeth, give rise to profuse salivation. In many cases of disease of the mouth attention is directed to the mouth at the time of the general inspection by the animal moving its jaws in an abnormal manner, for instance as is seen in the sucking action of the mouth in cattle affected with foot and mouth disease. Dogs with foreign bodies in the mouth, paw at the mouth with the fore feet, and, owing to the acute discomfort, become frenzied.

Injuries to the tissues of the mouth are revealed by a careful inspection. Before it is possible to inspect the mouth thoroughly it may be necessary to adopt measures of restraint. In horses, cattle and sheep the use of a mouth gag is advisable. In dogs and cats a narcotic, or even a general anæsthetic may be necessary before a thorough examination is possible ; especially is this desirable if the condition of the mouth is acutely painful.

The odour of the mouth and breath should be appreciated. In the horse the mouth normally has a smell that is not unpleasant. Unpleasant odours may arise locally from diseased tissues ; the abnormal smell may be indicative of general ill health, or the smell may arise in a more remote organ such as the lung. A sour smell with a sticky feeling of the mucous membrane frequently accompanies chronic indigestion or general debility. One of the most offensive smells encountered in veterinary practice is that which originates in gangrene of the lung in the horse. In any animal, but particularly cattle, the odour may be related to the foodstuffs ; thus the smell of turnips is often predominant in the breath of cattle. The smell of acetone in the breath of a cow may be a useful point in the diagnosis of acetonæmia (post-parturient dyspepsia). In the dog malodour may arise from gross encrustations of the teeth with tartar resulting in the retention of food material at the gum margins. Ulceration of the mouth is always accompanied by an offensive smell. In acute nephritis in the dog the breath invariably has a fœtid odour.

Toxæmia, whether of gastric, intestinal or other origin, leads to the appearance on the teeth of a dirty brown film associated with an intensely unpleasant smell. Frequently a well-marked gingivitis (inflammation of the gums) is also present under these conditions.

TONGUE.—Examination of the tongue will show various lesions of that organ. In cattle the tongue is inspected for evidence of foot and mouth disease in the form of vesicles, or ulcers following the rupture of vesicles ; the tongue is palpated to determine the presence of actino-bacillosis (wooden tongue). In the dog the tongue may be coated with a whitish film in cases of indigestion, but in severe cases of alimentary toxæmia and uræmia the tongue may be so discoloured as to justify the application of the term copper-coloured. As an injury to the tongue produces pronounced symptoms referable to the mouth, this organ must be examined with a view to detecting evidence of laceration, puncture, etc.

EYE

Apart from local diseases involving the eye that call for a special detailed examination, it is necessary to examine the eye with a view to the observation of any deviations from the normal that may have their origin in diseased conditions involving the body in general. Both eyes must always be examined. Examination of the eye in relation to the central nervous system is described in the chapter dealing with the nervous system.

The surface of the eye in normal health is moist and clear, the prominence of the eye varying in the different species ; it is most marked in cattle. There is a considerable variation in the different breeds—thus the eyes of a pekingese dog are always prominent, and those of a bull terrier tend to be rather sunken. Familiarity with these variations can readily be acquired by inspection of normal animals. Undue prominence of the eye is nearly always due to a local condition of the eye, such as glaucoma.

Conditions of the eye wherein the eye appears sunken in its socket and a red rim or space is visible between the eye and the periphery of the orbit may be seen in chronic wasting diseases where there has been a complete loss of fat. A similar sunken appearance may be noticed when there is a spasm of the external muscles leading to retraction of the eye ; this is seen in tetanus.

The surface of the eye may lose its normal bright moist condition in diseased states associated with dehydration of the body tissues. The surface of the eye may be obscured by the presence of conjunctival discharge ; in order that the eye may be properly examined any discharge must be removed with a swab of cotton wool moistened with clean water.

Lesions involving the cornea, such as keratitis and corneal opacity, may be due to a local injury, but these lesions also occur as clinical signs of specific diseases, such as canine distemper, equine influenza, malignant bovine catarrh, swine fever, etc. The general symptoms and clinical signs, in addition to local signs involving the eye, will enable the clinician to determine whether a lesion is of local or general significance. Local conditions may involve only one eye; general conditions usually involve both eyes, though in varying degree of severity.

The response of the pupil to light should be noticed in both eyes. Grossly dilated pupils in the presence of bright light are readily noticed. Failure of the pupil to react to light may be due to local disease in the eye or to involvement of the central nervous system leading to interference with reflex activity. Such involvement of the central nervous system may result from encephalitis or other diseases of the central nervous system. Reflex activity of the pupil may be seriously diminished by the action of drugs acting centrally, such as narcotics, and by drugs acting locally, *i.e.*, myotics and mydriatics. The action of atropine as a mydriatic may persist for several days after administration.

The state of the lens may be a useful indication of the degree of circulatory efficiency. In many old but healthy dogs a certain degree of haziness is present in the lens. In dogs suffering from chronic nephritis it is frequently found that the lens of each eye is opaque. In diabetes mellitus in the dog opacity of the lens is frequently present.

The state of the third eyelid (membrana nicitans) should always be observed, especially in horses. Protrusion of the third eyelid across the surface of the eye is one of the earliest signs of tetanus. In early cases of tetanus this may be noticed if the animal is walked towards the observer, or if the animal be made to raise its head sharply by either chucking it under the chin or by startling it or by threatening it or waving a handkerchief in front of its face. Local inflammatory conditions leading to protrusion of the third eyelid usually involve one eye only. Œdema of the harderian gland, leading to eversion of the third eyelid in the dog, may be bilateral, but inspection will reveal the swollen gland that is causing the eversion. The third eyelid may be evolved in the œdema already described as occurring in the effusive form of equine influenza.

EXAMINATION OF EXTERNAL SURFACES OF BODY

When the examination of the conjunctiva, nose, mouth and eyes has been completed it will be found convenient to examine the external surfaces of the body.

Various parts of the body are palpated to find out whether the body heat is maintained, elevated or depressed. This examination cannot take the place of an accurate determination of the temperature by means of a clinical thermometer, but it is profitable as a means of determining the general state of the body's reaction to disease. Several parts of the body must be palpated since a local inflammatory condition might produce heat in one part though the rest of the body surface was cold. In horses the ears and lower parts of the limbs are palpated. In cattle the ears, horns, if present, and lower parts of the limbs are handled; the muzzle should also be examined, in healthy cattle it is cool and moist. In dogs changes in the surface temperature of the skin are less pronounced and therefore not easily appreciated. The dog's nose is, however, a sensitive index of the body heat; normally it is cool and moist. A hot dry nose is a constant feature of many febrile conditions in the dog. Changes in the temperature of the surfaces of the body are only appreciable if they are considerable in degree. It is possible to recognise the heat of an intense fever, or the cold clammy feeling of a horse suffering from severe shock and exhaustion.

The appearance of the skin and coat has already been noticed during the first inspection of the patient. The coat should now be handled. This normally can be smoothed down with the hand to lie flat with a bright appearance; in chronic disease the coat becomes dull and lacks lustre; in severe acute conditions accompanied by fever the coat is harsh and staring. In chronic cachectic conditions the nutrition of the coat is disturbed and the hair or wool can be pulled out without causing pain. The skin is handled to ascertain if it is soft and pliable; in a healthy thriving animal it can be easily raised from the underlying tissues by grasping it with the hand. In many diseases the skin feels hard and is tightly adherent to the underlying tissues, giving rise to the condition known as "hide-bound." This is due to the loss of fat from skin and underlying connective tissues and in some diseases is also a result of tissue dehydration. The most convenient place to palpate the skin, to determine its pliability and freedom from the underlying tissues, is the loose fold of skin behind the elbow.

In female animals the mammary glands should be examined for evidence of mastitis, such an examination being of particular importance in cows and heifers.

PULSE

The exact point in the clinical examination when the pulse is taken may be left to the preference of the practitioner, but it is necessary that it should be taken before carrying out any painful manipulation that will cause reflex acceleration of the pulse. If the animal has been excited as the result of preliminary handling, or if there has been difficulty in catching it, time should be allowed for the animal to quieten down so that the pulse may return to the state that existed prior to these disturbances. These precautions are important in all animals but require special attention in highly strung nervous animals, otherwise a wrong impression may be formed in regard to the pulse, due to reflex disturbance of it.

The sites for taking the pulse vary in the different domestic animals. In the horse the most convenient sites are (1) the external maxillary artery just as it turns round the lower border of the jaw to become the facial where it runs alongside the corresponding vein and the parotid duct ; (2) the median artery at the upper extremity of the foreleg as it passes down the leg in company with the corresponding vein and median nerve ; in this site the artery is palpated through a thin layer of the superficial pectoral muscle as well as the skin. In the first site there is skin only, but if the horse is moving its head or jaw the movement may interfere with accurate pulse-taking at this point. In cattle the median artery as described for the horse is the common site for pulse-taking, but many clinicians use the facial artery on the lateral aspect of the man-dible. An alternative, though not so satisfactory, site is to palpate the coccygeal arteries on the under side of the tail. In sheep the site is the femoral artery high up inside the thigh where the artery emerges from the groin and passes down the thigh near the surface ; this site may also be used in quiet cows. In pigs, dogs and cats the femoral artery is also used. Additional alternative sites in horses and cattle are the digital arteries, and very rarely palpation of one of the large arteries per rectum.

It is essential that the student should practise pulse-taking in the various animals until he makes himself skilled at finding the pulse and estimating the rate, rhythm and character. Further, he must make himself familiar with the variations in the normal pulse associated with the different species and breeds. He will require to learn the alterations in the pulse that accompany physiological variations. This knowledge can only be acquired by the student for himself if he diligently practises taking the pulse in all types of animals under all available conditions.

The features to be noted in taking the pulse are the *rate*, *rhythm* and *character*. It is not sufficient merely to count the number of impulses per minute.

Alterations in the *rate* of the pulse are caused by exercise, excitement and fear, but the pulse rate should rapidly return to normal if these influences are removed. Pain causes a reflex acceleration of the pulse. Increase of the pulse rate takes place in many disease conditions, other than those involving the circulatory system. Febrile diseases, acute abdominal disturbances, *e.g.* volvulus and acute intestinal obstruc-tion and inflammatory conditions, whether suppurative or non-suppurative, all cause an increase in the pulse rate.

The *rhythm* is of very considerable importance. In horses and cattle in normal health the pulse is very regular and disturbances of the rhythm in these animals are usually of considerable significance. In horses accustomed to hard work it may be found that after a period of rest one beat of the heart is regularly dropped. This missing beat is restored on exertion and is not again dropped until the horse has been rested for some time. It is often found that in such animals the rhythm is that of every fifth beat being dropped. At rest this rhythm of a dropped beat is constant and regular, and when the dropped beat is restored after exertion the rhythm is also regular. This condition of a regularly dropped beat in a resting horse must be regarded as normal if the beat is restored and the rhythm remains normal after exertion.

In the dog some irregularity of the pulse rhythm is normal, there being variations both in the number of beats in any given unit of time and in the interval between each beat ; variations in the force are also noted. These irregularities can readily be appreciated on examining a dog's pulse. They must be differentiated from gross irregularities of rhythm, such as occur in cardiac disease and extreme toxæmic conditions.

The *character* of the pulse is, in some respects, of more importance than the rhythm or rate. Assessment of the character of the pulse entails an estimation of (1) the force of the impulse, (2) the degree to which the pressure wave is maintained, and (3) the form of the pressure wave. For example, the beat may be quick, strong and abrupt, but not sustained, or long, slow and rather soft, or very fast, thin and thready. In assessing the character it is necessary to determine if this is maintained over a reasonable period of time, or if there are variations in the character during that time.

The relationship of the pulse rate to the respiratory rate should be observed. In normal health there is a fairly definite ratio between the pulse rate and the respiratory rate in an animal at rest. In large horses at rest a respiratory rate of 14 and a pulse rate of 42 is found, giving a ratio of 1 : 3 for this class of animal in these conditions. In lighter classes of horses this ratio may vary from 1 : 4 to 1 : 5. In disease the ratio may be very greatly disturbed. In simple fevers not involving the respiratory system the ratio may be little disturbed, but in acute respiratory disease, *e.g.* pneumonia, the respiratory rate may so increase that it approximates the pulse rate, reducing the ratio to a little less than 1 : 1.

The following average pulse rates are given as a guide to the approximate rate that may be expected in each animal. As has already been explained these rates may be subject to quite considerable variations. In fast-working horses in a hard condition the pulse after a period of rest may be found to be quite slow, *e.g.* 32-36 beats per minute. In young animals the pulse is much faster than in the adult.

Animal.	Average pulse rate per minute.
Horse	40
Cattle	50-60
Sheep	70
Pig	60
Dog	80-100
Cat	100

ABNORMALITIES OF THE PULSE.—The following are some of the abnormalities of the pulse that are encountered. These serve to illustrate the value of the pulse in diagnosis. In a horse a strong bounding pulse with a rate of about 80 is found in the early stages of acute laminitis. In a dog a strong incompressible pulse, not materially abnormal in rate, is characteristic of chronic interstitial nephritis. A soft pulse is generally found present in animals affected with a slowly developing focus of sepsis. A fast soft pulse is encountered in the later stages of pleurisy with effusion. In the terminal stages of a fatal attack of colic, *e.g.* acute impaction or volvulus, the pulse is very fast—120 per minute or more— barely perceptible to the fingers, and if the character of the pulse is compared at intervals it will be realised that it is rapidly losing strength and so the term " running down " is applied to this type of pulse. In acute endocarditis the pulse is quick, wiry and irritable, and it is frequently possible to appreciate a vibration or thrill passing along the column of blood in the artery, this being caused by the manner in which the heart contracts as a result of the irritation to which its lining membrane is being subjected. An irregular fluttering pulse, varying in rate, rhythm and character, is encountered in severe cardiac palpitation.

TEMPERATURE

In the domestic animals the temperature is taken by inserting the thermometer into the rectum. In order to facilitate introduction of the thermometer through the anal sphincter it is useful to moisten the thermometer or lubricate it with a little soft paraffin or liquid paraffin. Suitable restraint should be adopted, as the animal may resent the intro-duction of the thermometer, especially if the tip of the thermometer catches on a fold of mucous membrane.

As a general rule the most suitable thermometer is the half-minute, blunt-nosed type with a magnifying scale. The mercury in the thermo-meter must be shaken down and the thermometer examined to make sure that the mercury has gone below the lowest temperature likely to be recorded.

The domestic animals do not have definite normal temperatures ; considerable variations will be found in the temperature of normal animals under different conditions.

The average normal temperatures are as follows :

Animal.	Temperature.	
Horse	100·5° F.	
Cattle	101·5° F.	Range 100-102·4.
Sheep	103·0° F.	,, 102-104.
Goat	103·0° F.	
Pig	102·6° F.	
Dog and cat . . .	101·5° F.	Range 101-102·5.
Birds	105·0° F.-107·0° F.	

The horse presents fewer fluctuations in temperature due to normal physiological actions than any of the other domestic animals. Strenuous exertion in hot weather will cause a rise in a horse's temperature, but the temperature rapidly returns to normal on cessation of the exertion. A pronounced variation in the temperature of healthy cattle is not only diurnal in character, but variations occur according to the physiological activity and also the environmental conditions. Cows in the later stages of pregnancy have an elevated temperature : though this is usually in the neighbourhood of 103° F. to 103·5° F., temperatures of 105° F. may be recorded in cows normal in every way except that they are very heavy in calf. Heavily fed fattening cattle when replete after a full meal show a rise in temperature of one or two degrees. Hot stuffy buildings cause a slight rise in temperature, especially in fat cattle or cows. If cattle loose in a courtyard or field are chased, when they are being caught, it will be found that the temperature rises proportionately to the amount of chasing that has taken place. Similarly cattle that have been driven even slowly over a considerable distance or hurried over a short distance will be found to have an elevated temperature. The temperature should return to normal once the animals have had a period of rest. The temperature of sheep, owing to the insulating qualities of the fleece, is very susceptible to conditions that entail an increased heat production. Sheep also are sensitive to climatic conditions involving a higher temperature than that to which they are normally accustomed. The heat-regulating mechanism of the dog is such that it is not able rapidly to get rid of excess heat produced by muscular activity ; consequently sharp elevations of temperature occur after vigorous exertion. Temperatures of 105° F. and over have been recorded in greyhounds shortly after they had run a race. A dog that has walked to a veterinary surgeon's premises, especially if the dog is young, active and frisky, will be found to have a rise in temperature varying according to the extent of the exercise entailed in this walk. In hot weather it is found that dogs' temperatures are higher than under cooler conditions. These factors must, therefore, be kept in mind when assessing the significance of an abnormal temperature in any of the domestic animals.

An elevated temperature is one of the clinical signs of fever. The significance of such an elevated temperature is that it serves as an index of the extent to which the body defences have been mobilised to resist an invader. As this mobilisation is proportional to the intensity of the invasion, the temperature gives a rough guide to the severity of the illness affecting the animal. It must be realised that individual animals differ in the degree to which they react to any given infection. It may be that this varying reaction is due to a difference in the degree of immunity that each possesses for such a particular infection. Apart from specific immunity clinical experience shows that there is a great individual variation in susceptibility to all infections.

Acute fevers are accompanied by a sharp elevation in temperature :

in chronic febrile conditions the temperatures may be only a little above the normal : subacute fevers occupy an intermediate position. Excessively high temperatures are recorded in the acute form of anthrax, in acute encephalitis and meningitis, and in heat stroke. Subnormal temperatures are present in the later stages of chronic wasting diseases, in marked exhaustion and in coma, whether arising from toxæmia, hypocalcæmia, or the effects of narcotics and anæsthetics. An animal will survive very much longer with a subnormal temperature than it will with an excessively high temperature. Persistent subnormal temperatures indicate either a lowering of the animal's resisting powers or that its resistance has been exhausted.

An elevation in temperature may be one of the earliest signs of the onset of disease. In outbreaks of equine influenza, cases can be detected in their earliest stages if the temperature of all horses are taken prior to their going to work. Similarly in cattle an increase in temperature may be the first sign of foot and mouth disease.

The temperature is not a good diagnostic guide in colic in the horse ; owing to the muscular activity associated with the violence shown by horses suffering severe pain, there may be a great increase in heat production leading to an elevation in temperature that has no relation to the severity of the actual colic. A progressive elevation of temperature in a case of colic is a bad prognostic sign, as it indicates that in all probability an extending inflammatory process involves the gut.

SIGNIFICANCE OF PRELIMINARY GENERAL EXAMINATION

(1) INTERPRETATION OF SYMPTOMS AND SIGNS.—It is convenient to consider at this stage the varying indications as to the nature of cases that will have been obtained as a result of the preliminary general examination. It may be found that the facts of the case point strongly to the involvement of a particular system with the obvious implication that that system be the subject of a complete examination. On the other hand, this preliminary general examination may indicate the possibility that there is present one of the specific or contagious diseases ; then it is necessary to make such further examination as will prove or refute the suspected presence of that disease. It may be that the preliminary general examination merely indicates that the animal is ill but gives no very definite indication as to the character of the illness. In such a case the clinician proceeds to make a complete examination of the body systems as is described in the later parts of this work.

The manner in which the preliminary general examination may be interpreted is illustrated by the following examples.

(a) A six-year-old heavy draught gelding in good condition used for farm work has been idle for a few days. During the last twenty-four

C

hours the animal has been dull and listless and has refused all food. It has passed only very small quantities of hard, dry dung at increasingly long intervals, and there has been no passage of fæces for the last eight hours. The horse is seen to be standing in a dull manner, with its head held low, the eyes partially closed giving a sleepy appearance. The mucous membranes are found to be very slightly icteric, giving them a dull almost dirty appearance. The mouth is pasty and the breath rather sour. The body surfaces are normally warm. The pulse and temperature are normal. In this clinical picture the lack of appetite, reduction of peristalsis with an absence of fever suggests the possibility of a functional derangement of the alimentary tract, the general trend of the case being to suggest a subacute condition. The next step in the examination of this case must be a thorough examination of the digestive system and abdomen.

(b) A five year-old steeplechaser in training has recently showed inability to sustain exertion, now has a poor irregular appetite and is losing condition. Even at rest the respirations are somewhat accelerated. The mucous membranes are slightly congested. There is an obvious pulsation in the jugular vein. The arterial pulse at rest is approximately 60, but the force is weak and the rhythm irregular. This clinical evidence indicates the need of a more detailed examination of the circulatory system.

(c) A nine-year-old fox terrier has been sick at irregular intervals for the past two years, of late the vomiting has become more frequent. During the past few weeks the animal has shown an increasing degree of thirst, frequent copious urination has also been noticed by the owner. The mucous membranes are normal but there is a good deal of mucoid discharge in the inner canthus of each eye. Opacity of the lens is present in both eyes. The animal is in poor bodily condition, the skin is dirty and scurfy. The pulse is very strong and is with difficulty compressed with the fingers; it is normal in rate and rhythm. The possibility of this being a case of chronic interstitial nephritis associated with increased blood pressure necessitates a more extended examination of the circulatory and renal system including analysis of a specimen of urine and if necessary blood urea estimation.

(d) A three-year-old male poodle is presented with a history of listlessness, inability to sustain exertion, the appetite has been capricious for some weeks. Examination shows the dog to be in a state of emaciation hidden by its coat. The mucous membranes are very pale, the pulse is fast and of poor quality, the heart sounds are very loud. The picture presented is one of acute anæmia the nature of which must be investigated. If anæmia due to blood loss can be eliminated, the enquiry is directed to detecting evidence of failure in blood production. This entails a hæmatological investigation.

(*e*) In a group of two-month-old calves three are noticed to be off their food, coats rather harsh and staring, coughing fairly frequently and breathing rather heavily. The mucous membranes are slightly injected, and there is a muco-purulent discharge from the eyes and nose. The pulse is accelerated by about one-third, the temperatures vary from 104·5° F. to 105° F. These symptoms and signs clearly indicate a febrile disease, probably involving the respiratory organs in the chest, therefore a physical examination of the chest is required.

(*f*) A dairy cow gave birth to her third calf about a month ago. After milking well her milk yield has dropped, her appetite is irregular and the fæces are pale and pultaceous. She has lost some condition and is slightly hidebound. Respirations, mucous membranes and pulse are normal. The clinical evidence points to a disturbance of the digestive system of which a detailed examination must now be made. It will be necessary to eliminate the possibility of the condition being caused by a disturbance of metabolism, *e.g.* acetonæmia (post-parturient dyspepsia).

(*g*) A two-year-old bullock is found to be suffering from acute abdominal distension. The history will reveal whether the animal was grazing when this developed or if it was on indoor feeding. Further examination will be directed to determining the nature of the distension, *e.g.* gaseous (tympany), solid matter (impaction) or fluid. It will then be necessary if the animal is tympanitic to decide if it is a case of simple bloat or one of frothy bloat. If simple bloat the cause may be excessive fermentation or there may be an œsophageal obstruction. If it is a case of impaction is it due to ingestion of dry food that has absorbed moisture and formed a dense mass with which the rumen cannot deal, or is there some displacement such as torsion of the abomasum ?

(*h*) A recently calved cow is seen to be passing highly-pigmented reddish-brown urine. Three main points in differential diagnosis should be cleared up in the course of the preliminary general examination : (1) Is there a febrile reaction? (2) Has the cow been grazing on a tick-infested pasture? and (3) Is the discoloration of the urine due to blood (hæmaturia) or blood pigment alone (hæmoglobinuria). The answers to these three questions will indicate the possibilities of the case being (*a*) an acute hæmolytic anæmia with hæmoglobinuria arising from infection with *Babesia bovis* (a protozoan blood parasite) transmitted by the tick *Ixodes ricinus*, or (*b*) an acute hæmolytic anæmia with hæmoglobinuria encountered in various parts of the world in newly calved cows ; the ætiology of this condition bovine post-parturient hæmoglobinuria is not clearly understood, or (*c*) chronic cystic hæmaturia due to a lesion in the bladder, or (*d*) pyelonephritis. Further clinical investigation will be directed to confirming the possibilities suggested by the preliminary general examination.

(*i*) A group of cross lambs going with their dams on a good pasture are quite suddenly affected with profuse diarrhœa and there have been one or two deaths. The history is suggestive of acute intestinal helminthiasis. Investigation is then directed to examining fæces samples for worm egg burden and if possible the identification of particular genera of parasitic helminths. If the carcasses of the dead lambs are available these can be subjected to a post-mortem examination, the worm burden can be estimated and the distribution among the various genera assessed.

(j) A group of pedigree Blackface ewes were brought down from the hills in early December and were placed on a low ground pasture where they received supplementary feeding. After a fortnight a ewe was found dead and several more deaths occurred during the subsequent ten days. The only satisfactory approach to this problem is by post-mortem examination which should be made on an animal as soon as possible after death. In order to complete the differential diagnosis it may well be necessary to submit material for laboratory examination, as for instance to establish the presence of enterotoxæmia.

In pigs the difficulties of interpreting symptoms and clinical signs are considerable. Many specific febrile diseases of the pig closely resemble each other. Sometimes the history is such that there is a strong suggestion that the disease affecting the pigs may be one of these specific diseases, but as a diagnosis can seldom be based on the history, symptoms and clinical signs, a post-mortem examination is required. It may be that there already is at least one pig dead, but if not, in order that a diagnosis may be made, an ailing pig is destroyed and a post-mortem examination made.

The history, symptoms and clinical signs disclosed by the preliminary general examination may not give any clear indication of the nature of the case under investigation; when completed an examination of the body systems, though indicating certain abnormalities, may still fail to elucidate the nature of the malady. In this type of case the assistance of some of the aids to diagnosis is sought. The results of urine analysis may point to disturbances not only of the urinary system but also of digestion and metabolism. Differential blood counts or biochemical examination of a sample of blood may suggest the nature of the pathological processes present in the case.

In all animals emaciation, anæmia and possibly diarrhœa may be caused by helminth infestations; if these are suspected further steps must be taken to establish the existence of a measure of infestation sufficient to cause the illness.

(2) FEVER, ITS CHARACTERISTICS AND SIGNIFICANCE.—The presence of fever will have been recognised during the preliminary general examination of the patient. Fever represents part of the general reaction of the patient's body to the entrance of infection. The clinical syndrome of fever is characterised by a relatively constant group of symptoms and

clinical signs. It is important that the existence of this syndrome should be recognised and its significance appreciated. Though it may not be possible in the early stages of a specific infective fever to do more than determine the presence of febrile symptoms, it must be understood that even as a tentative diagnosis " fever " is unsatisfactory and of little value, as it merely indicates the existence of a bodily reaction, and the presence of this has already been realised when the animal was seen to be ill.

Though varying in degree some febrile symptoms are constant in their appearance, other symptoms and clinical signs differ according to the causal disease. The symptoms and clinical signs in the early stages of fever are more similar in all cases than those in the later stages when the disease process has advanced sufficiently to produce the more specialised signs arising from involvement of local organs. These specialised signs will be discussed in detail when dealing with systematic examination of the individual systems of the body.

The general signs of fever may be conveniently discussed as a group at this point. A rise of temperature (pyrexia), though an essential feature of fever, is only one of the many symptoms and signs that together constitute the clinical syndrome of fever. As has already been explained, the temperature constitutes an index of the severity of the body reaction. The term pyrexia is used to describe rises in temperature falling within a moderate range ; the term hyperpyrexia is applied to excessively high temperatures, such as those over 106° F. If seen soon after the onset of illness, during the stage when the temperature is rising, the animal is shivering. Once the body has adjusted its heat regulation to the new temperature level, shivering usually ceases. It will, however, recur if the animal is taken from a warm atmosphere to a cold one.

The coat is staring and there is a general appearance of malaise. Many animals are very dull ; but in some fevers the animal appears for a time to be morbidly excited, as is the [case in some forms of meningitis and encephalitis. The appetite is impaired or all food may be refused. Constipation is a constant concomitant of fever, except in those inflammatory conditions of the alimentary tract that are manifested by diarrhœa. Rumination is invariably disturbed and frequently entirely suspended. Reduction in the milk yield is inevitable and is approximately proportional to the severity and duration of the febrile reaction. The mucous membranes are injected, the muzzle is dry. The mouth may have an unpleasant odour. It is often rather sticky and the tongue may be coated or furred. The external surfaces of the body feel hot. The surfaces of the body may be moist with sweat. Pulse and respiration are accelerated ; in the absence of complications, e.g. pneumonia, this acceleration is proportional to the severity of the fever and the relationship between pulse and respiratory rates is not materially altered. As a result of the increased loss of fluid by other routes the urine in febrile animals is reduced in volume, but is concentrated, with an increased specific gravity. In herbivorous animals there is a change of reaction from alkalinity to acidity ; in other animals an increased acidity is found. The percentage of nitrogenous compounds in the urine is considerably increased.

The symptomatology of fever is more readily appreciated when it is realised that acute fever pursuing a regular course passes through certain stages.

(1) The stage of development commences at the time of INFECTION when the causal organism gained entrance to the body. The period of INCUBATION is that during which no symptoms are shown but the causal organism is multiplying in the body or elaborating its disease-producing toxin. The PRODROMAL period is characterised by the appearance of only very slight symptoms that usually are indefinite in character, though indicating the commencement of illness.

(2) The stage of full development is introduced by the period of INVASION when the symptoms and signs characteristic of the disease develop. The period when the symptoms are at their greatest intensity, is known as the FASTIGIUM. This period merges with the AMPHIBOLIC a period of uncertainty during which the prognosis is in doubt ; the amphibolic period is popularly known as the " crisis."

(3) The stage of resolution is introduced by a period of DEFERVESCENCE. The disappearance of the febrile symptoms may take place rapidly by *crisis* or more slowly by *lysis*. Defervescence by lysis is more common in the domestic animals than defervescence by crisis. Finally during a period of CONVALESCENCE the damaged and diseased tissues are, as far as possible, restored to normal and the animal regains its strength.

CHAPTER III

DIGESTIVE SYSTEM AND ABDOMEN

General Symptoms and Signs in all Species
Horse :—Regional Anatomy—Detailed Clinical Examination—Rectal
Examination—Classification of Colic—Differential Diagnosis of
Various Types of Colic—Alimentary Disturbances in Foals
Cattle and Sheep :—Regional Anatomy—Detailed Clinical Examination
Pig :—Regional Anatomy—Clinical Examination
Dog and Cat :—Regional Anatomy—Clinical Examination—Radio-
logical Examination
Liver :—Regional Anatomy—Clinical Examination—Jaundice—Canine
Virus Hepatitis

THE great anatomical and physiological differences that exist between
the different domestic animals make it impossible simultaneously to
discuss the clinical examination of the alimentary tract of them all. It
is, therefore, necessary to discuss separately the examination as it is
applied to each species. Certain general methods may be considered
before dealing with each species.

In the preliminary general examination attention has already been
directed to the state of the appetite. It is necessary to distinguish between
lack of appetite (*anorexia*) and inability to take food due to difficulty in
prehension and mastication or inability to swallow food. Difficulties of
prehension are associated with lesions in the mouth, and an examination
of the mouth, if not already made, will reveal the lesion. This examination entails inspection and palpation of such parts as the lips, gums,
teeth, cheeks and tongue. In some cases the sense of smell is of considerable assistance in locating the site and determining the nature of a
lesion in the mouth. Diseased teeth and necrotic bone are both responsible for very unpleasant smells. Painful conditions of the pharynx
and the associated lymph glands—principally submaxillary and retropharyngeal—may interfere with free movement of the lower jaw and so
make prehension and mastication difficult and painful. *Dysphagia*, or
difficulty in swallowing, may arise from painful pharyngeal conditions.
New growths or foreign bodies may obstruct the pharynx. Difficulty
in swallowing may be caused by an obstruction in the œsophagus. The
methods of examination of the pharynx and œsophagus vary in the
individual species and will be discussed later.

The enquiries made when ascertaining the history of the case should
have revealed the degree of peristaltic activity of the bowel. This information may be confirmed by an inspection of the fæces. The character of
the fæces is of importance. The fæces may be normal, unusually

fluid or excessively hard. Hard fæces from constipated animals have a firm glazed surface to which some mucus is usually adherent. The fæces may have an offensive smell and may contain either changed blood that has passed down the bowel or fresh blood shed from the terminal portion of the rectum.

The abdomen may appear empty, normally full or distended. Distension of the abdomen may arise from a number of causes : food, flatus, fœtus, fluid, fæces, or foreign body. The differentiation between fullness due to repletion after a meal and impaction is based on the knowledge that an excessively replete animal is not ill though temporarily uncomfortable. An animal with impaction is ill. Obviously there are border-line cases where repletion, due to over-engorgement with food, passes on to impaction. Distension due to flatus is such that percussion of the abdomen produces a resonant or drum-like sound. Pregnancy, whether simple or multiple, will only lead to acute distension of the abdomen in the later stages when the presence of the fœtus or fœtuses can usually be appreciated by direct clinical methods. Ascites (dropsy of the peritoneal cavity) is recognised by the production of a percussion wave in the fluid. A hand is laid flat on one side of the abdomen and the other side of the abdomen struck sharply. In small animals the clinician can do this himself ; in larger animals an assistant is required. The wave created in the fluid by the impact travels across the abdomen and impinges on the hand held flat on the abdominal wall. The impact of the wave on the far side of the abdomen can be detected aurally by means of a stethoscope. Percussion of the abdomen will produce a dull non-resonant sound in the area occupied by the fluid ; the normal resonance of the abdomen can be demonstrated by percussion in the upper part of the abdomen if that is not occupied by fluid. Alterations in the position of the animal alter the position of the fluid in the abdomen and the areas of dullness and resonance are altered correspondingly. Such alterations are more easily produced in small animals that can be conveniently laid on the side and turned on the back during the course of the examination. If the abdominal cavity is greatly distended with fluid the weight drags down the abdomen so that the lower part is round and prominent, but there is a hollow area on each side of the body below the lumbar vertebræ. In any case of doubt an exploratory puncture of the abdominal cavity should be made with a view to withdrawing some of the fluid should any be present. The fluid causing distension of the abdomen may not be free in the peritoneal cavity, but may be contained in a closed sac, when percussion with the animal in varying positions reveals that the fluid does not move freely throughout the peritoneal cavity but remains localised. Distension of the abdomen by fluid enclosed in a sac within the peritoneum is a clinical feature of hydronephrosis, hydrops amnii and any advanced cystic condition.

Distension of the abdomen with fæces will only occur when there is a most marked degree of constipation. Such a measure of constipation is extremely rare in animals. Foreign bodies before leading to distension of the abdomen must attain a considerable size in proportion to the animal and are limited mainly to large tumour growths.

Palpation of the abdomen is of limited value in the horse, though pain and tension may be revealed. In cattle much useful information may be obtained by palpating the rumen through the abdominal wall, and some information may be obtained by palpation of the abdominal wall over the site of abomasum. In sheep palpation of the abdomen may prove quite useful. In pigs it is unfortunately of little value. It is only in the dog and cat that deep palpation through the abdominal wall is possible, and in these animals this form of palpation constitutes an essential part of the clinical examination of the abdomen. In foals, calves and lambs, especially in the very young, a fairly extensive examination of the abdomen by palpation is possible.

Percussion is of value in all animals, though the information gained varies in the different species.

Auscultation is useful in all animals to reveal the state of peristaltic activity.

EXPLORATORY PUNCTURE OF THE ABDOMEN.—The peritoneal cavity may be tapped to confirm the suspected presence of fluid and to obtain samples of the fluid for bacteriological examination. In the larger animals the operation is performed with a small bore trocar and cannula, in the smaller animals a hypodermic needle 1 to $1\frac{1}{2}$ inches long and 0·9 to 1·4 mm. in diameter is used. The site selected is the abdominal floor near the midline so as to avoid the large vessels of the abdominal wall. If the animal is in a standing position the pressure of fluid is usually sufficient to cause it to flow from the needle, the fluid being collected in a sterile receptacle held below the needle ; if necessary the fluid may be withdrawn into a sterile syringe.

HORSE

REGIONAL ANATOMY

The soft palate in the horse is greatly developed, extending from the hard palate to the epiglottis with which it comes in contact. Thus a complete membranous curtain separates the mouth from the pharynx, except during the act of swallowing. The presence of this membranous curtain prevents direct inspection of the pharynx in the horse.

At its commencement the œsophagus is in the middle line of the neck ; in the middle third of the neck it passes to the left side where, if containing solid material, it can be palpated.

The stomach of the horse is relatively small and is situated high up in the abdominal cavity, immediately behind the diaphragm and liver and mainly to the left of the median plane.

The first part of the duodenum has a relatively short mesentery, but the second part is more loosely attached to the abdominal roof. The other portions of the small intestine have a very loose mesentery, and in

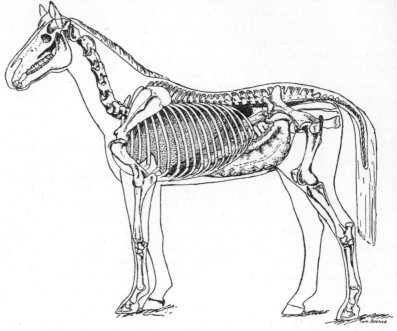

FIG. I.—Horse.   Thorax and Abdomen.   Left side.

consequence vary very much in position. The small intestine lies principally on the left side, but coils may be found in contact with the abdominal floor and even the right side.

The large intestine is formed by the cæcum, the large colon, the small colon and the rectum. The cæcum of the horse is very large ; it resembles a comma in shape. The rounded base of the cæcum lies in the right iliac and sub-lumbar region ; the more pointed extremity lies on the abdominal floor behind the xiphoid cartilage. The ileo-cæcal orifice and the cæco-colic orifice lie close together on the concave curvature of the base.

The first part of the large colon, the right ventral colon, commences at the cæco-colic orifice and sweeps downwards and forwards from a position approximately behind the lower end of the last rib. Sweeping across the abdominal floor from right to left forming the sternal flexure, the colon turns back to form the left ventral colon. This passes upwards and backwards, reaches the entrance to the pelvis where the pelvic flexure of the colon is formed by a sharp forward and upward turn that leads to the left dorsal colon. Not only is there this acute turn at the pelvic flexure of the colon, but there is also a sudden diminution in the lumen of the bowel at this point. The left dorsal colon passes forward

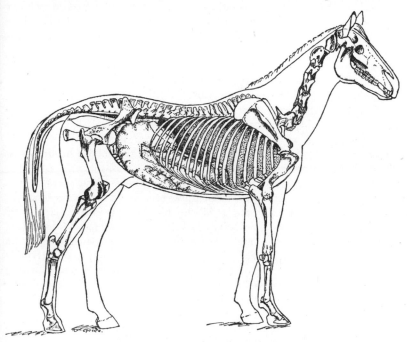

FIG. 2.—Horse. Thorax and Abdomen. Right side.

immediately above the left ventral colon to which it is attached. Passing across to the right it forms the diaphragmatic flexure and continues to form the right dorsal colon. The right dorsal colon runs upwards and to the left and with a sudden narrowing of the lumen becomes the small colon, this point being approximately below the last two ribs on the left side.

The small colon is from ten to twelve feet in length; its coils are intermingled with those of the small intestine. The small colon terminates in the rectum.

Longitudinal bands are present on both the large and small colon. The presence of these bands enables the clinician to recognise the colon when it is palpated in the course of a rectal examination, as both the bands and sacculations caused by them can be felt.

Clinical Examination

THE MOUTH.—A detailed examination of the mouth will be required if the symptoms and clinical signs already recognised point to an involvement of it. Thus salivation, difficulty in feeding or chewing may have been noticed. A horse with unevenly worn teeth may allow the food to drop out of its mouth. A not uncommon cause of debility in horses is uneven wearing of the molar teeth leading to the development of projections and prolongations on the teeth. Such a horse cannot properly chew its food and in consequence malnutrition develops. Inspection of the mouth may be performed by opening the mouth and grasping the free portion of the tongue with the hand, the hand holding the tongue preventing closure of the mouth. This method does not permit a detailed examination of the mouth. To enable the mouth to be more thoroughly examined it is necessary to make use of a mouth gag. Two forms of gag are in common use, namely Varnell's and Haussman's ; details of these are to be found in text-books dealing with animal management.

PHARYNX.—Owing to the amount of lymphoid tissue present the pharyngeal mucous membrane is an important site of tissue reaction to infection. Inflammatory changes in the pharynx are made evident by coughing, nasal discharge, difficulty in swallowing, heat, pain and swelling of the pharyngeal region and frequently a defensive reaction in the associated lymphatic glands. The pharynx can be palpated externally to determine the presence of pain, heat or swelling. When palpating the pharynx it is always well to palpate the associated lymphatic glands, namely the sub-maxillary, the sub-parotid and the suprapharyngeal.

As has already been stated, inspection of the horse's pharynx through the mouth is not possible. It is possible to inspect the mucous membrane of the pharynx to some extent by means of an instrument known as the rhino-laryngoscope. This instrument is passed up the nose ; by means of a small electric light and mirrors within the instrument the mucous membrane of a small area of the pharyngeal wall is illuminated and an image of the area can be seen. By moving and rotating the instrument other areas can be inspected. It is also possible with this instrument to inspect the larynx and vocal cords. Many horses show little resentment to the passage of this instrument, but if necessary a narcotic or anæsthetic may be administered to facilitate the introduction of the instrument through the lower meatus of the nose.

ŒSOPHAGUS.—Difficulty in swallowing or regurgitation of food may indicate œsophageal involvement, but may also be associated with gastric disorder. Inflammatory processes involving the œsophagus almost invariably arise from trauma caused either by mechanical damage or by the action of chemical irritants.

Choking may result from an attempt to swallow any substance of a character that the œsophagus cannot convey to the stomach. Choking with sugar-beet pulp is not uncommon in horses. The horse attracts attention as it is uneasy and unable to feed properly. It may attempt to swallow some food, but immediately shows signs of discomfort and the bolus of food is returned from the œsophagus and ejected through the nostrils. This regurgitation of food causes so much pain that the horse squeals, arching the neck as the food is expelled.

If the obstruction should be located in the cervical part of the œsophagus it may be palpated on the left side of the neck where the œsophagus passes dorsal to the trachea. If in the thoracic portion of the œsophagus, and also if in the cervical portion, the obstruction may be located by passing the stomach tube. After the stomach tube enters the œsophagus it should be pushed gently down until it comes in contact with the obstruction. By noting the length to which the tube has penetrated when it reaches the obstruction it is possible to estimate approximate position of the obstruction.

Spasm of the œsophagus most commonly occurs in the cardiac portion, being in fact a cardiospasm. In this condition spasmodic contraction of the œsophageal muscle prevents the passage of a bolus of food to the stomach. The food is expelled by a peristaltic wave passing up the œsophagus. Cardiospasm is only observed when the horse is feeding or attempting to feed. After chewing some food the normal swallowing effort is made, the horse stops feeding, arches his neck, and a reverse peristaltic wave is seen passing up the neck, the food material, mixed with saliva and mucus, being ejected through the nose. The spasm of the œsophagus is painful and the horse may show signs of considerable distress. Passage of the stomach tube will assist differentiation from obstruction of the œsophagus. The stomach tube should be lubricated thoroughly with some bland oil so that it may pass easily through the portion of the œsophagus constricted by the spasm.

COLIC.—The term " colic " is applied rather indiscriminately to the symptoms shown by a horse that is suffering abdominal pain. Such pain may arise from stomach, small intestine or large intestine and is known as " true colic." The pain may, however, be caused by lesions in the urinary system, or any of the other abdominal organs, and also in organs or tissues outwith the abdominal cavity. Colic arising from organs other than the stomach or bowel is spoken of as " false colic " ; sometimes its origin is definitely indicated, e.g. renal colic. An outstanding example of " false colic " arising from pain in tissues outwith the abdominal cavity is the subacute pain that accompanies the early painful stages of pleurisy in the horse.

Acute peritonitis is accompanied by pain, but the severity of the pain is apparently dependent on the cause of the peritonitis even more than its extent. Thus acute intestinal obstruction (acute impaction) is in its later stages associated with an intense local peritonitis and some measure of generalised peritonitis. The pain in acute impaction is severe, the horse in consequence being very violent. Acute generalised peritonitis following trauma may only cause dull pain ; the horse stands stiffly and shows marked disinclination to move.

In the mare, symptoms of colic may arise from violent uterine contractions ; this form of colic may be seen after the fœtal membranes have been removed manually and appears to develop more frequently following retention of the placenta after an abortion than after parturition at full term.

Colic is in effect the outward manifestation of pain affecting the viscera. Horses indicate the presence of colic by a group of characteristic symptoms. If the animal is feeding when the attack commences he will stop and will not normally take food again till the spasm has passed. Horses in the throes of intense pain may chew at pieces of straw, or hay, or even dry fibrous sticks. Inspection of the animal will readily reveal that it is not feeding. Pawing and scraping with the fore feet are seen. The horse lies down but may be no sooner down than he springs up again. If there is severe distension of the abdomen the horse lies down with caution, often hesitating in a crouching position before finally allowing his body to reach the floor. When he does let the body touch the ground the pressure on the abdomen causes him such pain that he gives a deep groan. While lying the horse may roll and kick. If free in a loose box he may do himself little harm. If he is in a stall he may get into an awkward position with the feet fixed tightly against the side of the stall, making access to the head difficult and dangerous. Many horses, if suffering severe pain, appear to be oblivious to damage they inflict on themselves by their violence ; severe bruising, especially of the head, is a distressing result in these cases. The horse postures as though attempting to urinate, and the attendant may erroneously assume that the horse is suffering from some disorder of the urinary system. In severe colic the horse often backs his hind quarters into a corner or against some fixed object and stands pressing firmly against it.

Regurgitation of foodstuffs up the œsophagus and the ejection of food material through the nose is seen in gastric distension and in rupture of the stomach. It appears that following rupture of the stomach the cardiac sphincter relaxes, and the material in the stomach passes through the open sphincter up the œsophagus. The enormous distension of the stomach with green foul-smelling fluid in acute grass sickness causes the fluid to overcome the sphincter and pass up the œsophagus, the material trickling from the nostrils in a fairly steady stream.

Intense pain in the anterior portion of the abdomen, especially if accompanied by gastric distension pressing on the diaphragm, is to some extent reduced if the horse sits upright on its haunches like a dog. The presence of this symptom is always associated with serious illness and may be seen shortly before a fatal ending.

Sweating, in patches or all over the body so that the horse is literally bathed in sweat, is partly an index of the severity of the pain and partly an indication of the reaction of that individual horse to pain. Horses in fat or soft condition tend to sweat more profusely in colic than horses in hard working condition; excitable, highly bred horses tend to show most violence.

Respiration is reflexly stimulated by the pain of colic. In the later stages of an acute abdominal catastrophe toxæmia along with shock and exhaustion, due to continued pain, cause grave disturbances of respiration. Thus in volvulus the breathing has a sobbing character that is most distressing to the observer. Increased abdominal pressure interfering with the movements of the diaphragm may produce pronounced dyspnœa.

The pulse rate rapidly accelerates during spasms of pain. If the pain is of the spasmodic type the pulse will return to normal during the intervals between the attacks of pain. If the pain is continuous the pulse continues to increase in rate and may in an hour or two reach a rate of 80 per minute or more. Should the case be of a nature that allows the rapid development of toxæmia, the depression of the circulation is more marked and the pulse may continue to increase in rate and lose strength until shortly before death the rate may be 120 per minute and the impulse becomes so weak that it is almost imperceptible. By the time this stage is reached the animal is suffering severely from shock and exhaustion, and the body surfaces have a cold clammy feeling.

The appearance of the visible mucous membranes varies according to the nature and cause of the colic.

The temperature is not of assistance in the diagnosis of colic; it may, however, be of some assistance in prognosis, a progressive rise in temperature indicating a serious and possibly fatal case.

Owing to the great thickness and strength of the abdominal wall in the horse there is a distinct limitation on the amount of information regarding the contents of the abdominal cavity that can be obtained by examination through the abdominal wall. This information can be supplemented by that obtained from a rectal examination. The details observed during the preliminary general examination are of particular importance in the differential diagnosis of the various forms of equine colic.

STOMACH.—Palpation of the horse's stomach is not possible. Palpation of the left flank immediately behind the last rib will be found to be of very little assistance since the stomach does not lie sufficiently near the surface to enable any accurate location of the seat of the maximum intensity of pain. These factors create difficulties in the diagnosis of gastric disorders in the horse. The clinician must largely depend on indirect symptoms.

Acute continuous pain with considerable reflex acceleration of the pulse is a feature of gastric impaction and gastric tympany. Quick shallow respiratory movements with injected mucous membranes occur when the movements of the diaphragm are restricted by a distended stomach. By sitting on his haunches the horse allows his stomach to fall away from the diaphragm. Profuse sweating indicates the severity of the horse's discomfort. Distension of the abdomen giving rise to a drum-like resonance on percussion may affect the left side principally if tympany is confined to the stomach. For a short time after the onset of pain due to gastric distension, small quantities of fæces may be passed, but complete stasis develops rapidly.

Regurgitation of foodstuff and its passage down the nose suggest the likelihood of impaction or distension of the stomach with semi-fluid or fluid material. Eructation of gas occurs when the stomach is distended with gas. If the stomach tube is passed gas or fluid may escape by it, indicating the nature of the cause of the gastric distension. If food material is impacted in the stomach, some of it may be removed by pumping in through the stomach tube half to one gallon of saline solution and then allowing this to siphon out. But as the saline does not enter or leave the stomach with any appreciable degree of force it may merely flow on to the surface of the impacted food material and then pass back out of the tube without removing any appreciable amount of the impacted material.

It may appear that the severity of the pain is temporarily abated after the expulsion of food, fluid or gas from the stomach. Disappearance of pain unaccompanied by any improvement in the general symptoms indicates a deterioration and not an improvement in the horse's condition. If, after a period of some hours, the pain abates gradually, but the pulse continues to increase in rate and lose volume, and at the same time the surfaces of the body become cold, the animal is suffering from the secondary effects of the gastric condition, e.g. exhaustion and an increasing degree of toxæmia.

On the other hand, if, after an intense spasm of pain evidenced by extreme violence, there is a sudden disappearance of pain with at the same time every evidence of shock and the ejection of gastric contents through the nose, it must be appreciated that the stomach wall may have ruptured.

No positive evidence is found by rectal examination in gastric disorders of the horse. Such negative information is, however, of value in the differential diagnosis of acute colic of the horse.

Depraved appetite (pica) is a symptom commonly associated with chronic indigestion in the horse. In young horses during the period when the permanent teeth are in process of eruption some degree of indigestion is not uncommon. Helminthiasis (worm infestation) may cause some disturbance of appetite.

A sour pasty condition of the mouth, a rather slow soft pulse, some nausea shown by yawning, sour butyric smelling soft fæces, and a depraved appetite are characteristic features of indigestion following malnutrition ; clinical examination of the mouth and a fæcal worm egg count are necessary steps in differential diagnosis.

INTESTINE.—Inspection of the abdomen will have revealed distension that may be due to intestinal tympany. External palpation of the abdomen is of very limited value in the horse, but pain and tension are revealed by palpation. In some cases the fullness due to an impaction in the left ventral colon can be appreciated by palpation of the flank. Percussion is of value in demonstrating resonance due to tympany. Extreme dullness due to overloading of the bowel with solid foodstuffs can rarely be demonstrated by percussion. Auscultation of the abdomen will show whether the peristaltic sounds are normal ; their absence indicates intestinal stasis and abnormally loud peristaltic sounds may indicate increased peristaltic activity, but the volume of the sound may depend on the character of the foodstuff.

Emphasis has already been laid on the necessity of determining the character and quantity of the fæces. The horse normally defæcates several times a day. The character of the fæces varies according to the foodstuffs, but in any horse the fæces should normally be formed. The fæces of a pony are usually drier and firmer than those of a horse. The character of the fæces provides a useful index of the degree of peristaltic activity. The main points to be observed in regard to the character of the fæces are consistency, colour and smell. Hard dry fæces are passed in very small amounts in the period immediately preceding the appearance of clinical signs of impaction. At a later stage hard pellets may be found lying within the rectum, but no fæces are passed by the animal. Such hard pellets have a glazed surface often covered with a film of mucus. A few hard pellets are found in the rectum in acute grass sickness. Soft fæces resembling those of a cow in consistency, having an unpleasant sour smell, are passed in chronic indigestion.

Fluid fæces containing mucus and epithelial debris are passed in muco-enteritis that may develop as a result of excessive dosage with a purgative. Following septic absorption from a focus of infection, e.g. chronic metritis following parturition, muco-enteritis may develop. Diarrhœa is a symptom of intestinal irritation. Once any substance has passed from the stomach it can only be expelled from the body by passing throughout the length of the bowel to the exterior. If the substance is irritant in character the bowel responds by an increase in the peristaltic rate. In consequence absorption time in the bowel is reduced and there may be increased secretion from the glands of the bowel in response to

D

the irritant ; so the food residue reaching the terminal part of the colon is of greater volume and has a much higher fluid content.

Hæmorrhagic fæces are passed whenever there is a break in the continuity of the lining of the bowel wall that allows the escape of blood into the lumen. If the blood is being lost into the anterior part of the bowel it is invariably dark in colour. The term melæna is used to describe the passage of fæces dark in colour due to the presence of changed blood pigment. The amount of blood varies from a small quantity shed from a minute ulcerated area to the great volume lost in cases of acute hæmorrhagic enteritis.

The term dysentery is used to describe an inflammation of the intestine attended by pain and straining with the passage of fæces containing blood and mucus.

If large quantities of blood are present in fæces they are readily detected by inspection ; smaller quantities easily escape notice if the fæces are not tested for occult blood.

Benzidine Test.—A thin suspension of fæces is made with distilled water, 5-10 c.c. being sufficient. This is boiled to destroy any enzymes and allowed to cool. To 2 c.c. of a saturated solution of benzidine in glacial acetic acid is added 3 c.c. of 3 per cent. hydrogen peroxide and 2 or 3 drops of the fæcal suspension. A clear blue colour develops if blood is present.

In carnivores, before carrying out this test, red meat and vegetables may be withheld for two or three days. But if the blue colour develops within thirty seconds the presence of blood may be assumed irrespective of the constituents of the diet.

There is a tendency to discontinue using the Benzidine Test because of the possible carcinogenetic actions of benzidine.

Guaiacum Test.—A small quantity of fæces is thoroughly mixed with 10 c.c. of glacial acetic acid. An equal quantity of ether is added and the mixing repeated. In about 2 c.c. of the resulting mixture there are placed 5 drops of freshly prepared tincture of guaiacum, and to this is added slowly 10 per cent. ozonic alcohol (10 c.c. 20 vol. hydrogen peroxide alcohol to 100 c.c.) until a blue or green colour develops or a definite excess has been added without any colour appearing.

Occultest.—This test for blood pigment in urine can be applied to a suspension of fæces as a test for occult blood (see page 311).

RECTAL EXAMINATION.—When the symptoms and clinical signs observed up to this point are co-related it will often be found that a rectal examination must be performed in order to obtain further information.

In making a rectal examination suitable restraint must be used. It may suffice for one assistant to lift up a foreleg while another holds the tail. The application of a twitch is sometimes useful in quietening a troublesome patient. If it is thought that the horse is likely to give trouble it may be wise to apply side lines or service hobbles—for details see standard works on animal management. The hand and arm should be thoroughly lubricated with soap and water or some bland emollient. It is a good plan to fill the edges of the finger nails with soap. It will be found that though the majority of horses resent the introduction of the hand through the anal sphincter, once this initial difficulty is overcome little resentment is shown to any further part of the examination unless the manipulation causes pain. If on introducing the hand the rectum is found to be full of fæces these must be removed.

The state of the rectum is then examined. Normally the wall of the rectum is applied to the arm with a gentle but firm pressure. The rectum may be ballooned when for any reason the intestinal musculature has lost tone. This may result from complete intestinal stasis from any cause, such as necrosis of a portion of the bowel wall following obliteration of its blood supply by volvulus. Artificial ballooning of the rectum may be produced by the repeated introduction and withdrawal of the hand and arm during the removal of fæces from the rectum. The hand and arm may be tightly gripped by the rectal wall and the animal may strain against the operator in any acutely painful condition in the abdomen, the principal alimentary causes being acute impaction and volvulus before the occurrence of necrosis.

When the hand and arm have been introduced into the rectum the comparatively restricted portion of the abdominal cavity within the operator's reach should be systematically examined. In the normal animal except for the initial resentment caused by the introduction of the hand through the anal sphincter, little discomfort is caused, and exploration of the abdomen should give an impression that there is a complete absence of pain or discomfort.

Many of the portions of the bowel can only be clearly defined by palpation when they are distended with gas or delineated by an impaction. One portion of the bowel that can nearly always be palpated with facility is a portion of the small colon lying anterior and ventral to the brim of the pelvis. This loop of the small colon can be identified as it contains fæcal masses sufficiently formed in character to be recognised by palpation and also because the longitudinal bands and sacculations enable the clinician to distinguish it from a loop of small intestine.

The pelvic flexure of the colon is appreciated on the left side just within the anterior entrance to the pelvis ; the tip of the pelvic flexure may traverse the middle line. Passing the hand forward and to the left the longitudinal bands of the double colon may be appreciated. If the pelvic flexure is the site of an impaction, the latter is felt as a mass varying in consistency from that of dough to that of a firmly flexed human knee. If an impaction is present the bands of the colon tend to be tense.

To the right, extending from the posterior part of the lumbar region in an anterior and ventral direction, is the mass of the cæcum ; this can only be clearly appreciated when it is distended.

As far forward as can be reached in the lower part of the abdomen the coils of the small intestine can be felt as indefinite objects that can easily be pushed out of the way. If distended with gas the loops of the small intestine may be definitely identified. If the small intestine is the site of volvulus the loop that is cut off from its blood supply and from the lumen of the rest of the bowel becomes acutely distended with gas, and can readily be felt as a resilient mass. It is only very exceptionally that the twisted portion can be felt, but the displacement caused by volvulus may be such that portions of mesentery are rendered tense and can be felt as cord-like structures traversing the abdomen. These can be distinguished by their position and form from the longitudinal bands of the colon that may be rendered tense by the distension of the bowel in tympany.

If the horse is not too large it may be possible to palpate the junction of the large and small colon in the region ventral to the last two ribs on the left side, but this region is in many horses beyond the reach of the operator.

It is usually possible to recognise the bladder by passing the hand forward along the floor of the pelvis ; when empty the bladder lies mainly within the pelvis, but as it fills it projects beyond the brim of the pelvis. If empty it may not be possible to identify the bladder clearly. If pain were arising from distension of the bladder caused by obstruction of the urethra, the bladder would be sufficiently distended to make it easily recognisable. The left kidney may be palpated in small horses ; in large animals it is usually out of reach.

In the mare the uterus and ovaries may be examined.

If the operator has a long arm he may be able to palpate the posterior margin of the spleen far forward on the left side ; if the spleen is grossly enlarged it may be more easily felt and the margin may feel thicker than in the normal ; gross distension of the stomach may bring the spleen back within reach.

Dorsally the pulse may be felt in the abdominal aorta and the aorta may be traced back to its bifurcation into the great vessels leading to the hind limbs. The internal inguinal ring on either side may be palpated. If the internal inguinal ring is the site of hernia the portion of bowel entering the ring may be felt.

It is only in exceptional cases that intestinal calculi can be palpated when making a rectal examination. They are felt as extremely hard masses.

During the exploration of the abdomen attention must be directed to the detection of pain in any area, the distension of any portion of the bowel with gas or impacted food material and the presence of any evidence of abnormal displacement of a portion of the bowel.

When the rectal examination has been performed it is possible to analyse the symptoms and clinical signs with a view to forming a diagnosis of the nature of the colic.

CLASSIFICATION OF COLIC

The colics of the horse other than gastric distension are divisible into four main groups according to their cause. First, there is spasmodic colic that is the result of violent irregular peristaltic movements. These may arise as a result of irritation of the alimentary tract by unsuitable foodstuffs, or may be associated with general muscular fatigue in a horse that has had a heavy day's work, or may be the consequence of an excessively hungry horse bolting his food, or may develop shortly after changes in the food supply. In very many cases of spasmodic colic there is a certain degree of intestinal tympany.

Second, there is tympanitic colic (or simply tympany); this is due to distension of a hollow viscus following the rapid production of gas from foodstuffs that ferment readily. Any food such as cut grass, especially if rich in clover, or damaged or defective foodstuffs, are likely to lead to tympany. Distension of a hollow viscus with gas under tension stimulates spasm, which not only causes pain but also prevents the passage of gas along the lumen of the intestine.

Third, obstructive colic (or impaction) is that form of colic which is caused by the development within the lumen of the gut of a mass of ingesta that is sufficiently dry and firm to cause an obstruction within the bowel. In many cases the impaction is to be regarded as a symptom of antecedent stasis, but in other cases it develops as an immediate result of engorgement or the ingestion of indigestible foodstuffs such as old dry straw. Obstructive colic associated with impaction may involve either stomach or colon. It is chiefly the large colon that is involved, and the most common site is the pelvic flexure. The junction of the large and small colon is the next site in order of frequency, but impaction there is much less common; the small colon is seldom the site of a definite impaction. Impaction of the cæcum is a comparatively rare condition. Impaction of the small intestine is rare with the exception of so-called "sand colic" developing as a result of the ingestion of considerable quantities of sand. Under obstructive colic it is necessary to include colic associated with intestinal calculi.

Fourth, colic that is due to mechanical causes outside the bowel causing obstruction of its lumen. In this category are included a number of conditions. Volvulus (twist) involves in descending order of frequency the double colon, the small colon, the middle portion of the small intestine, the remainder of the large colon and the ileum. Volvulus of the duodenum is exceedingly rare owing to its short mesentery limiting the movement necessary to produce a volvulus. Volvulus is uncommon in foals. Intussusception (invagination or telescoping) of the bowel is not common in adult horses but is encountered in foals. The invagination usually commences in the small intestine but may extend till a considerable portion of the small intestine has passed into the large bowel ; owing to the anatomical relationships of the ileo-cæcal and cæco-colic orifices in the horse, intussusception of the small intestine through the ileo-cæcal orifice passes into the cæcum. Intussusception of the cæcum within itself may extend into the colon (*i.e.* cæco-colic intussusception). Strangulated hernia or incarcerated hernia leads to colic by interfering with the blood supply to the strangulated or incarcerated portion of bowel and may also obliterate the lumen of that part of the bowel. Scrotal hernia is the most common type ; diaphragmatic hernia occurs occasionally ; umbilical hernia seldom leads to acute incarceration or strangulation ; hernia of a loop of bowel through a normal opening in the mesentery or through a tear in the mesentery is seen occasionally. Other forms of hernia such as inguinal, femoral and perineal are fortunately rare in the horse. In the category of mechanically caused colic it is necessary to include those cases that develop from the effects of peritoneal adhesions. Such cases are not common in the horse.

Differential Diagnosis of Various Types of Colic

Bearing this general classification in mind, the symptoms and clinical signs can now be discussed individually. An analysis of these is given in the table on p. 56.

PAIN.—The onset is sudden and the pain is intense in character, but intermittent in spasmodic colic. The onset is sudden, and the pain is intense and continuous in acute gastric distension and in acute intestinal tympany. The onset is sudden, the pain, though at first fairly acute, increases in intensity and is continuous in character till shortly before death in volvulus, strangulated hernia and intussusception. The onset is slow and the pain only dull in subacute impaction. The onset is gradual and the pain at first not severe, but gradually increases in intensity and persists until shortly before death in acute impaction.

. PULSE.—In general it may be stated that if the pulse is little altered in rate and character the colic is not of an acute nature. But if the pulse rapidly increases in rate and at the same time becomes thin and thready the colic is acute and may prove dangerous to life. The pulse is undisturbed in subacute impaction of the colon. The pulse may be rather slow and intermittent in chronic indigestion. A slow intermittent pulse is encountered in indigestion associated with dental changes in young horses. The pulse is accelerated immediately after the onset of pain in gastric distension and continues to increase in rate until the condition is relieved. The pulse is accelerated, but the increase in rate and the diminution in strength are relatively slow in acute impaction, and it may be twenty-four to thirty-six hours before the pulse reaches a rate of over 100 per minute and assumes a thin thready character. The pulse is accelerated and the increase in rate and loss of strength are rapid in both acute tympany and volvulus. The pulse is increased in rate but is soft in character in septic conditions in the abdomen.

VISIBLE MUCOUS MEMBRANES.—There is little change in the appearance of the mucous membranes in spasmodic colic. The mucous membranes have a dirty appearance due to mild jaundice in chronic indigestion. The mucous membranes are dull in subacute impaction. A dull red appearance of the mucous membranes is seen in acute impaction ; the injection of the mucous membrane increases in intensity during the progress of the case. Intense injection of the mucous membrane is present in volvulus and other acute mechanical interferences with the abdominal viscera. Pallor of the mucous membranes is seen in shock and hæmorrhage arising from severe trauma to the viscera, such as rupture of the stomach or rupture of the intestine.

RESPIRATIONS.—The respirations are normal in subacute impaction. The respirations may be rather slow in chronic indigestion. Acceleration of the respiratory rate is noticed during the paroxysms of pain in spasmodic colic : as soon as the paroxysm passes the respiratory rate returns to normal. The respiratory rate is markedly increased in acute impaction and volvulus : in the latter stages the respirations become sobbing in character. Marked dyspnœa accompanies acute gastric distension. Short shallow accelerated respirations are present in diaphragmatic hernia. Physical examination of the chest may show a dull area corresponding to the position of the organs that have passed into the chest.

ABDOMINAL DISTENSION.—Obvious distension of the abdomen is usually due to tympany ; percussion giving a resonant note will confirm that the distension is due to flatus. Gross symmetrical distension of the abdomen occurs in intestinal tympany and in the tympany that follows volvulus. In gastric tympany, uncomplicated by intestinal tympany, distension of the abdomen is not marked and may involve the left side more than the right.

SWEATING.—Sweating accompanies severe pain. Individual horses vary in their reaction to acute pain, but profuse generalised sweating is only seen in acute conditions. If the surface of the body is wet with sweat but feels unnaturally cold, the condition is a serious one that may readily prove fatal as this combination points to marked shock.

MUSCULAR TREMORS.—Muscular tremors leading to trembling of the whole body is evidence of exhaustion developing during the course of a severe colic.

FÆCES.—The continued passage of fæces negatives the presence of

TABLE I

	Spasmodic Colic	Gastric Distension	Intestinal Tympany	Intestinal Impaction		Volvulus
				Subacute	Acute	
Pain	Sudden intense Intermittent	Sudden intense Continuous	Sudden intense Continuous	Absent or only very slight	Onset slow. Intensity increasing. Continuous	Sudden intense Continuous
Pulse	Accelerated only during spasms	Accelerated	Accelerated	Normal	Accelerated	Accelerated
Mucous membranes	Little change	Injected	Injected	Dull	Moderately injected	Injected
Respirations	Accelerated only during spasms	Dyspnœa	Dyspnœa	Normal	Accelerated dyspnœa may develop	Accelerated dyspnœa develops
Abdominal distension	Absent	Present but not marked	Marked	Absent	Present but not marked	May develop due to tympany
Sweating	Occurs if pain very severe	Occurs	Occurs	Does not occur	Occurs	Usually generalised
Faeces	No passage during attack	May be passed	No passage	No passage	No passage	No passage
Regurgitation and eructation	Absent	Frequently occurs	Absent	Absent	Absent	Absent
Rectal examination	Negative	Negative	Pain and straining. Distended bowel may be felt	No pain or straining. Impaction may be felt	Pain and straining. Impaction may be felt	Pain and straining. Distended loops of bowel may be felt
Temperature	Not elevated	Elevation of temperature may occur as case progresses, but elevation is not of diagnostic significance				
Muscular tremors	Absent	Occur in the later stages of fatal cases				

any intestinal obstruction. Passage of fæces in small amounts at long intervals is evidence of intestinal stasis but may also follow abstention from food. Entire absence of fæces is evidence of either stasis or intestinal obstruction. An effective response to purgative drugs unaccompanied by any amelioration in the animal's condition may be evidence of impaction of the cæcum. Soft or fluid unpleasant smelling fæces indicate intestinal putrefaction with its concomitants of intestinal irritation and toxic absorption. The passage of flatus through the anus may indicate that there is no obstruction to the lumen of the bowel. If the passage of flatus is followed by a reduction in the severity of the pain it is a good prognostic sign, but if no such improvement is seen it is possible that the gas being voided has been formed behind an obstruction in the lumen of the intestine.

REGURGITATION AND ERUCTATION.—These acts are associated with gastric involvement. Passive regurgitation may indicate rupture of the stomach or relaxation of the cardiac sphincter from any other cause. The passage of the stomach tube may give evidence of the cause of gastric distension.

TEMPERATURE.—The temperature is of relatively little value as a diagnostic aid in the early stages of colic. A rise in temperature at a later stage usually indicates the onset of inflammatory changes in the bowel wall.

RECTAL EXAMINATION.—The findings are entirely negative in gastric distension. There is no evidence of pain in subacute impaction until the impaction is palpated, when the animal may groan. The consistency of the impaction may be estimated. There is evidence of acute pain accompanied by straining in acute impaction, acute tympany and volvulus. In acute impaction if the obstruction is palpated the pain is intensified and it will be appreciated that the impaction is of a firm character. In acute tympany distended loops of bowel may be felt and the bands on the colon may be tense. In volvulus the distended loop of bowel that is shut off from the rest of the gut may be felt and also tense bands of mesentery. The distinction between very acute tympany and volvulus is often difficult and it may be necessary to delay expressing a definite opinion until the progress of the case has been observed.

MISCELLANEOUS.—Any external evidence of hernia should be looked for, and if it is the cause of colic the hernia is usually hot, swollen and painful. Other evidence of hernia may have been found in rectal examination. It is well to remember that strangulated scrotal hernia is a not uncommon cause of colic in stallions. Epileptiform convulsions in foals are frequently found in post-mortem examination to have been associated with intussusception.

RECURRENT COLIC.—Recurrent colic may be the result of the reappearance of the etiological factor originally responsible for the colic. Thus a horse fed on old oat straw may develop an impaction of the colon that responds to treatment. It may be realised that the oat straw has been the causal factor and so the feeding of it is discontinued. But if at a later date feeding of oat straw is again practised the horse may again develop an impaction.

On the other hand, recurrent colic may be due to some abnormality in the alimentary tract.

Calculi are recognised as an important cause of recurrent colic in the horse, though less common nowadays due to the improved methods of preparing animal foodstuffs. The circumstances under which calculi cause colic are not always clear. Large calculi are sometimes found on post-mortem examination in animals that have shown no symptoms during life and have died from some other cause or have been destroyed. It is unusual to find more than one very large calculus in any animal and then the calculus may be found in a diverticulum of the bowel. If small, calculi may be passed in the fæces and their presence may have been observed. It is often found that the smaller calculi are multiple ; lying within the gut they appear to do little harm until they are moved from the part that they have hitherto occupied. The presence of a calculus in any part of the colon gives rise to some irritation. Increased peristaltic activity for any reason may result in the movement of the calculus. If the calculus has been propelled into another portion of the colon it acts there as a mechanical irritant, and if there is any disproportion between the size of the calculus and the diameter of the bowel the calculus may become impacted leading in effect to an acute intestinal obstruction. If this obstruction should occur at the pelvic flexure of the colon the calculus can be palpated per rectum. Large single calculi, if containing a high proportion of mineral material, by their weight tend to cause a sacculation in the wall of the portion of the colon in which they develop. Whether a large calculus can be felt per rectum is entirely dependent on the site it occupies in the bowel and, as has already been stated, only a comparatively small part of the whole abdomen can be explored by a rectal examination. The history of the feeding the animal has received may assist in diagnosis ; an excessive quantity of dry bran has been incriminated as encouraging calculus formation, and millers' horses fed largely on mill sweepings have been found to show a high incidence of intestinal calculi.

Adhesions between the visceral and parietal layers of the peritoneum are a relatively rare cause of colic, but usually there is a history of recurrent attacks of colic extending over a prolonged period. Such cases appear to be more frequent in geldings, and it is possible that they owe their origin to a local peritonitis developing from infection that has gained entrance to the peritoneal cavity at the time of castration. It may be possible—though very rarely—to determine by rectal examination the presence of peritoneal adhesions; these should be sought, especially in the inguinal region. Adhesions tend to become firmer and less elastic as they become older, and in consequence the attacks of colic become more frequent and more severe. Ultimately symptoms, suggestive of volvulus, but lacking the intensity associated with complete torsion, develop and death results. It may be found that peritoneal adhesions limit the expansion of the bladder and in consequence abnormal frequency of urination is observed.

Helminth infestations may lead to recurrent colic by irritation of the intestinal mucous membrane. Verminous aneurisms in the cranial mesenteric artery caused by the larvæ of *Strongylus vulgaris* interfere with the blood supply to the bowel, and if the interference is sufficiently serious a severe attack of colic may result. The inflammatory changes in the aneurism may result in intermittent interference with the blood supply causing recurrent colic. Further invasions of larvæ may stimulate the inflammatory process in the vessel wall leading to a reappearance of the symptoms. Recurrent colic due to verminous aneurism develops rather slowly but is persistent in character and responds slowly to treatment. Details of the steps necessary for differential diagnosis are described in the chapter on clinical helminthology.

ALIMENTARY DISTURBANCES IN FOALS

In young foals there are some conditions that merit special mention.

RETENTION OF THE MECONIUM.—The foal shows signs of abdominal discomfort and is disinclined to suck. Digital rectal examination will reveal the hard pellets of retained meconium.

INDIGESTION.—The foal does not suck, the abdomen is somewhat distended and palpation is resented. Eructation and regurgitation may occur. A not infrequent sequel to indigestion in the foal is an acute attack of diarrhœa.

DIARRHŒA.—It is frequently observed that foals suffer from an acute attack of diarrhœa immediately after the mare has been in œstrus. Persistent diarrhœa in foals may be due to an infestation with *Strongyloides westeri*, the infective larvæ of this parasite penetrating the skin of the foal when it is lying on an infested pasture.

INTUSSUSCEPTION.—Very often there is a history that the foal has not been thriving and there have been attacks of indigestion and diarrhœa. Suddenly the foal becomes acutely ill, showing evidence of acute abdominal pain accompanied by intense straining. With intensification of the symptoms the foal may manifest general convulsions, death usually occurring shortly after their appearance.

The diagnosis of diseases of the liver is described at the end of this chapter.

CATTLE AND SHEEP

REGIONAL ANATOMY

CATTLE.—The muzzle formed by the central part of the upper lip and the surface between the nostrils is devoid of hair and in the healthy animal is kept cool and moist by a clear watery fluid secreted by glands lying immediately under the skin. There are no incisor teeth in the upper jaw ; their place is taken by a dense layer of connective tissue covered by horny epithelium forming the dental pad. The anterior two-thirds of the hard palate is marked by a number of prominent transverse ridges ; the posterior part of the hard palate is smooth.

The soft palate is not so long as in the horse but it completely separates the cavity of the mouth from the pharynx. It is therefore not possible to inspect the pharynx. The cavity of the mouth is wide and it is relatively shorter than in the horse. In adult cattle it is possible for a man with a hand of average size to explore the mouth and pharynx and entrance to the œsophagus. The œsophagus is wide, and owing to the wall being relatively thin it is capable of considerable dilatation. An important relation of the œsophagus within the chest is to the mediastinal lymph gland that lies dorsal to it immediately before the œsophagus passes through the diaphragm. The œsophagus terminates in the œsophageal groove that opens into the common cavity of the rumen and the reticulum. The rumen and reticulum are the first and second of the three fore stomachs or œsophageal dilatations. From the end of the œsophageal groove there runs a groove along the ventral wall of the omasum, the third of the fore stomachs ; this groove terminates in the abomasum or true stomach.

In adult cattle the rumen is the largest of the four compartments that form the complex bovine stomach ; the capacity of the rumen varies from 30 to 50 gallons and represents approximately 80 per cent. of the total volume of the three fore stomachs and the true stomach. In the newly-born calf the capacity of the rumen is less than half that of the abomasum ; by the time the calf reaches an age of ten weeks the rumen has attained a size twice that of the abomasum. The rumen occupies almost the whole of the left side of the abdominal cavity, a small area in the most anterior part being filled by the reticulum. The rumen reaches the middle line of the abdomen and may even extend over to the right side of the middle line. The position occupied by the rumen makes it possible to palpate, percuss and auscultate it over the entire area of the left flank covered by the abdominal muscles. The rumen is divided by pillars into a dorsal and a ventral sac and a dorsal blind sac and a ventral blind sac. These pillars correspond with grooves on the outer surface of the rumen.

The reticulum is the smallest of the fore stomachs and is smaller than the abomasum; its capacity is approximately 5 per cent. of the whole. The reticulum occupies the most anterior part of the abdominal cavity lying in immediate contact with the diaphragm almost entirely in the middle line and reaching as far forward as the 6th or 7th rib, the posterior part lying immediately above the xiphoid cartilage. The reticulum is separated from the rumen by an almost vertical ridge,

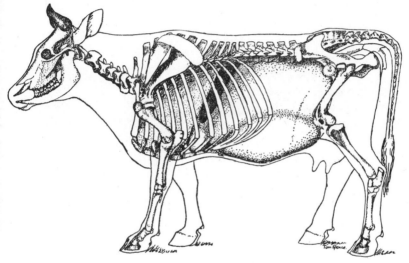

Fig. 3.—Cow. Thorax and Abdomen. Left side.

the rumino-reticular fold. The lining membrane of the reticulum is raised into folds which form the boundaries of spaces or cells giving it a honeycombed appearance.

The capacity of the omasum is about 8 per cent. of the total capacity of all four compartments. The omasum is situated almost entirely on the right side of the middle line of the abdomen; its left surface is in contact with the rumen and reticulum and its right surface reaches a small area of the abdominal wall under cover of the 8th, 9th and 10th ribs at their lower thirds. The omasum lies above the abomasum. The interior of the omasum is filled with approximately a hundred longitudinal folds of mucous membrane; these arise from the dorsal wall and each lies in close apposition with its immediate neighbours.

The mucous membrane of the rumen, reticulum and omasum is covered with thick stratified squamous epithelium.

The abomasum, or true stomach, has a capacity equivalent to approximately 7 per cent. of the total capacity of all the compartments. The greater curvature of the abomasum lies on the abdominal floor on the right of the middle line, extending from immediately behind the xiphoid cartilage to the level of the last rib. The left or visceral surface of the abomasum is in contact with the ventral sac of the rumen ; the anterior extremity lies against the reticulum. The right or parietal surface comes in contact with the abdominal wall in an area extending from the lower end of the 7th rib to the level of the 10th or 11th rib. The lesser curvature

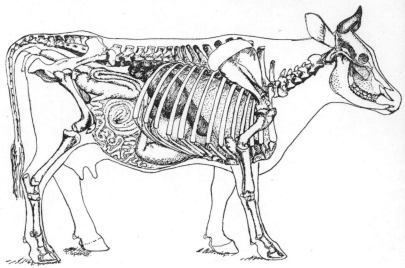

Fig. 4.—Cow. Thorax and Abdomen. Right side.

faces dorsally and is in contact with the omasum. The mucous membrane of the abomasum is glandular and has the appearance of a true gastric mucous membrane ; it is arranged in a series of loose folds.

On account of the large bulk of the rumen and the space occupied by reticulum, omasum and abomasum, the intestine in cattle lies almost entirely on the right side of the body.

The duodenum commences at the level of the 11th rib and passes dorsally forwards till it reaches the visceral surface of the liver. After forming a sigmoid curve in the region of the right kidney the duodenum passes back almost to the level of the coxal tuber. It then turns completely and runs forward to the commencement of the free portion of the small intestine in the neighbourhood of the right kidney. The free portion of the small intestine is arranged in very short coils and it occupies the space bounded by the rumen on the left, the omasum and abomasum anteriorily, the colon dorsally and to the right and the abdominal wall ventrally.

The large intestine in cattle has not the great size of its counterpart in the horse, but it is complex in disposition. The ileum enters the colon at a point on a level with, and slightly medial to, the lower end of the last rib ; for a short distance before its termination the ileum passes along and is attached to the medial surface of the cæcum. The cæcum passes backwards and upwards from its commencement at the junction of ileum and colon, the posterior end of the cæcum lies just within the pelvis at the right side. The colon runs forward and then turns dorsally and backwards in the sublumbar regions to a point near the last lumbar vertebra. It again turns and runs forward to enter the spiral part of the colon. This part consists of a double loop of colon coiled into a flat spiral lying between two layers of mesentery ; the spiral lies against and facing the right side of the abdominal wall. The portion of the colon that leaves the spiral passes forward and then turns backwards to pursue a course dorsal to the last part of the duodenum ; passing through a sigmoid curve the colon terminates in the rectum. The bovine rectum is of smaller diameter than its equine counterpart. The peritoneum extends into the pelvis as far as the first coccygeal vertebra. In healthy animals the retroperitoneal portion of the rectum is encased in fat.

SHEEP.—Apart from the relatively larger size of the abomasum the alimentary canal of the sheep closely resembles that of the bovine.

CLINICAL EXAMINATION

THE MOUTH.—Examination of the mouth in cattle may be performed without a gag or, if it is preferred, a gag may be employed. The animal's head is held by grasping the muzzle with the thumb in one nostril and the forefinger in the other. If preferred, a pair of bull holders may be applied to the nose ; this has the advantage of giving a firmer hold of the nose than can be achieved by the hand alone. If the nose is held up the animal has much less power of resisting the examination than if it is allowed to get its head lowered so that it can press forward. Additional purchase on the head can be secured by turning the head round so that the neck is flexed to whichever is the more convenient side. In animals with horns the restraint is aided if an assistant grasps the animal's horns and so steadies the head.

Owing to the absence of incisor teeth in the upper jaw it is possible to introduce the hand between the anterior portion of the upper and lower jaws, and by depressing the lower jaw the mouth is opened. The tongue may then be grasped and the mouth inspected. It is desirable to move the head into varying positions so that light may play on the parts being inspected. It is often necessary to turn the animal round so that it faces a source of daylight ; if artificial light is being used the source should be such that the light can be directed into the mouth.

It is possible in adult animals to pass the hand between the molar teeth if the fingers are extended and lying close together with the thumb flexed into the palm of the hand, and passing over the dorsum of the tongue the hand enters the pharynx. In passing the hand through the mouth it will be found more convenient if the hand is held so that the plane formed by the fingers lies at right angles to the hard palate.

The use of a gag facilitates the examination of the mouth and the passage of the hand through the mouth. For this purpose the most convenient form of gag is that known as " Drinkwater's Gag." This is in the form of a wedge with a groove on each surface into which the molar teeth fit, when the gag is pushed between the upper and lower jaws.

Examination of the mouth should include attention to the following points. Evidence of vesication and ulceration on the dental pad, gums, cheeks, lips, tongue or palate that would suggest the presence of foot and mouth disease. The vesicle of foot and mouth disease contains clear fluid and it is a simple vesicle without septa ; the vesicle ruptures readily and leaves a sharply defined, relatively superficial ulcer with a bright red floor. Induration of the tongue, with ulceration of the dorsum, showing as a shallow crater with ragged edges and a dirty brown floor, is a characteristic of actinobacillosis of the tongue. This disease may involve the cheeks, leading to swelling and induration. Enlargement and distortion of the jaw with loosening of the teeth is present in actinomycosis of the jaw-bone. If the lesion has ulcerated a thick yellow discharge containing granules and having a nutty odour may be observed.

The presence of foreign bodies, either sharp objects penetrating the soft tissues or larger masses such as a piece of turnip wedged between the teeth, give rise to symptoms that may appear alarming ; the significance of these symptoms is appreciated when the foreign body is discovered on examining the mouth.

Necrosis of the buccal mucous membrane develops in malignant bovine catarrh. Ulceration of the buccal mucous membrane is seen in mucosal disease of cattle (possibly not a single disease entity and therefore sometimes termed the mucosal complex). The ulcers are small, very superficial and heal rapidly. A form of superficial necrosis of the mucous membrane of the tongue is sometimes seen in imported Irish cattle. In this condition the horny epithelium is raised from the underlying tissue and can be stripped off, leaving a dirty brown surface. The layers of epithelium that have been removed show translucent dots corresponding to the sites of the lingual papillae ; this appearance has been compared to that of a gas mantle. Diphtheresis of the buccal mucosa occurs in calf

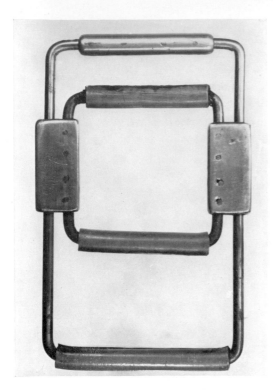

Fig. 5.—Mouth Gag for sheep.

Fig. 6.—Mouth Gag for sheep in use.

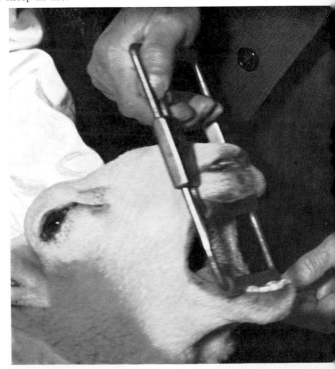

diphtheria, the lesions being particularly noticeable in the inside of the cheeks. An offensive smell in the mouth is a notable feature of calf diphtheria.

A partial examination of the mouth in sheep may be made without the aid of a gag. Such an examination is sufficient to demonstrate the presence of lesions of foot and mouth disease ; these are found particularly on the dental pad. If a more complete examination of the mouth is required a gag must be inserted. The use of a gag is essential if a proper examination of the teeth is to be made. A simple but effective form of gag for sheep is shown in figs. 5 and 6.

Examination of the mouth in either cattle or sheep should include inspection of the teeth. Dental abnormalities may interfere with prehension, but it is usually during the process of chewing the cud that the outward manifestations of dental disease are readily seen in ruminants. Inspection will show that the animal is not performing the normal rhythmic grinding movements and that food is allowed to drop out of the mouth.

In some cases it is actually the teeth that are affected ; in other instances, though the teeth are sound, they have become loose and have deviated from their normal alignment.

In sheep the condition known as " broken mouth " is one involving the incisor teeth ; either the incisor teeth are actually broken or they have been lost. Involving the central pairs of incisors more than the later pairs, there is a tooth-less gap. In such a sheep there is some interference with grazing and the sheep would have difficulty in eating roots such as turnips. This condition of broken-mouth in sheep is widespread but is much more troublesome in certain areas, *e.g.* the north-east of Scotland. Infection of the sockets of the incisor teeth in sheep is troublesome in some areas and may result in the loss of some or even all the incisor teeth. The organism most commonly involved is *Actinobacillus lignieresi.* In some districts the cheek teeth in older sheep become loose and their altered position causes the sharp edges to press into the cheek or tongue. Inherited abnormalities of conformation may lead to the development of dental defects interfering with chewing. Thus if the lower jaw is relatively more narrow than usual in proportion to the upper jaw in a sheep, the upper cheek teeth wear with a long slant on the mesial aspect and the lower teeth wear with a long slant on the later aspect. Effective chewing of the ingested food and more particularly effective chewing of the cud is not possible in such a sheep, and if the animal is going on a rough grazing, especially in winter, there may be serious loss in condition. This condition is known colloquially as " scissors-mouth " and the appearance of the condition in a high proportion of home-reared female sheep of the same age group suggests the possibility of a hereditary factor.

E

In chronic fluorine poisoning in cattle and sheep (often termed fluorosis) the incisor teeth show mottling and pitting of the enamel; deformity of the incisor teeth is sometimes seen. The lesions are only seen in the permanent teeth and in those teeth formed while the animal is ingesting excessive amounts of fluorine compounds. In similar circumstances the cheek teeth are defective and the defect is one of poor wearing quality with the result that the teeth are worn down in a very uneven manner—a process known as selective abrasion. When selective abrasion is advanced the animal is unable properly to chew the cud. The lesions of dental fluorosis are shown in figs. 7 and 8. It is probably true to say that the lesions involving the incisor teeth are fairly characteristic of dental fluorosis. The same cannot be said of the process of selective abrasion of the molar teeth especially in so far as it involves sheep. A severe degree of selective abrasion of the first molar has been encountered in sheep of three years old and upwards. There were no lesions of fluorosis in the incisor teeth. It appears that the poor wearing qualities of the first molar in these sheep resulted from a period of severe malnutrition during the first winter of their life.

While the lesions of dental fluorosis are sufficiently characteristic if involving back incisor and cheek teeth to justify a tentative diagnosis being advanced, it is wise to confirm this by analysis of tooth and bone for fluorine content. Even though the ingestion and absorption of excessive amounts of fluorine compounds may long since have ceased, if excessive fluorine has been incorporated in teeth and bone, it is retained almost indefinitely. (See Chapter XIX).

In adolescent animals the shells of the deciduous teeth may not be shed normally, their retention interfering with chewing. Actinomycosis of the jaw causes alteration in the position of the cheek teeth and in some cases actual loss of teeth.

PHARYNX.—Examination of the pharynx in cattle is made by external palpation and, if necessary, manual exploration of the cavity through the mouth. The examination is conducted with the object of finding evidence of inflammatory changes in the wall of the pharynx, enlarged lymphatic glands and the presence of foreign bodies. Inflammatory changes in the pharyngeal mucosa cause irritation that provokes coughing. External manipulation of the pharyngeal region will show if there is local pain, heat and swelling, with possibly inflammatory involvement of the associated lymphatic glands. Manual exploration of the cavity of the pharynx may be necessary to assist differential diagnosis.

Enlargement of the retropharyngeal lymphatic glands may cause snoring respiration; if the enlargement has attained considerable dimensions these glands may be palpated externally; if the enlargement is of a lesser degree it may only be appreciated when the glands are palpated through the pharyngeal wall from within the cavity of the

Fig. 7.—Dental Fluorosis in Sheep

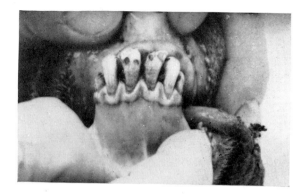

Incisor Teeth. Pitting and stippling of enamel.

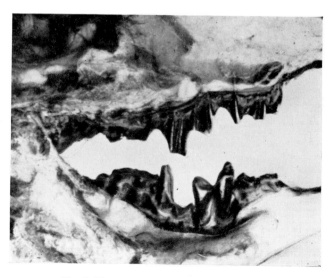

Cheek Teeth. Marked selective abrasion.

Fig. 8.—Dental Fluorosis in Cattle

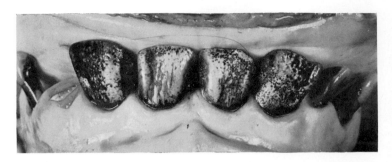

Incisor Teeth.   Pitting and stippling of enamel of first two pairs of
permanent incisors.

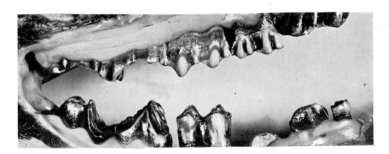

Cheek Teeth.   Marked selective abrasion of molars and separation
of lower molars I and II.

pharynx. Enlargement of these glands may be due to any pyogenic infection or possibly tuberculosis.

The foreign bodies most commonly found in the pharynx are pieces of turnip or other roots. They may be in the pharynx itself or just within the capacious entrance to the œsophagus.

Examination of the pharynx in sheep is limited to an external examination, owing to the small dimensions of the mouth.

ŒSOPHAGUS.—In spite of the large size and powers of dilatation of the œsophagus, choking is very common in cattle. The process of predigestion that takes place in the rumen results in the production of a considerable volume of gas; this in the normal animal is voided through the œsophagus by eructation. If the œsophagus is obstructed the gas cannot escape; in consequence tympany of the rumen is an important feature of œsophageal choking in cattle. If the foreign body is spherical it acts as a ball valve and completely obstructs the egress of gas; in consequence tympany may develop very rapidly and may become very acute. If the foreign body is irregular in outline gas may be able to pass by its edges and so escape; in such a case tympany does not develop so rapidly and is not so acute. In addition to tympany it will be observed that the animal is salivating and is making expulsive coughing efforts to dislodge the foreign body.

Enlargement of the posterior mediastinal lymph gland may by pressure on the œsophagus prevent the normal expulsion of gas from the rumen and thus there develops tympany, which, though varying in intensity, is usually subacute. When tympany is due to pressure on the œsophagus by an enlarged mediastinal gland it is probable that it will be recurrent. Enlargement of this gland is commonly due to actinobacillosis or tuberculosis.

Recurrent tympany in young bulls usually between six and nine months, and especially of the beef breeds, appears to be most troublesome in those animals which are still suckling a cow, either the dam or a nurse cow, at an age when they might normally be expected to be fending for themselves. Repeated post-mortem examinations have failed to reveal any lesion to account for the tympany other than what seemed to be a failure of the development of the rumenal papillæ. This may be a result of continued ingestion of milk making it unnecessary for the young animal to eat sufficient roughage to stimulate development of the rumen, thus suggesting that the problem is a managerial one. It has been suggested that a hereditary factor may be involved, but the available evidence in favour of that hypothesis is by no means conclusive. As might be expected in these cases clinical examination fails to reveal any lesion that could cause the recurrent tympany which may be sufficiently acute to require relief with a stomach tube.

If a foreign body is obstructing the cervical portion of the œsophagus it may be palpated on the left side of the neck, except when it is in the entrance to the œsophagus, when it may only be possible to palpate it from within the pharynx.

If the foreign body is in the thoracic portion of the œsophagus it will be necessary to pass a probang to confirm a tentative diagnosis. Before passing the probang it is essential that adequate precautions be taken to prevent the animal getting its head down and plunging forward. If it succeeds in doing so it may strike the free end of the probang against some fixed object and so drive the probang through the œsophageal wall. An effective method of preventing this accident is to secure the animal's head over some fixed object. A special form of gag with a hole in the centre, through which the probang is passed, may be used, but it is frequently found that the animal does not so actively resent the passage of the probang if the instrument is passed over the dorsum of the tongue without a gag. The end of the probang usually enters the œsophagus without any difficulty and the introduction of it is continued until the end comes in contact with the foreign body. If the lumen of the œsophagus is constricted by external pressure from an enlarged gland, the probang will pass this point with difficulty and considerable pressure may be necessary to force the dilated end of the probang through the constriction. Once it is passed less pressure will be needed to move the probang ; on withdrawal a similar difficulty will be experienced. It will be possible to locate the site of the obstruction by measuring the distance to which the probang was passed when it came in contact with the obstruction or constriction of the œsophagus.

Oesophageal choking of sheep is not common ; in these animals a smaller type of probang can conveniently be employed if it appears from the symptoms and clinical signs that its use is necessary.

ABDOMEN.—Cattle and sheep, unlike horses, do not as a rule become violent when suffering from digestive disturbances ; they tend rather to become dull and depressed. Colic as an outward manifestation of pain is in cattle principally due to mechanical interference with the bowel such as occurs in intussusception, to irritation of the urinary passages as in cystitis, and to acute inflammatory conditions of the bowel wall such as acute anthrax.

Prior to this stage in the examination of the animal information has been obtained regarding the animal's appetite, rumination and defæcation ; the state of the abdomen will have been noticed when making the preliminary general examination of the animal.

Cattle suffering from digestive disturbances very often grunt. This grunt may be provoked by palpation and manipulation of the abdomen ; it may also be evinced when the animal either lies down or gets up or walks. Continuous grunting is not common unless the animal is lying, thereby increasing the pressure on a distended or painful abdomen.

Grunting must be distinguished from the plaintive murmuring sound that some cows make for various reasons, but not necessarily on account of discomfort. Further details of the diagnostic aid obtained from noticing the character of the grunt will be given later in this section. Cattle suffering abdominal pain often grind their teeth, producing a most unpleasant crunching sound ; grinding of the teeth in this way nearly always occurs in acute abomasitis (true bovine gastritis).

Examination of the bovine abdomen should be carried out with a view to determining the state of the rumen, reticulum and abomasum. Direct examination of the omasum is not possible ; there appears, however, to be every reason to believe that the functional activity of the omasum is dependent on that of the rumen and reticulum. It seems that only very rarely, if ever, does any disease affect the omasum alone.

It must be admitted that the physiological mechanism governing the movements of the rumen, reticulum and omasum are as yet imperfectly understood, but the clinician has at his disposal adequate means of ascertaining the state of functional activity of these organs. An important criterion of normality is the act of rumination. Interference with rumination is one of the earliest symptoms of digestive disturbance from any cause. A careful study of the act of rumination in a normal animal should be made by all students before approaching the subject of digestive disturbance in the bovine. The posture of a ruminating animal is one of repletion, comfort and contentment. The animal assumes a comfortable position and the facial expression is placid and peaceful. At regular intervals a bolus of food is brought up from the rumen into the mouth with a slight lifting movement of the abdominal muscles. As soon as the bolus enters the mouth a single stroke of the jaw drives it between the molar teeth and thereafter the chewing of that bolus is done on one side of the mouth only. The chewing is done in a rhythmic methodical manner at no great speed. Each bolus is chewed on an average from fifty to sixty times. The student should find no difficulty in distinguishing between normal rumination and grinding of the teeth to which reference has already been made. If a bovine is seriously disturbed or alarmed while ruminating, the function is usually at once stopped. It might well be said that the act of rumination is the essential criterion of normality in the ruminant digestive system. The outstanding difference between the act of rumination in cattle and the same function in sheep is that sheep chew the cud much more rapidly.

RUMEN.—In the course of the digestive processes that take place in the rumen considerable quantities of gas are formed. These accumulate in the dorsal sac of the rumen and are got rid of by belching. If for any reason the gas cannot thus be voided, its accumulation in the rumen causes tympany. Examination of the rumen is carried out by inspection, palpation, percussion and auscultation. Inspection has already been discussed under the preliminary general examination ; it will have revealed any gross abnormality such as distension. Palpation of the rumen is performed by the tips of the fingers or the flat of the hand on the left flank, commencing immediately below the ends of the transverse processes of the lumbar vertebrae ; palpation should be continued down into the lower third of the abdomen. Firm pressure with the fingers is necessary to overcome the natural resistance of the abdominal wall in order that the state of the rumen may be ascertained by means of the tactile sense of the fingers. In the normal animal palpation reveals a resilient tone of the musculature of the underlying viscus. In the upper third firm digital pressure causes the abdominal wall and the wall of the rumen to yield slightly, and it will be realised that this portion of the rumen is not distended with either food or gas. Palpation of the middle third shows that the food material fills the rumen to a level approximating to the upper margin of the middle third. This part of the rumen is moderately firm and definitely resilient to pressure. The lower third of the rumen is more resistant to pressure owing to the weight of foodstuff bearing down on the wall of the organ and the abdominal wall. If firm pressure is maintained with the fingers over the upper third of the rumen it is possible to estimate the frequency, regularity and strength of the ruminal movements. If the rumen is abnormally full and the contents feel like a mass of stiff dough impaction is present. Impaction of the rumen is not common. It occurs when a large quantity of dry food has been eaten and then a considerable quantity of water has been drunk, causing the dry food to swell and form a firm mass that the rumen cannot disperse. It also occurs when an animal has ingested such quantities of acorns that the rumen contents consist of little but acorns. A lack of resilience and impression of lifelessness is conveyed to the fingers in atonic conditions of the rumen. A feeling of tenseness is appreciated if the rumen is tympanitic.

In the event of the wall of the rumen lacking tone, the upper part of the dorsal sac may not be in close apposition to the abdominal wall in the sub-lumbar fossa. Palpation in this region will give the impression of such a separation between the wall of the rumen and the abdominal wall.

When a distended abomasum has become displaced to occupy a position on the left of the rumen, the rumen is slightly separated from the abdominal ; this abnormality can be appreciated by palpation in the sub-lumbar fossa. Intraperitoneal tympany gives a similar feeling of space between the abdominal wall and that of the rumen. Intraperitoneal tympany seldom, if ever, accompanies traumatic reticulitis, since the bovine peritoneum appears to respond rapidly to irritation and localises any infection carried through by the foreign body.

Gas may enter the peritoneal cavity from the rumen following puncture of that organ with a trocar and cannula to relieve tympany.

Percussion of the rumen requires to be carried out with some force in order to produce a sufficiently clear response. In the normal animal very slight resonance in the upper third indicates that this part of the rumen contains relatively little food material ; the sound in the middle third changes from very slight resonance on its upper border to complete dullness on the lower part due to the food material in the rumen ; the lower third is completely dull. A reduction of the very slight resonance in the upper third to almost complete dullness is present in impaction of the rumen ; a less pronounced change is seen in completely atonic conditions of the rumen. Increased resonance is indicative of tympany of the rumen ; in severe cases the distension with gas may be so acute that a clear drum-like note is produced on percussion. If the gas produced by fermentation in the rumen is free in the upper part, the percussion note attains its greatest resonance ; if, on the other hand, the gas is mixed throughout the fermenting mass so that this is leavened and fills the rumen (frothy bloat), there will be an abnormal degree of resonance extending down into the middle third, but the resonance is not so pronounced as when the gas is free in the upper part of the organ. Very occasionally as a result of changes in the microbial population the rumen becomes distended with evil-smelling fluid. Percussion then gives a dull note and the presence of fluid can be demonstrated by the wave-like motion produced by vigorous palpation or percussion. The presence of such fluid can be confirmed by passing the stomach tube and siphoning off some of it. The cause of the changes in the microbial population of the rumen are not always easy to determine ; in some cases it was found in association with overdosage of sulphapyridine.

Auscultation of the rumen should be done with a stethoscope ; while the ear may be applied directly to the flank the results obtained are not so satisfactory, and the operator runs the risk of acquiring skin parasites from the patient. The rhythmic churning movements of the rumen produce a sound that on auscultation clearly conveys the impression that the semi-solid contents of the rumen are being turned over and so mixed. These waves of movements occur at regular intervals, varying according to the nature of the food. The frequency of these waves varies from two to three in a minute. If the activity of the rumen is reduced these waves of sound are less frequent and not so loud. A complete absence of such sounds is noted in absolute stasis, whether due to severe impaction of the rumen or atony from any cause, but in such circumstances a weird collection of indistinct splashing sounds may be heard. These appear to be caused by movement of the ingesta by the contraction and relaxation of the diaphragm.

It is important that the clinician should appreciate that not only does auscultation provide valuable information as to the activity of the rumen, but as the movements of the rumen are directly related to those of the rest of the alimentary tract it is possible by auscultation of the rumen to form a reasonably accurate estimate of the degree of functional activity of the rest of the alimentary tract. The movements of the rumen—and reticulum —serve several purposes. First there is the constant process of mixing the contents and secondly there is the need to secure eructation of the gas evolved during the digestive processes taking place in the rumen. Thirdly movements of the rumen are an essential part in the process of returning boluses of food material to the mouth there to be further triturated in the process of chewing the cud.

RETICULUM.—The situation of the reticulum in the concave dome of the diaphragm, low down and far forward in the abdomen under cover of the ribs, prevents direct examination of this organ. Impaction of the reticulum does not occur. Tympany of the reticulum without tympany of the rumen cannot take place, owing to the open and direct communication between reticulum and rumen.

The reticulum is a frequent site for the lodgement of foreign bodies. A blunt foreign body may lie in the reticulum without causing any harm, but if the object is sufficiently large it may be pressed into the wall of the organ by the action of its musculature ; necrosis of the wall of the reticulum results when the foreign body will enter the peritoneal cavity, carrying with it infection that sets up a local peritonitis. Sharp, and especially pointed, foreign bodies pierce the mucous membrane readily, and may rapidly penetrate the wall of the reticulum. During the period of penetration the irritation of the wall produces a digestive disturbance that is of a subacute character. If the process of penetration is not continuous the symptoms of digestive disturbance may be intermittent. The length of time, during which the digestive symptoms alone are noticed, varies very greatly ; a period of little more than twenty-four hours is not uncommon, but in other cases this has been known to extend to five and a half months. The diagnosis of a foreign body injuring the wall of the reticulum is largely dependent on the elimination of the various possible causes of a subacute and rather indefinite digestive disturbance. Following penetration of the wall there develops between the reticulum and diaphragm a localised area of peritonitis. The occurrence of traumatic peritonitis is manifested by a sudden loss of appetite, a painful grunt and cessation of peristalsis. The temperature may be elevated. The association of pain with the region of the reticulum is necessary in diagnosis of traumatic peritonitis. Penetration of the reticulum may take place on any part of its ventral or anterior aspect and if in the upper anterior aspect the foreign body may pass on through the diaphragm to enter the pericardial sac, there setting up a septic pericarditis. Penetration of the posterior wall of the reticulum appears to be much less common.

Indirect pressure exerted over the site of the reticulum may cause the animal to grunt if pain is present in the reticulum. This indirect pressure may be achieved by pinching the spine in the thoracic region. This causes the animal to crouch and the tension on the abdominal wall increases the pain so that the animal gives a grunt or groan. Pressure on a level with the xiphoid cartilage of the sternum in the lower third of the chest, especially if forceful, makes the animal grunt and move backwards and forwards ; if desired this pressure may be exerted on either side of the chest simultaneously by the clinician and an assistant. Another method of applying indirect pressure is to press up under the posterior part of the sternum with one hand and down on the corresponding part of the spine with the other.

It has been claimed that an area of dullness over the region of the reticulum can be demonstrated by percussion, but it is very doubtful if this can be done.

Williams (1955) by combining auscultation of the reticulum with palpation of rumen was able to establish a co-relation between movements of the reticulum and the rumen. Auscultation of the reticulum is carried out at the costo-chondral junction of the seventh rib—a point to be found approximately a hand's breadth behind the point of the elbow. Considerable practice is required if the reticular sounds are to be recognised and it may often be very difficult to interpret them. When the reticulum contracts the liquid ingesta in it are forced over the reticulo-ruminal fold, creating a " mild swishing " sound which lasts for two to three seconds. This is followed by sounds recognisable as caused by the movement of fluid and are due to fluid ingesta flowing back into the reticulum as it relaxes. The movements of the rumen are assessed by placing the hand in the sub-lumbar fossa.

By means of this examination Williams was able to show that the cycle of reticulo-ruminal movement started with contraction of the reticulum ; after an interval of two to three seconds the dorsal sac of the rumen was felt to reach its maximum contraction followed by relaxation. After a pause of about thirty seconds the dorsal sac was involved in a second phase of contraction. It was observed that eructation of gas accompanied the second phase of contraction but did not accompany the primary contraction following on reticular contraction. Though in the majority of cases the rhythm is one primary or reticulo-ruminal wave of contraction followed by one wave of contraction involving the rumen alone, the rhythm may vary between 2 : 1 and 1 : 2.

Williams then applied these observations to the diagnosis of traumatic reticulitis. He showed that the grunt in this condition is associated with contraction of the reticulum and that the phase of reticulo-ruminal contraction could be distinguished from that involving the rumen alone by the absence of eructation during the reticulo-ruminal phase of contraction. Thus with the hand in the sub-lumbar fossa the movements of the rumen can be identified ; observation will show at which stage the cow eructates and occurrence of a grunt can be co-related with the phase of reticular contraction. The identification of a reticular grunt is then a useful piece of clinical evidence when taken in conjunction with other points already observed in the general examination of the patient.

REFERENCES

WILLIAMS, E. I. (1955).   *Vet.*, *Record*, vol. lxvii, pp. 907-911 and 922-927.
WILLIAMS, E. I. (1955).   *ibid.*, vol. lxviii, pp. 835-839.

Mine detectors have been used in the differential diagnosis of traumatic reticulitis and traumatic pericarditis. Positive results are only obtained if the foreign body is metallic. When taken in conjunction with strongly suggestive clinical signs positive results obtained by the mine detector may be accepted as confirmatory evidence. It must, however, be borne in mind that many adult cattle harbour metallic foreign bodies in the reticulum and that these foreign bodies do the animals no harm. So an indication by the mine detector that a foreign body is present does not justify an assumption that the animal is suffering from truamatic reticulitis. Furthermore, the mine detector may fail to indicate the presence of the foreign body. The value of X-rays in the diagnosis of traumatic reticulitis is to some extent governed by the need to have a plant with very considerable power and also the need to have available an adequate grid to obviate the scatter of X-rays. The mobile unit in ordinary use has not sufficient power for this purpose. A positive result with X-rays would be useful for clinical evidence but a negative result would not necessarily exclude the presence of a penetrant foreign body.

Differential blood counts have been of only limited value in the differential diagnosis of traumatic reticulitis. The increase in total white cell count is, as a rule, not very marked, the figure falling within one standard deviation above the normal. There is some shift in the distribution of the cells, the percentage of neutrophils increasing by as much as one tenth of the normal at the expense of the other white blood cells. The proportion of non-lobulated (younger forms) to lobulated (older forms) shows an increase. Unfortunately these changes are not always clear cut and in any case they only indicate a defensive reaction and are in no way specific of traumatic reticulitis.

On the other hand a differential blood count may prove useful in deciding whether in a particular case a foreign body has penetrated the diaphragm and reached the pericardium. When infection has reached the pericardium there is an immediate strong defensive reaction. This is reflected by a total white cell count of as much as 20,000 to 30,000 (normal 7,000$\pm$2) with a marked increase in the percentage of neutrophils. This percentage may reach a figure of 70 in contrast to the normal of 30$\pm$9·8 and the proportion of non-lobulated to lobulated cells shows a marked increase in favour of the non-lobulated cells.

Subacute but persistent digestive disturbances in the ruminant may be associated with chronic inflammatory processes involving the wall of the reticulum, the wall of the rumen or the œsophageal groove. These are quite commonly caused by *Actinobacillus lignerieresi*. The associated lymphatic tissue in the posterior mediastinum is often affected. The signs are those of inappetance, irregular or suspended rumination with possibly subacute but persistent tympany of the rumen. Rumen movements are suspended or feeble. Attempts to provoke evidence of pain as described as occurring in traumatic reticulitis do not evince any response. Agglutination tests with *Actinobacillus* antigen have not proved entirely dependable and there are no characteristic changes in the blood picture. A tentative diagnosis of actinobacillosis of the rumeno-reticular tissue may justify treatment with iodides or sulphonamides, though an apparent recovery does not necessarily confirm the diagnosis.

The diagnosis of liver abscess in cows is beset with many difficulties. The signs are somewhat similar to those of a slowly developing case of traumatic reticulitis or actinobacillosis. The blood picture in liver abscess may show little change or may suggest a chronic defensive reaction (see Chapter XIX). There is no rise in temperature as may be found in traumatic peritonitis. The presence of liver abscess can only be established satisfactorily on post-mortem examination.

OMASUM.—As was mentioned on page 69 direct examination of the omasum is not possible and its functional activity must be presumed from the clinical evidence of functional activity of the rest of the alimentary tract. Lesions of the omasum can be demonstrated in cattle plague (rinderpest), malignant catarrh, the mucosal disease complex, and hyperkeratosis.

ABOMASUM.—The position of the abomasum on the abdominal floor on the right side behind the xiphoid cartilage permits of forceful palpation being employed to determine the presence of pain. This can be done in an upward direction with the clenched fist ; pain caused by this procedure is shown by the cow emitting a sharp painful grunt. Owing to the strength of the abdominal wall in this region and the great weight of the viscera and their contents resting on the floor of the abdomen, more detailed palpation is not possible in adult bovines. Neither percussion nor auscultation is of assistance in the investigation of diseased states involving the abomasum.

It should be borne in mind that the functional activity of the rumen is directly related to the condition of the abomasum. Inflammatory conditions of the abdomen in adult cattle are manifested in part by atony of the rumen and suspension of rumination. Attention has already been drawn to the grinding of the teeth by which cattle give expression to the discomfort caused by abomasitis. Inflammatory conditions of the abomasum are accompanied by febrile symptoms.

Displacement in association with dilatation of the abomasum is most commonly, though not always, encountered in dairy cows. It appears that there may be a relationship between this condition and the later stages of pregnancy, but such a relationship is apparently not an essential feature of the ætiology. The clinical picture is that of a cow which has lost its appetite and is not ruminating. After a period of starvation the animal starts to feed and may again ruminate. But the appetite is again lost and rumination ceases. The fæces tend to be rather pale in appearance. A mild degree of ketosis is present and can be regarded as a starvation ketosis. Examination of the abdomen shows a rather flaccid rumen and it may be necessary to push in the abdominal wall in the sub-lumbar fossa before the rumen can be felt. In some cases it is possible to find a bulging cylinder mass impinged between the rumen at the abdominal wall just under the margin of the last rib. Auscultation over the last two ribs may reveal a splashing tinkling sound quite unlike rumenal sounds. Rectal examination may show the rumen extending further over to the right side than is normal. These signs are strongly suggestive of dilatation and displacement of the abomasum, but an exploratory laparotomy may be required before the diagnosis can be confirmed.

Impaction of the abomasum appears to be a relatively uncommon condition. The clinical picture is that of an animal completely off food, with a distended abdomen in obvious discomfort. Accurate palpation through the abdominal wall is extremely difficult ; at the best it may be possible vaguely to feel a large ill-defined firm mass when palpating deeply in the right side. It is possible that by rectal examination the outline of the impacted abomasum may be felt far forward in the abdomen. Exploratory laparotomy is necessary before the diagnosis can be confirmed.

Torsion of the abomasum has been recorded by Neal and Pinsent (1960) and may be a sequel to dilatation. The animal is in great pain and distressed ; the pulse is fast and weak ; the temperature may be subnormal. The abdomen is distended and tympanitic but there is no tympany of the rumen and the site of tympany is located on the right side. Vigorous palpation on the right side may produce splashing sounds, auscultation showing high-pitched sounds comparable to that heard on the left side in displacement of the abomasum. Considerable resonance over the last rib may be demonstrated by percussion. Rectal examination may reveal the greatly distended abomasum pressing back into the posterior part of the abdomen. Exploratory laparotomy is indicated as a prelude to diagnosis.

REFERENCE

NEAL, P. A., and PINSENT, P. S. N. (1960). *Vet. Record*, vol. lxx, pp. 175-180.

Ulceration of the abomasum in cattle has been observed in cases of displaced abomasum including those complicated by peritoneal adhesions.

The time relationship between ulceration and displaced abomasum is not clear. The clinical picture of displaced abomasum is not materially different when ulceration is present. Ulceration of the abomasum is associated with parasitic gastritis in both cattle and sheep. It may be that cases of abomasal ulceration in cattle are a sequel to parasitic gastritis. These cases are most often encountered in cattle between one and two years old. The animal is losing condition, its appetite is irregular and rumination is performed irregularly. There is either intermittent diarrhœa or persistent looseness of the fæces. Examination of the fæces for Johne's bacilli and evidence of helminthiasis is negative. Hæmatological investigations show a mild degree of anæmia and little else. No response is obtained with symptomatic treatment to correct the diarrhœa. While the possibility of ulceration of the abomasum may be suspected in life it cannot be confirmed except by post-mortem examination.

Ulceration of the abomasum in calves associated with fungal infections present a picture of a fairly brief fatal illness in which diarrhœa is the leading symptom. Diagnosis is dependent on demonstrating the fungal infection of the abomasal ulcers by post-mortem examination. It is obviously of importance to establish the diagnosis in these cases in order that steps may be taken in relation to hygiene and management to prevent the occurrence of further cases.

Ulceration of the abomasum occurs in the course of specific diseases such as cattle plague, malignant catarrh, the mucosal complex and hyperkeratosis.

Parasitic gastritis may cause serious disturbances in young cattle. This condition is associated with diarrhœa, anæmia and emaciation. Further details of diagnosis are discussed in the chapter on clinical helminthology.

In young calves fed on milk the rumen is smaller than the abomasum and the latter is the more important viscus from a clinical standpoint until the relative enlargement of the rumen and the consumption of solid bulky food results in the development of the function of rumination. During this early period of life gastric catarrh, associated with intestinal catarrh, is an important clinical condition. Disease of this type falls into the general group known as " white scour." In very young calves acute septicæmia of a very fatal type is common, a high percentage of these cases being due to B. coli. The susceptibility of calves to septicæmia of this type is increased if there be a lack of vitamin A. A mother's colostrum is normally rich in antibodies, and it is well known that failure to allow calves an adequate supply of colostrum results in a high incidence of illness.

During calfhood foreign bodies in the abomasum may cause severe indigestion. This may develop during or immediately after feeding. A certain amount of tympany is present in these cases ; the fæces are clay-like in consistence and have a sour smell ; epileptiform convulsions are also observed.   In very small calves deep palpation of the abdomen is possible ; this may be performed with the calf standing on its feet, when it will be found convenient to place one hand on each side of the abdomen. Alternatively the calf may be laid on its side and the abdomen palpated from the upper side, or one hand may be slipped under the abdomen and with the other hand pressing downwards deep bi-manual exploration may be performed.

It is important to realise that epileptiform convulsions in calves preceding death may be due to lead poisoning, vitamin E deficiency or low blood magnesium.   In these cases there are not the signs of gastro-intestinal disturbance.   The discovery on post-mortem examination of a foreign body in the abomasum does not necessarily establish that it is the cause of the epileptiform convulsions and death.   It is necessary to eliminate the possibilities mentioned before concluding that a foreign body in the abomasum is responsible.   Enquiry as to the methods of husbandry may indicate the likelihood of vitamin E deficiency or hypo-magnesæmia.   Blood samples can be taken from animals of the group exposed to the same environment and diet, in order that the status in relation to blood magnesium can be determined.   (See page 370).   The position in regard to lead poisoning should be investigated, with regard to possible sources of lead and tissue from the dead animal and blood and fæces from other animals at risk should be sent for analysis.   (See page 373).

INTESTINE.—The state of the intestine is largely reflected in the character of the fæces.   In intestinal stasis the increased absorption time renders the fæces drier and harder ; the firm fæcal masses often have a glazed appearance due to a coating of mucus.   Diarrhœa is a symptom of intestinal irritation.   This may be dietetic in origin and represents the attempt of the intestine to remove as rapidly as possible any irritant in the foodstuff.   Diarrhœa is very frequently a symptom of specific disease. Acute diarrhœa occurs in anthrax, when the fæces may contain large quantities of blood.   Hæmorrhagic fæces are passed in bovine pasteurellosis (hæmorrhagic septicæmia).   In bovine coccidiosis large clots of blood may be voided along with fluid fæces.   Chronic diarrhœa in the bovine is a symptom of Johne's disease, liver fluke infestation and round worm infestation of the alimentary tract.   Johne's disease, owing to the long incubation period, occurs in cattle of more than eighteen months.   The disease is characterised by loss of condition, anæmia and œdema of the intermaxillary space.   The fæces are fluid and contain gas bubbles. Diagnosis is confirmed by the demonstration of *Mycobacterium para-tuberculosis* in the fæces, the method being described in the chapter dealing with clinical bacteriology.   Liver fluke (*Fasciola hepatica*) infestation occurs in any age from young store cattle to old cows.   The cattle have been grazing on damp pastures where conditions are favourable for the parasite and its intermediate host the snail *Limnœa truncatula*.

Clinical signs are only observed in cattle if a fairly heavy infestation with liver fluke is present. The persistent profuse fluid diarrhœa causes a rapid loss of condition. Diagnosis is dependent on the demonstration of the eggs of the liver fluke in the fæces.

Round worm infestations of the alimentary tract may occur in any age of cattle. Permanent pastures and overstocking are contributory factors in the development of a measure of infestation sufficient to cause clinical signs which closely resemble those of fluke infestation. In order to establish a diagnosis of round worm infestation it is necessary to determine the presence of a substantial number of eggs in the fæces. The methods of demonstrating and counting the eggs of liver fluke and round worms in the fæces are described in the chapter on clinical helminthology.

As it is not always possible to distinguish clinically between Johne's disease, liver fluke infestation and round worm infestation, a useful practice is, as a routine, to examine fluid fæces from cases of persistent diarrhœa for *Mycobacterium paratuberculosis*, liver fluke eggs and round worm eggs.

In addition to " white scour " or coli-septicæmia mentioned on page 77 outbreaks of diarrhœa in calves may be causedby *Salmonella* infections, the presence of which can only be established by a bacteriological examination. (See page 329). Adult carriers of *Salmonella* infection can be detected by means of the agglutination test. (See page 330).

Palpation of the right side of the abdomen does not prove helpful in the diagnosis of digestive diseases of cattle with the possible exception of distension of the abomasum.

By means of the process of ballottement it may be possible to demonstrate distension of the abomasum. Ballottement is useful in the diagnosis of pregnancy in its later stages. Percussion of the right side of the abdomen would reveal the presence of intestinal tympany ; the condition of intestinal tympany is however rare in cattle, and a resonant note to percussion in the right side would be more likely to arise from acute distension of the abomasum with gas, a condition possibly associated with torsion of the abomasum. Percussion in the right side of the abdomen may demonstrate an increase in the area of dullness due to enlargement of the liver, but the degree of enlargement would have to be very substantial before this could be appreciated. Auscultation of the right flank will give information as to the state of intestinal activity and will reveal abnormal sounds arising from an abomasum distended with a mixture of fluid and gas.

Rectal Examination in Cattle.—Rectal examination as an aid to the diagnosis of digestive diseases of cattle is not performed so frequently as in horses. The information regarding the state of the rumen obtained by rectal examination adds little if anything to that already obtained by palpation through the left flank. The position of the reticulum and

TABLE II

Scheme for the Differential Diagnosis of the Causes of Acute Distension of Abdomen in Cattle.

			Diagnosis	*Corroboration by*
ACUTE DISTENSION OF ABDOMEN	TYMPANITIC	RIGHT SIDE	Severe Gaseous Distension of Abomasum or Torsion of Abomasum	Auscultation, Percussion, Ballottement, Rectal Examination, Laparotomy
		LEFT SIDE — Lower Resonance	Frothy Bloat...........	History of Feeding. Evidence by Probang or Trocar and Cannula
		LEFT SIDE — Higher Resonance	Choke (Cervical or Thoracic Oesophagus)	Palpation of Neck, Passage of Probang
			Acute Tympany of Rumen...............	History of Feeding, Evidence by Probang or Trocar and Cannula
	NON-TYMPANITIC	RIGHT SIDE	Impaction of Abomasum	Auscultation, Palpation, Ballottement, Rectal Examination, Laparotomy
		LEFT SIDE	Impaction of Rumen	History of Feeding, Palpation, Auscultation

In female exclude any complications of pregnancy such as hydrops amnii.

(Dilatation and Displacement of Abomasum see Table III.)

omasum in the anterior part of the abdomen renders it impossible to examine them by means of a rectal examination. Only when it is grossly distended can the abomasum be felt on rectal examination. It will be found that rectal examination in cattle provides valuable information in cases showing symptoms of colic, in cases of dull pain with straining, and in cases of recumbency associated with evidence of toxæmia.

The temperature will have been taken during the preliminary general examination; a rectal examination should not be made in a bovine animal that is acutely ill and showing symptoms of colic if the temperature is found to be acutely elevated. These symptoms may indicate that the case is one of anthrax, when a considerable risk would be run by the person making the rectal examination.

Symptoms of colic are present in cattle suffering from certain urinary diseases, and a rectal examination may indicate either renal or bladder conditions that could cause the acute pain.

Mechanical interference with the bowel, such as " gut tie " and intussusception, cause colic in cattle, and diagnosis of these conditions is facilitated by rectal examination. Gut tie may result from castration by traction when the *ductus deferens* has been severed high up in the inguinal region so that the lacerated end retracts within the abdominal cavity and becomes attached by an inflammatory adhesion to the parietal peritoneum. The band thus formed in the abdominal cavity forms with the parietal peritoneum a space through which a loop of small intestine may pass, there becoming incarcerated when strangulation may follow.

Intussusception of the small intestine is sometimes encountered in cattle of all ages. In addition to symptoms of a digestive disturbance and intestinal obstruction, pain is shown; this varies in degree from acute colic to dull discomfort, the pain being persistent. Straining is acute in many cases; the animal may remain recumbent and cannot be raised to its feet. It may be possible, through the rectum, to palpate the sausage-like intussusception lying fairly far forward in the abdomen to the right of the median plane. Unless necrosis of the invaginated portion of the bowel has occurred, palpation of the intussusception will cause considerable pain. On withdrawing the hand and arm from the rectum they may be found to be covered with mucus and extravasated blood so mixed that the material has been described as resembling red currant jelly.

Acute septic metritis with closure of the *os uteri* causes a profound toxæmia that frequently renders the cow so comatose that she becomes recumbent and superficially appears to resemble a case of milk fever. This condition develops within a few days of parturition. Though in the early stages there is an increase in the temperature, the heat-regulating centre may be so depressed that the temperature is normal or subnormal. Owing to the closure of the *os* no purulent material is escaping through

F

TA

Scheme for Differential Diagnosis of D

	NO DIARRHŒA				
Appetite	Milk Yield	Rumination	Fæces	Temperature	Grunt
Depressed or Lost	Depressed	Suspended	Stasis Dry firm	Often raised	Clearly audible Related to reti contraction
Irregular but still feeding to some extent	Slight progressive reduction	Irregular, i.e. intermittent	Reduced in quantity but not abnormal	Normal	Very little if an
Refuses food for a period then eats for a period and again loses appetite	Progressive reduction	Only takes place occasionally	Pale soft	Normal	Absent
Lost for concentrates otherwise depressed may be depraved	Marked reduction	Suspended or irregular	Firm, dry dark glazed scanty	Normal	Absent

	DIARRHŒA				
Type of Diarrhœa	Class of Animal	Grazing or Indoors	Appetite	Temperature	Mouth
Acute persistent	Particularly young stock	Grazing or been grazing recently	May persist	Normal	Normal
Chronic following recurrent sub-acute attacks	2 years or older seldom under 2 years	Indoors or grazing	Often persists	Normal	Normal
Acute persistent	Any age other than calves	Indoors or grazing	Usually lost	Elevated in early stages later may be sub-normal	Small superfici ulcers in mouth These heal rap and may be mi
Sub-acute persistent later becoming profuse	Most common in store cattle, but may involve adult cattle	Usually in winter or spring following grazing on wet or poorly drained pastures	Persists until later stages	Normal	Normal
Chronic sub-acute diarrhœa, fæces often pale	Most frequent in young stock	Indoors or grazing	Depressed	Normal	Normal

ances of Cattle Without Distension of Abdomen.

NO DIARRHŒA				
umen Activity	Pain	Ketosis	Possibility	Further Investigation Required
epressed	Provoked by pressure referable to reticulum	Not present	Traumatic Reticulitis	Rumenotomy
ome reduction	Not present	Not present	Actinobacillosis of reticulum and/or Oesophageal groove	Laparotomy or Rumenotomy " Test therapy "
epressed. May e space between dominal wall d rumen	Not present	Mild degree of ketosis may be present, i.e. starvation ketosis	Dilated and displaced abomasum	Auscultate over last two ribs on left side for abnormal gurgling tinkling sounds. Laparotomy
epressed	Not present	Marked Confirm by test of milk	Acetonæmia	Confirm history in relation to parturition eliminate displaced abomasum in sub-acute cases

DIARRHŒA				
Intermaxillary space	Mucous Membranes	Bodily Condition		
ormal		Some loss	Parasitic gastro-enteritis	Examine fæces for worm eggs. In older and adult cattle eliminate Johne's disease
Iay be marked dema	Rather pale	Progressive emaciation	Johne's disease	Examine fæces for clumps of acid-fast bacteria. Complement fixation test on blood sample
ormal	Dirty	Rapid loss	Mucosal Complex	Examine blood sample for evidence of leucopœnia
dema	Pale watery	Considerable loss over some weeks	Liver fluke infestation	Examine fæces for fluke eggs; one negative sample does not exclude. Consider locus and suitability of ground for intermediate stage. In group postmortem examination of worst affected may be justified for confirmation
ormal	Pale	Poor	Abomasal ulceration	Can only be diagnosed with certainty by post-mortem examination

the vagina.   The distended uterus can be palpated if a rectal examination is made.

SHEEP.—The principal difference in the examination of the abdomen of the sheep and that of cattle is that the organs are very much less bulky. The smaller size permits deep palpation in much the same manner as has been described for calves, but in adult sheep the contents of the rumen are sufficient in quantity to limit the extent of such an examination in the same way as in the case of older calves.   The abdomen of young lambs can be thoroughly explored by deep palpation.

Diarrhœa is a leading symptom in a number of important conditions in sheep.   In lambs in the first fortnight of life diarrhœa may be a symptom of the less acute form of lamb dysentery, a fatal toxæmia due to *Cl. welchii* (type B).   Diagnosis is established if a post-mortem examination shows acute enteritis and a varying degree of ulceration in the small intestine. If the post-mortem findings are indefinite, a bacteriological examination of the intestinal contents is carried out to demonstrate the presence of the specific toxin produced by *Cl. welchii* (type B).   In older lambs, and in sheep of any age, persistent diarrhœa may be due to worm infestation ; in these cases a fæcal worm egg count is made, with a view to establishing the degree of infestation.   If a large number of sheep are involved, a post-mortem examination of a badly affected sheep will provide useful confirmatory evidence.   Johne's disease, owing to the prolonged incubation period, only causes persistent diarrhœa in sheep over eighteen months old ;   diagnosis is dependent on the microscopic demonstration of the causal organisms in the fæces or in a smear made from a portion of the intestinal wall.   Unlike cattle, however, sheep with Johne's disease may reach a severe stage of emaciation without showing any diarrhœa.

Liver fluke infestation in sheep, if severe, causes profuse diarrhœa and progressive emaciation.   Œdema of the intermaxillary space may be seen and there may be a substantial degree of ascites.   The mucous membranes become very pale.   The condition is more troublesome in the late winter or early spring.   The incidence increases after a wet summer.   Geographical conditions such as poorly drained land and soil conditions favourable to the intermediate host *Limnea truncatula* influence the incidence of this disease.   The demonstration of fluke eggs in the fæces confirms the presence of adult flukes in the bile ducts of the liver. Post-mortem examination of a badly affected sheep will confirm the diagnosis both as regards mature and immature flukes.

Pulpy kidney in lambs and enterotoxæmia in older sheep due to *Clostridium welchii* type D though essentially related to an intestinal lesion is manifested by a very severe rapidly fatal toxæmia without any outward evidence of the intestinal lesion such as diarrhœa.

PIG

REGIONAL ANATOMY

The pig has a capacious mouth. The stomach is large, the greater curvature reaches the abdominal floor behind and to the left of the xiphoid cartilage ; if distended the stomach may extend to a point midway between the xiphoid cartilage and the umbilicus.

The small intestine is very long. The large intestine is about six times the length of the animal's body. The cæcum is eight to twelve inches in length ; from the anterior part of the left lumbar region it runs downwards, backwards and medially ; the apex lies approximately midway between the brim of the pubis and the umbilicus nearly on the middle line of the abdomen. The bulk of the colon is arranged in the form of three spiral coils lying on the floor of the abdomen. The terminal part of the colon commences on the right side of the body, passing forward till it reaches the region of the stomach where it crosses the abdomen and then runs backward to terminate in the rectum.

CLINICAL EXAMINATION

MOUTH.—In young pigs, if the animal is held by an assistant, the mouth may be opened with a smooth flat piece of wood, or pieces of bandage or tape may be applied to the upper and lower jaw, and by traction on these the mouth may be opened sufficiently to inspect its cavity. In larger pigs it will be necessary to secure the animal against a wall by means of a gate or door held by assistants. A rope may then be applied to the upper jaw with a running noose ; if this is held securely the lower jaw may be depressed with some stout object such as a piece of a broom handle, or a piece of rope may be applied to the lower jaw.

PHARYNX.—Examination of the pharynx in the pig is limited to external palpation, and owing to the thickness of the skin and subcutaneous fat in the normal animal it is not possible to obtain by this examination any very accurate information, other than evidence of discomfort and unusually easy provocation of coughing.

ABDOMEN.—Owing to the thickness of the abdominal wall in all but very emaciated pigs, palpation of the abdomen is of very limited value. Differential diagnosis of digestive disturbances in the pig is beset with such difficulty that in many cases a satisfactory diagnosis can only be made after a post-mortem examination has been made.

The pig is an animal in which loss of appetite is a symptom of any acute illness in spite of the voracious and omnivorous appetite with which this animal is usually credited. The onset of any of the infectious diseases affecting the pig may be manifested by a complete loss of appetite. Thirst is another symptom often noticed in pigs, especially if they are suffering from febrile disease; the craving for liquid may be so intense that the animal will drink any fluid however filthy. Even pools of urine on the floor of the sty will be taken if no other fluid is available.

Vomiting occurs in the pig; it is evidence of gastric irritation. Such irritation may be due to the ingestion of irritant material or it may be caused by one of the specific diseases of the pig, for example, swine fever.

Constipation in pigs may be due to an unsuitable diet that either does not contain sufficient roughage or is of a character that leads to the formation of unusually hard dry faeces. A not uncommon cause of constipation is lack of exercise; brood sows kept entirely indoors are particularly liable to develop constipation from this cause.

Diarrhœa may be a symptom of specific disease such as swine fever, swine erysipelas or necrotic enteritis and it is an important symptom of catarrhal enteritis in young pigs, arising from the intestinal irritation of a heavy infestation with *Ascaris lumbricoides*. Any intestinal irritant in the diet may cause diarrhœa. Eversion of the rectum may occur in pigs as a complication of diarrhœa resulting from the straining that follows excessively frequent evacuation of faeces. Eversion of the rectum may thus be a sequel to helminth infestation in young pigs; it is also seen as a symptom of enteritis due to chronic swine fever. Eversion of the rectum is seen in sows following parturition, and arises from straining consequent upon pelvic irritation.

Distension of the abdomen giving a pot-bellied appearance is seen in young debilitated pigs; the debility may be caused by helminth infestation or by a chronic wasting disease such as chronic swine fever or necrotic enteritis. Epileptiform convulsions or fits in young pigs are commonly a sequel to ascarid infestation. The condition known as gut œdema of pigs, usually encountered in store pigs shortly after they have been put on a new ration, is essentially a condition involving the digestive system. It is, however, manifested by clinical evidence of a more general character. In addition to loss of appetite there may be œdema of the eyelids and evidence of interference with posture and locomotion. Diagnosis can only be established with certainty by post-mortem examination.

DOG AND CAT

REGIONAL ANATOMY

DOG.—The shape of the mouth varies according to the breed of the dog. In all dogs it is possible, if the mouth is opened widely, to inspect the whole of the buccal cavity.

A well-developed elongated tonsil is present in a clearly defined sinus situated between the anterior and posterior pillars of the fauces.

The stomach of the dog is large in relation to the size of the animal. The cardiac portion of the stomach, lying on the left side of the abdomen, forms a large rounded sac when full. The pyloric part, lying on the right side of the abdomen, forms a small cylinder ; the size of this part does not vary greatly according to the amount of the food in the stomach. When empty the stomach does not reach the abdominal floor and lies

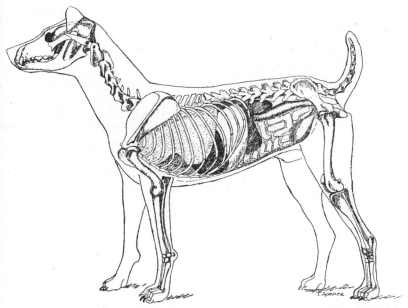

FIG. 9.—Dog. Thorax and Abdomen. Left side.

under the cover of the costal arches. When fully distended the greater curvature may reach the abdominal floor behind the xiphoid cartilage and may even extend backwards to a point half-way between the xiphoid cartilage and the umbilicus.

The duodenum runs backwards from the pylorus high up in the abdominal cavity on the right side ; a small part makes contact with the right flank. On a level with the sixth or seventh lumbar vertebra the duodenum turns medially and passes forward medial to the left kidney, to terminate in the jejunum. The mesentery of the duodenum is short, anchoring it comparatively firmly in the abdomen. The second part of the duodenum, that passes forward medial to the left kidney, is connected to the mesentery of the colon by a fold of peritoneum. The free portion of the small intestine has a long mesentery, and except for the terminal portion of the ileum is disposed in coils filling the abdominal cavity from behind the stomach to the pelvis ; many of these coils come in contact with the abdominal wall.   The terminal part of the ileum runs forward in the sublumbar region on the right side and joins the colon at the ileo-colic orifice, which lies on a level with the last rib.

The cæcum forms a type of spiral, the flexures forming this being held in place by the peritoneum which attaches one to another and also attaches the cæcum to the terminal part of the ileum.   The cæcum extends from the level of the last rib to the second or third lumbar vertebra. It lies approximately midway between the median plane of the body and the right abdominal wall.   The colon is somewhat variable in its position. It consists of a part running forward, followed by a transverse part crossing the abdomen from right to left and ending in a portion that runs backwards to communicate with the rectum.   The disposition of the colon is comparable to that in man, the three parts corresponding respectively to the ascending, transverse and descending colon.   Radio-logical studies of the dog's colon show that very frequently, when viewed dorso-ventrally, the path of the colon describes the figure of a question mark (?).   The rectum of the dog is almost completely covered with peritoneum, this tissue being reflected back to the level of the first coccygeal vertebra.   The so-called anal glands of the dog are two sacs, one on each side of the anus, with a small opening at the junction of the rectum and anus.   The glands contain a dirty grey evil-smelling material that is greasy in character.   Normally they are no bigger than a hazelnut, but if impacted with secretion may be larger.

CAT.—The alimentary system of the cat follows the general plan of the dog.   The stomach is large and is not so completely under cover of the ribs as in the dog.   The anal glands described in the dog are not present in the cat, but a number of small glands disposed around the anus have independent openings.

CLINICAL EXAMINATION

THE MOUTH.—In the dog, owing to the great length of the oral rim, it is possible, by retracting the lips, to inspect the outer aspect of the incisor, canine and premolar teeth, and the corresponding parts of the gums and lips.   Many dogs show no resentment to this procedure if it is done quietly and gently.

The mouth may be opened by grasping the upper jaw with a hand placed over the nose so that the thumb lies on one side and the fingers on the other ; pressure with the thumb and fingers pushes the lips between the upper and lower teeth, thereby forcing open the mouth and at the same time protecting the fingers against the animal's teeth.   It will be necessary to depress the lower jaw if it is desired to open the mouth widely; this may be done by pressure with a forefinger on the lower incisor teeth. A small proportion of dogs resent handling of the mouth, and care is required that the dog does not bite the fingers. The application of a piece of tape to the upper jaw and a similar piece to the lower jaw provides a method of opening the mouth that avoids placing the fingers too close to the mouth. In examining the mouth it is necessary that the dog be securely held by a competent assistant; the examination can be carried out with greater speed and will cause the animal much less distress if the animal is properly held. In the case of vicious dogs or animals suffering acute pain in the mouth a narcotic or short-acting anæsthetic should be administered.

In cats the mouth may be opened by grasping the head firmly with one hand placed so that the thumb and fingers lie in front of the ears; with a finger of the other hand or a blunt instrument such as a spatula placed between the canine teeth the lower jaw may be depressed. As in dogs a narcotic or anæsthetic may be required in the case of troublesome animals.

The condition of the mucous membrane of the tongue, gums and cheeks should be noticed; this is normally of a bright red colour. The tongue may be covered with a thin white film during attacks of indigestion. A copper-coloured discoloration of the tongue is observed in severe toxæmic conditions, such as acute nephritis. The tongue is coated with a dark brown evil-smelling film in acute gastritis and acute intestinal obstruction. Gingivitis is commonly observed as a symptom of alimentary toxæmia. Necrosis and ulceration of the gums and buccal mucosa in general and necrosis of the tip of the tongue develop during the course of acute nephritis, leptospiral jaundice, and also in cases associated with a deficiency of the anti-pellagra factor of the vitamin B complex. The term " Stuttgart disease " has been somewhat loosely applied to toxæmia in the dog associated with persistent vomiting, necrosis of the buccal mucosa and tongue. The disease originally described as occurring in Stuttgart appears to be that caused by *Leptospira canicola*.

The condition of the teeth should be observed. In healthy dogs these are clean and the enamel is a clear white colour. Gross encrustations of tartar cause damage to the gums and consequent oral sepsis. Distemper during puppyhood, at the time when the permanent teeth are being formed, may interfere with the enamel formation and the teeth are seen to possess an enamel tip, but part of the enamel is absent; the dentine thus exposed is of a dirty yellowish-brown colour and is uneven in texture, and the surface is rather lower than that of the enamel. An evil-smelling brown film covers the teeth in the alimentary form of distemper, in acute gastritis and any acute form of intestinal toxæmia. Blue translucent deciduous teeth are seen in puppies suffering from acute calcium deficiency.

Foreign bodies wedged between the teeth may cause intense discomfort to the animal, and in consequence alarming symptoms of acute nervous excitement may develop. Inspection will reveal the presence of the foreign body. Sharp foreign bodies may penetrate the soft tissues of the mouth. Frequently part of the foreign body projects above the surface of the tissues, but if completely buried in the tissues the reaction to the trauma caused by the penetration of the foreign body will be noticeable. A radiological examination of the mouth will reveal the presence of the foreign body if it is sufficiently opaque to X-rays to show up in contrast to the tissues surrounding it.

PHARYNX.—In the dog and cat the pharynx may be inspected if the mouth is opened and the tongue is depressed. Depression of the tongue is resented by most animals, but if the procedure is carried out expeditiously in a good light it will be found possible in many cases satisfactorily to examine the pharynx. In those animals that resent the examination, it will be necessary to resort to the use of a narcotic or anæsthetic if a detailed examination of the pharynx is desired. Such an examination will be necessary if the presence of a foreign body in the pharynx is suspected. Small light-coloured objects, as for instance a small spicule of fish bone, are not always easily seen in the pharynx of a cat ; thorough inspection in these cases is obviously of great importance.

While inspecting the pharynx, the tonsillar tissues can also be inspected. The inspection of the pharynx and tonsillar tissue will show evidence of inflammatory changes and of tumour growths, the latter frequently originating in the lymphoid tissue of the tonsil. It may not be possible to distinguish by inspection between chronic inflammatory changes and tumour formation.

Following inspection of the cavity of the pharynx, the external surfaces of the pharynx should be palpated, with a view to determining the presence of pain, heat and swelling. The associated lymphatic glands should be palpated in order that any involvement of them may be appreciated.

ŒSOPHAGUS.—Examination of the œsophagus is concerned principally with the diagnosis of the presence of foreign bodies in the lumen. If the foreign body is in the cervical portion, careful palpation of the course of the œsophagus will enable its presence therein to be determined. A foreign body in the œsophagus often gives rise to a train of rather suggestive symptoms ; these are ability to swallow fluids but inability to swallow solids. Small pieces of meat may be taken greedily but after the lapse of a short space of time the meat is rejected. Passage of a soft rubber sound will be prevented by the foreign body and the length to which the sound can be passed will indicate the position of the foreign body. A very common site of the obstruction is that part of the œsophagus between the base of the heart and the diaphragm. Decomposition of the foreign body and necrosis and sepsis of the wall of the œsophagus give rise to evil odours ; particles of tissue adhering to the sound will convey the odour when the sound is withdrawn.

Radiological examination of the œsophagus will assist the diagnosis if this is in doubt.

The lumen of the œsophagus may be inspected with an œsophago-scope. This instrument is preferably passed on an animal under deep narcosis or light anæsthesia.

VOMITING.—Though vomiting in the dog and cat is a constant symptom of gastric derangement, it is also frequently a symptom of disease conditions in other organs in the abdomen and may, on occasion, be caused by disease of organs outwith the abdominal cavity. Therefore, before discussing in detail the examination of the abdomen in these animals, it is necessary to consider the various conditions that may cause vomiting in these animals.

Overloading of the stomach is relieved by vomiting ; young animals vomit more readily than adults. Vomiting is so common an occurrence in puppies and kittens that, if unaccompanied by any other evidence of disturbance of health, it is only of significance as an indication of overeating. Inflammatory conditions affecting the gastric wall induce vomiting by local irritation of the nerve endings, reflexly stimulating the vomiting centre ; thus vomiting is a symptom of all types of gastritis. Vomiting is caused by irritant drugs, *e.g.* arsenic, phosphorus and many anthelmintics. The presence of a foreign body in the stomach may induce vomiting either by irritation of the gastric wall or by obstruction of the pylorus. The vomiting so induced is in some cases continuous, but in others it may be intermittent in character.

The presence of intestinal affections is commonly indicated by vomiting. Enteritis uncomplicated by gastritis seldom causes vomiting unless the inflammatory process is acute. Complete obstruction of the small intestine rapidly causes severe and continuous vomiting. The obstruction may be due to the presence of a foreign body, or it may result from intussusception, or the occlusion of the lumen may be due to a tumour or inflammatory growth developing either in the wall of the bowel or in neighbouring structures. Since intussusception does not always cause complete occlusion of the lumen of the intestine the condition may not be manifested by vomiting.

Obturation of the colon does not immediately cause vomiting and several days usually elapse before this occurs. When vomiting arises from a fæcal impaction of the terminal part of the colon the vomitus may consist of material resembling fæces in character, this being known as stercoraceous vomiting.

Diseased conditions of organs other than those of the alimentary tract frequently lead to vomiting. Involvement of organs such as the liver and pancreas may cause vomiting. Acute nephritis, chronic nephritis and suppurative nephritis all cause vomiting in consequence of the toxæmic state that develops as a result of the interference with efficient excretion by the kidneys. Toxic vomiting in cystitis may be caused by absorption through the bladder wall of the products of the bacterial activity therein. Acute metritis and chronic endometritis in bitches frequently cause toxic vomiting. Vomiting may be caused reflexly by irritation of the peritoneum in inflammatory processes involving that tissue. Toxæmia due to absorption from septic peritonitis increases the severity of the vomiting. Pharyngitis, laryngitis and bronchitis may cause spasms of coughing that terminate in retching and vomiting. Cardiac disease of a severe character not infrequently causes attacks of vomiting, especially in the terminal stages.

DIARRHŒA.—In the dog diarrhœa may be a symptom of specific disease, as in the abdominal form of distemper. It may be caused by helminthiasis ; in tape-worm infestations the gravid segments are passed in the fæces, in round worm infestations the fæces must be examined microscopically to demonstrate the eggs. If the fæces are hæmorrhagic, it is desirable to determine whether the blood has been shed from the terminal part of the rectum, when it is bright red in appearance, or whether it has been shed further forward in the intestine, when it will be dark in colour, due to the changes that have occurred in its passage along the bowel. Intussusception occurs as a result of intestinal irritation ; its presence may lead to severe straining and the passage of considerable quantities of blood in the fæces.

ABDOMEN.—Clinical examination of the abdomen entails inspection, palpation and percussion.

Inspection of the abdomen has already been discussed under the description of the preliminary general inspection of the patient, the basis of differentiation of the causes of enlargement of the abdomen being there described.

Percussion of the abdomen will indicate the presence of tympany. Tympany may be generalised throughout the abdomen or may be local-ised in a particular portion of the viscera. If so localised careful per-cussion may indicate the site of the tympany in relation to organs involved. Percusson of the abdomen may reveal an area of complete dullness due to the presence of any large solid mass such as a large tumour. The process of producing a percussion wave as a means of determining the pre-sence fluid in the peritoneal cavity has already been described. (See p. 40).

Palpation is of great value in the diagnosis of diseases of the abdominal organs in the dog and cat. Palpation should be conducted in a firm but gentle manner. Vigorous palpation, especially if the abdomen is painful, will result in the animal tensing the abdominal muscles so that examina-tion of the abdomen is prevented. If the fingers are placed gently on the abdomen and pressure gradually increased the resistance of the abdominal muscles is overcome and the contents of the abdominal cavity can be explored. In acutely painful conditions the tense contraction of the abdominal muscles sometimes renders palpation of the abdomen difficult. Patient handling of the abdomen may render it possible to overcome this resistance. But as soon as the site of an acutely painful condition is approached by the fingers the abdominal muscles will contract. In small animals the examination may be made with one hand grasping the abdomen between the thumb and fingers. In larger animals it will be found more satisfactory to utilise both hands, one placed on either side of the abdomen and the pressure being made with the tips of the fingers. A considerable part of the abdomen can be palpated in most animals ; it is, however, not possible to palpate the anterior part lying under the cover of the ribs.

If empty the stomach cannot be accurately defined, but foreign bodies in the stomach can in a proportion of cases be palpated. Failure to palpate a foreign body does not necessarily exclude the possibility of one being present in the stomach. The presence of a foreign body in the small intestine can often be determined by careful thorough deep palpation of the abdomen. Pressure over the foreign body usually causes an increase in pain evidenced by tensing of the abdominal muscle. A radiological examination is often necessary to assist in diagnosis if the presence of a foreign body is suspected. Intussusception presents a cylindrical swelling that has been compared to a sausage in shape. The intussusception may be under cover of the ribs lying beyond the reach of palpation if the animal is standing in a normal horizontal position ; if the fore end of the animal is raised so that the long axis of the animal is vertical, the intussusception may fall back into that portion of the abdomen that lies within reach of the clinician's examination. Firm masses of fæcal material in the colon and rectum can in most cases be felt by deep palpation. The presence of hard faecal material in the rectum can be confirmed by a rectal examination.

Enlargement of the mesenteric lymph glands is appreciated as an indefinite swollen mass. Such an enlargement commonly involves the mass of glands lying in the mesentery of the ileo-cæco-colic region, and if of sufficient extent may interfere with the peristaltic function of the bowel, giving rise to the general symptoms of subacute intestinal obstruction evidenced principally by vomiting and toxæmia.

Inflammatory changes in the wall of the alimentary tract, i.e. gastritis and enteritis, cause pain which may be localised by palpation of the abdomen. Thus in gastritis the presence of pain in the left epigastric region may be demonstrated. Inflammatory processes involving the small intestine give rise to diffuse abdominal pain. Colitis gives rise to less acute pain that cannot be definitely referred to any particular organ.

The position and characteristic feeling of organs such as the kidneys and bladder should be borne in mind when palpating the abdomen ; the student should make himself familiar with these points by palpating the abdomen of animals of the different breeds and sizes.

Care will be required to distinguish between an enlarged uterus and the colon in female animals. Gross abnormalities such as enlargement of the spleen, the presence of a large hæmatoma arising from the spleen, or the existence of a tumour mass can all be appreciated by palpation. Consideration of the topographical anatomy of the abdomen in relation to the findings of palpation will render it possible in many cases to decide upon the site and probable nature of the mass that is being felt. Furthermore, the general clinical signs may already have indicated the probable involvement of a particular organ.

Rectal examination in the small domestic animals is carried out with the forefinger. Before doing so the finger should be anointed with soap or a bland substance such as soft paraffin or lard, but preferably the finger should be covered with a thin rubber finger-stall and this smeared with a little liquid paraffin or soft paraffin. The extent to which the rectum and pelvic organs can be examined is limited by the length of the finger. Hard fæcal material in the rectum will obstruct the introduction of the finger. Stricture of the rectum is not an uncommon sequel to fæcal impaction, and if present as an annular contraction of the rectum, passage of the finger beyond the stricture may be found impossible. In the male dog enlargement of the prostate gland interferes with the passage of fæcal material, especially if this material is hard in consistency. Enlargement of the gland, if acute, is revealed as a soft painful swelling ; if of a more chronic nature the enlargement is hard, fibrous in character and less painful.

The anal glands (or paranal sacs) should be examined. Frequently these are found distended with an accumulation of the unpleasant smelling dirty material secreted into these sacs. The contents of either of these glands may become infected and the subsequent suppuration may result in the production of an abscess involving the gland concerned.

RADIOLOGICAL EXAMINATION OF THE DIGESTIVE SYSTEM

Radiological examination of the digestive system is practically confined to dogs and cats.

MOUTH AND PHARYNX.—A radiological examination may be useful in cases in which the presence of a foreign body buried in the soft tissues is suspected, but will only show objects that are more opaque than the surrounding tissues.

ŒSOPHAGUS.—A radiological examination may be of great assistance in the diagnosis of obstruction of the œsophagus, whether due to a foreign body or due to constriction. If the foreign body is opaque to X-rays it will be seen by a direct radiographic examination. If not sufficiently opaque the administration of a radio-opaque substance such as bismuth carbonate will render the foreign body more obvious. For this purpose a fairly thick suspension of bismuth carbonate or barium sulphate in gum mucilage may be administered as a draught, or one or two small gelatine capsules filled with bismuth carbonate may be administered as pills, or a piece of worsted may be soaked in a suspension of bismuth carbonate

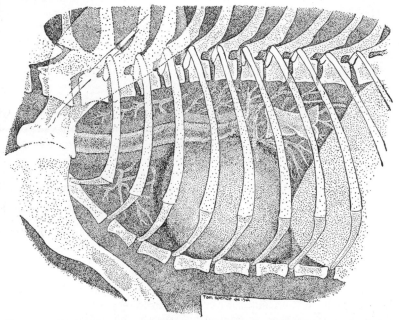

Fig. 10.—Dog. Drawing of Radiograph showing foreign body in posterior part of œsophagus. One-third actual size.

in gum mucilage, rolled into a ball and administered as a pill. The fluid suspension of bismuth used in the first method flows over the surface of the foreign body and sufficient of it is usually held up to reveal the outline of the foreign body. The foreign body prevents the passage of the pill in the second and third method, and it is seen arrested anterior to the point where the foreign body lies. In any of these methods the radiographic examination requires to be carried out immediately after the radio-opaque substance has been administered. In some cases it is practicable to administer the radio-opaque substance to the animal while it is in position under the X-ray screen, and the actual swallowing of the material may be observed. Constrictions of the œsophagus are shown up if the swallowing of a radio-opaque suspension is watched under the X-ray screen ; but if desired a radiograph may be taken.

STOMACH AND INTESTINE.—Foreign bodies in the stomach and intestine, if opaque to X-rays, are readily seen either by means of the fluorescent screen or by radiograph. The stomach and intestine must be free from any radio-opaque drugs, such as bismuth carbonate, if foreign bodies are to be demonstrated radiologically. If not radio-opaque they may be shown up in the stomach by giving a radio-opaque suspension and allowing time for this to leave the stomach when sufficient of the suspension may have been retained on the surface of the foreign body to delineate it. If a foreign body in the intestine is not causing a complete intestinal obstruction, this method of delineating the foreign body with a radio-opaque suspension may prove successful, but if there is a complete intestinal obstruction the suspension will not pass along the lumen of the bowel to reach and delineate the foreign body.

A radiological examination of the stomach and intestine may be of assistance in the diagnosis of indefinite cases of toxæmia that appear to be alimentary in origin. This examination may be done by means of the fluorescent screen. It is usually more satisfactory to conduct the examination by taking a series of radiographs. Such a series enable the clinician to compare the observations made over a period of time and provide much more detailed information than can be obtained from the transient pictures seen by fluoroscopy.

Food having been withheld for at least twelve hours, the examination should commence with a preliminary radiological examination before administering any opaque material. Then a radio-opaque suspension is administered by mouth for this purpose. If a prepared suspension is not available, 120 grains of bismuth carbonate, 120 minims of mucilage of tragacanth and four ounces of water are made into a uniform suspension, this quantity being sufficient for a medium-sized dog.

The first radiological examination, whether by radiographs or by fluorescent screen, should be carried out as quickly as possible after the radio-opaque suspension has been administered. Thereafter further radiological examinations are taken to study the flow of the radio-opaque material along the alimentary canal.

In a normal fasting animal the stomach begins to empty in a few minutes, and after about fifteen minutes the radio-opaque material can be seen passing along the coils of the free portion of the small intestine. Within an hour the bulk of the opaque suspension will have been expelled from the stomach and the material will reach the large intestine in less than four hours. If the animal defæcates normally all the opaque suspension will have been voided from the alimentary canal within twenty-four hours of its administration. If the animal is constipated, defæcation may be stimulated with a soap and water enema.

Delay in the stomach emptying may be due to stasis or rarely to pyloric spasm. Retention of some of the bismuth on the mucous membrane giving a mottled appearance may indicate ulceration.

In the early stages of enteritis, characterised by complete stasis, the stomach may be seen contracting when the opaque material flows into the duodenum, but due to the stasis the material is not accepted by the duodenum and when the stomach relaxes the opaque material flows back into the stomach. This appearance must not be interpreted as indicating an obstruction of the duodenum with a foreign body, when the stomach does not empty and the suspension is usually vomited a few minutes after its administration.

Rectal injection of a suspension of opaque material such as bismuth carbonate or barium sulphate can be used to demonstrate dilatation of the colon, and stricture of the terminal part of the colon or rectum. Stricture may follow damage to the wall of the rectum by a fæcal impaction, and dilatation then occurs anterior to the stricture.

Intussusception is not necessarily visible on a radiological examination of the abdomen and the administration of an opaque meal is of little assistance.

LIVER

Extensive lesions of the liver are frequently found on post-mortem examination of animals that have shown no symptoms during their life. It is clear that a normal animal is provided with a very considerable reserve of liver tissue. Localised lesions do not produce outward evidence of their presence until this reserve has been damaged and the liver rendered unable to perform the minimum degree of function required for bodily health.

Regional Anatomy

HORSE.—The greater part of the liver lies to the right of the median plane. The parietal surface is mainly in contact with the diaphragm, that of the right lobe lying below the upper halves of the 8th to the 15th rib, but separated from the ribs by the diaphragm and in the more anterior part of the area by the border of the right lung. The liver does not extend beyond the edge of the costal arch.

CATTLE.—The liver also lies to the right of the median plane. The parietal surface is mainly in contact with the diaphragm, but a small area is in direct contact with the upper third of the last two or three ribs. Occasionally a small area is in contact with the right flank.

SHEEP.—The liver lies to the right of the median plane. A small area may come in contact with the abdominal wall just beyond the lower part of the margin of the costal arch.

G

PIG.—Though the greater part of the liver lies to the right of the median plane the parietal surface extends beyond the costal arch and comes in contact with the abdominal wall for a small area on the left side of the body and a rather larger area on the right side.

DOG.—Only a small portion of the parietal surface of the liver makes contact with the abdominal floor behind the xiphoid cartilage, where owing to the rectus muscle of the abdomen it cannot be palpated.

CLINICAL EXAMINATION

Where possible an examination of the liver is directed to determine enlargement or alteration in the contours of the organ. The greater part of the examination of the liver is concerned with an investigation of the symptoms and signs of disturbance of liver function.

PHYSICAL EXAMINATION

In all animals except the dog and cat the position of the liver is such that examination by physical means is of very little value. In the dog and cat gross enlargement of the liver causes the margin to project beyond the edge of the costal arch, when the margin can be felt by deep palpation. If the enlargement of the liver is uniform the margin feels smooth and rounded. If due to tumour growth the edge of the liver may feel nodular. It is not possible with any degree of accuracy to demonstrate by percussion in the larger farm animals an increase in the area of dullness in the right side due to enlargement of the liver.

JAUNDICE

The term jaundice (icterus) implies staining of the tissues by bile pigment that is present in the general circulation in abnormal amounts. The pigmentation of jaundice is most easily seen in the visible mucous membranes but can also be seen in non-pigmented skin when the coat is parted. The existence of jaundice should have been detected during the preliminary examination of the patient. It is quite often found that the owner was unaware of the presence of jaundice.

Jaundice is an important piece of clinical evidence but is in itself not a diagnosis as there are a number of different causes of jaundice. The causes of jaundice are classified as

Pre-hepatic (Hæmolytic)
Hepatic (Toxic, Infective and Obstructive)
Post-hepatic (Obstructive)

Pre-hepatic or hæmolytic jaundice occurs where there is excessive destruction of red blood cells and the liver is unable to cope with the increased amount of bilirubin formed by the breakdown of hæmoglobin liberated from the red blood cells.

In the domesticated animals hæmolytic jaundice is encountered in piroplasmosis as seen in tropical and sub-tropical countries. In Britain hæmolytic jaundice is encountered in British Bovine Piroplasmosis (caused by *Babesia bovis* and transmitted by the tick *Ixodes ricinus*) and in Post-parturient Bovine Hæmoglobinuria, an acute hæmolytic anæmia of indefinite ætiology. Hæmolytic jaundice in other species of domesticated animals in Britain is uncommon. If hæmolysis is sufficient to cause jaundice the renal threshold for hæmoglobin will have been exceeded and a feature of the case is hæmoglobinuria.

Bilirubin formed by the breakdown of red blood cells (hæmobilirubin) and present in the circulation has not been acted on by the liver cells and so gives an indirect reaction to the Van den Bergh test when applied to serum. (See page 317). A small amount of bilirubin is produced during the formation of hæmoglobin and if hæmoglobin formation is unusually active an increase in bilirubin may be shown by the quantitative Van den Bergh test. In such circumstances traces of " bile pigment " may be found in the urine but are not significant of any abnormality.

Hepatic jaundice may result from damage to liver cells as a result of the action of either toxic or infective agents. These two types are exempli-fied by phosphorus poisoning in any species of animal and infection in the dog with *Leptospira icterohæmorrhagiæ*. In toxic or infective hepatic jaundice there is damage to the liver cells and in some cases there may be actual obstruction of the smaller bile channels so that the condition is a combination of toxic or infective and obstructive hepatic jaundice. Tumour growths in the liver may cause hepatic obstructive jaundice by pressure on bile ducts. In toxic and infective jaundice the Van den Bergh test may give a biphasic reaction, an immediate direct reaction due to absorption of conjugated bilirubin (cholebilirubin) from the liver cells and an indirect reaction due to increased bilirubin (hæmobilirubin). The test is thus not of any value in determining the presence of toxic or infective jaundice.

In acute cases of toxic or infective jaundice damage to the liver cells causes an increase in the blood transaminase figures. There is a greater increase in glutamic-pyruvic transaminase (G.P.T.) than in glutamic-oxalo-acetic transaminase (G.O.T.). (See page 37).

In obstructive jaundice conjugated bilirubin (cholebilirubin) accumu-lates in the blood a direct Van den Bergh reaction being obtained. In addition in obstructive jaundice there is absorption into the blood of bile salts, which can be demonstrated in the urine.

Post-hepatic jaundice is essentially obstructive in character. Obstruc-tion of the common bile-duct with gall stones is extremely rare in the domesticated animals, so also is occlusion of the duct lumen by an inflammatory process involving the duct wall. Tumour of the head of the pancreas in the dog may press on the common bile duct, involve the duct itself or involve the liver substances.

In post-hepatic obstructive jaundice bile is not passing into the duodenum. In consequence in animals other than herbivores the absence of bile is reflecting on the appearance of the fæces which are pale-coloured, evil smelling and putty-like in consistence. In herbivores the absence of bile is marked by the pigment of the foodstuffs and the odours associated with the digestive processes in these species. In post-hepatic obstructive jaundice a direct reaction is obtained with the Van den Bergh test and bile pigment and bile salts can be demonstrated in the urine.

The qualitative Van der Bergh test directed to determine an indirect reaction due to bilirubin (hæmobilirubin) or a direct reaction due to conjugated bilirubin (cholebilirubin) has not proved useful in the differential diagnosis of the various forms of jaundice, largely because of the difficulties arising from biphasic reactions. The test is however of value as a quantitative test in assessing the severity of jaundice.

Canine Virus Hepatitis.—Canine virus hepatitis, contagious canine hepatitis, Rhubarth's Disease is a virus disease of the dog. Apparently the infection is widespread in any area with a substantial dog population. Very many young dogs must pass through a symptomless reaction to infection and thereafter are immune. Some show a mild degree of malaise and recover spontaneously. In more severe cases the picture is one of a fulminating toxæmia resulting before long in death. Tenderness may or may not be appreciated in the liver region. Certain diagnosis is dependent on post-mortem examination and subsequent laboratory investigation. (See page 332). In these more severe cases the damage to the liver cells is acute and progressive. There is therefore a great increase in the liberation of transaminase and the increase in glutamic-pyruvic transaminase (G.P.T.) is very much greater than in glutamic-oxalo-acetic transaminase (G.O.T.). (See page 371).

This change in serum transaminase levels is indicative of acute liver damage but is not a specific indication of virus hepatitis.

An immediate direct Van den Bergh reaction has been observed in the acute cases of canine virus hepatitis, but the reaction has no specific significance in relation to diagnosis of this virus disease.

TESTS OF ANTITOXIC FUNCTION.—The glycuronic acid test gives an indication of the efficiency of the detoxicating function of the liver. In horses and cattle there is normally a considerable amount of glycuronic acid present in the urine. Its absence from urine in horses or cattle may be taken as evidence of liver dysfunction. In the dog there are normally only traces of glycuronic acid in the urine. In order to test the detoxicating function of the liver in the dog, ten grains of aspirin are given by mouth or three grains of camphor in oil are injected intramuscularly; the urine passed during the following twenty-four hours is collected and tested for glycuronic acid. For details of test for glycuronic acid see Urine Analysis (p. 315). If the detoxicating function of the liver is entirely arrested, conjugation of the aspirin or camphor with glycuronic acid does not occur. The absence of glycuronic acid in the urine after the administration of aspirin or camphor is therefore an indication of grave liver damage, but conjugation still occurs even when extensive damage to the liver tissue has taken place.

COAGULATION TIME.—The coagulation time is increased, due to the decreased fibrinogen content in hepatic insufficiency. The method of determining the coagulation time is described in the chapter on clinical hæmatology.

LÆVULOSE TOLERANCE.—The power of the liver to convert lævulose to glycogen is tested by administering lævulose in proportion to the animal's weight and observing the rate of disappearance of the lævulose from the circulation.

RADIOLOGICAL EXAMINATION

Radiological examination of the liver can only be carried out in the dog or cat. Owing to the rarity of gall-stones in the dog, cholecystography is seldom performed. To render the contents of the bile ducts and gall-bladder opaque to X-rays a solution of the sodium salt of tetrabromphenolphthalein is injected intravenously. A fluoroscopic examination or a radiograph sometimes shows enlargement of the liver shadow or distortion of its outline, but very frequently an X-ray examination fails to reveal any abnormality in liver disease.

PARASITISM

The presence of liver flukes is determined by the demonstration of the eggs of these parasites in the fæces of the host. The technique of examination of fæces for worm eggs is described in the chapter on clinical helminthology. Parasitic cysts in the liver can seldom be diagnosed except on post-mortem examination.

CHAPTER IV

RESPIRATORY SYSTEM

General Signs—Regional Anatomy
Clinical Examination of Respiratory System as a Whole :—Inspection—
    Respiratory Movements—Nasal Discharge—Cough—Lymphatic
    Glands
Physical Examination of the Chest—Palpation—Percussion—Ausculta-
    tion
Exploratory Puncture and Radiological Examination of the Chest
Analysis of Symptoms and Clinical Signs of Chief Respiratory Diseases

SOME of the general signs that suggest the presence of disease of the respiratory system have already been discussed ; these include cough, nasal discharge and alterations in the respiratory movements ; many respiratory diseases are accompanied by febrile symptoms.

Respiratory disease may be primary or secondary. Primary disease of the respiratory system is common in the domestic animals. Some cases are sporadic in character, others are of an infectious nature, *e.g.* equine infectious pneumonia. Secondary involvement of the respiratory system occurs when the defences of some other part of the body are overwhelmed and the infection reaches the respiratory system. Thus equine tuberculosis commencing in the abdomen may overwhelm the local lymphatic resistance, the infection becoming miliary in character, and in consequence there develops an acute and rapidly fatal tuberculous pneumonia. Secondary involvement of the respiratory system also follows conditions that result in a lowering of the tissue resistance to the invasion of commensals, *e.g.* broncho-pneumonia as a complication of canine distemper. In both sheep and cattle respiratory disease frequently arises as a result of infestation of the bronchi or bronchioles with parasitic helminths. The differential diagnosis of parasitic bronchitis is discussed in the chapter on clinical helminthology.

Respiratory disease in the domestic animals is not only of significance on account of the ill health and mortality caused by it, but is also of importance in those animals whose value depends on their respiratory efficiency. Animals whose respiratory efficiency has been impaired by serious respiratory disease are no longer capable of sustaining fast or strenuous exertion. Equally so an animal whose respiratory efficiency has been lowered may not be able so economically to convert food into milk or flesh as the animal with a normal respiratory system. Early accurate diagnosis may make possible the application of effective therapy in time to initiate a recovery before irretrievable damage has been done to the tissues. It should be appreciated that these principles of early diagnosis and treatment apply equally to diseases of the upper respiratory passages as well as to diseases of the lungs and pleura.

Diseases of the respiratory system are very easily spread, not only because many are infective in character, but also because the expired air contains the infective agent. The wide spread of the infective agent may be facilitated by coughing.

REGIONAL ANATOMY

HORSE.—The nostrils in the horse are capacious ; they are placed obliquely so that the openings look mainly in a lateral direction. The lower part of the mucous membrane of the nasal septum can be inspected. The nasal cavity on each side is divided into three meatus, the dorsal, the middle and the ventral ; these open into a common meatus bounded medially by the nasal septum. The posterior nares leading from the nasal cavity into the pharynx are elliptical in outline. The pharynx is completely separated from the buccal cavity by the long soft palate. The prolongation of the soft palate renders inspection, through the mouth, of the pharynx and larynx impossible in the horse. The ventricle of the larynx is a membranous sac lying lateral to the vocal cord and the arytenoid cartilage that makes contact with the medial surface of the thyroid cartilage. The ventricles communicate with the cavity of the larynx by an opening lateral and dorsal to the vocal cord.

The trachea is large in section, being slightly wider in the horizontal transverse section than in the dorso-ventral. The bifurcation of the trachea is situated approximately on a level with the 5th rib and is almost equidistant between the dorsal and ventral surfaces of the chest.

The lungs occupy the greater part of the thoracic cavity, being closely in contact laterally with the thoracic wall and medially with the other organs of the chest. The dorsal border of the lung extends from the 1st rib to the second last intercostal space (16th-17th rib). The anterior part of the lower border of the lung is interrupted by the cardiac notch. From the 6th rib the lower border passes upward and backward, being on a level with the costo-chondral junction of the 7th rib, and is approximately midway up the length of the 12th rib. The anterior portion of the chest is covered by the upper part of the foreleg ; when the leg is upright the posterior border of the area covered runs from the upper part of the 6th rib to the lower end of the 5th rib. On the right side the portion of the heart not under cover of the lung lies in front of the elbow and dorsal to the humerus. On the left side, the portion of the heart in contact with the chest wall is larger in area, forming the area of cardiac dullness (see Figs. 1 and 2, pp. 42 and 43).

CATTLE.—The nostrils are relatively small and owing to the thickness of the borders are not dilatable like those of the horse; the openings face laterally. The nasal cavity is shorter than in the horse, and in the posterior third the cavity is not divided owing to the abrupt termination of the nasal septum. The trachea is shorter and relatively smaller in diameter than in the horse.

The bronchus supplying the apical lobe of the right lung leaves the trachea opposite the 3rd rib; the bifurcation of the trachea into the two

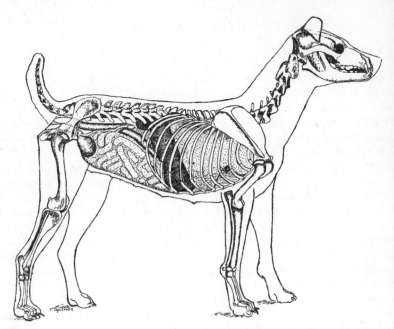

FIG. 11.—Dog. Thorax and Abdomen. Right side.

main bronchi lies on a level with the 5th rib. The lower border of the lung runs upwards and backwards in practically a straight line from the lower extremity of the 6th rib to meet the dorsal border at the second last intercostal space (see Figs. 3 and 4, pp. 61 and 62).

SHEEP.—The respiratory system of the sheep largely resembles that of the ox.

PIG.—The nostrils are small and, situated on the flat anterior surface of the snout, face forward. The nasal cavity is long and narrow. The trachea is relatively short. It possesses an extra bronchus supplying the apical lobe of the right lung, as in the ox. The dorsal border does not extend beyond the third last intercostal space and more frequently only reaches the anterior border of the fourth last intercostal space. The lower border of the lung runs in a more or less straight line from the lower end of the 6th rib to join the posterior end of the dorsal border.

DOG.—The nostrils are comma-shaped and the cavity of the opening is small. The nasal cavity varies in length and shape according to the breed. On opening the mouth and drawing forward and depressing the tongue, the cavity of the pharynx may be inspected and also the larynx. The upper and lower extremities of the trachea are practically circular on section ; the middle portion is flattened slightly in a dorso-ventral direction. The bifurcation of the two main bronchi forms a wide angle.

Owing to the chest wall being rounder in outline than in either the horse or ox, the lateral surface of the lungs are more convex. The dorsal border of the lung extends to the posterior margin of the second last intercostal space. The lower border of the lung is slightly curved ; it runs upwards from the ventral extremity of the sixth intercostal space to join the dorsal border at the 12th rib.

CAT.—The respiratory system of the cat closely resembles that of the dog.

CLINICAL EXAMINATION

INSPECTION

RESPIRATION.—The inspection carried out in the preliminary general examination may now require to be supplemented. The rate, the rhythm and the character of the respiratory movements must be carefully observed.

The rate may be observed by noting the excursions of the ribs and the abdominal wall, and also, chiefly in the horse, by observing the nostrils. It may be found convenient in certain cases to estimate the rate by listening to the passage of air in and out of the nostrils. The rate varies widely in the different domestic animals. The smaller the animal the faster is its respiratory rate.

Increase in the respiratory rate inevitably follows exertion. Excitement, especially in highly-strung animals, causes considerable disturbances of the respiratory rate. Badly ventilated stuffy buildings are a possible cause of an increase in the respiratory rate. Engorgement with food, particularly in fat cattle and pigs, causes an obvious alteration in the respiratory rate that is often accompanied by grunting. A constant concomitant of fever is an increase in the respiratory rate. The respiratory rate is increased whenever there is any interference with either the normal ventilation of the lungs or the gaseous exchange in the lung itself, causing defective oxygenation of the blood and an increase in the carbon dioxide tension in the blood.

Obstruction to the free movement of air may be located in the respiratory passages. Spasms of coughing interfere with normal respiratory movements and severe attacks of coughing may, especially if frequent and prolonged, cause considerable dyspnœa.   Interference with the respiratory movements, such as occurs in the muscular spasms of tetanus, or limitation of the excursion of the diaphragm due to abdominal distension, necessitates an increase in the respiratory rate to compensate for the reduced efficiency of the respiratory mechanism.   Disease of the lungs, whether acute or chronic, interferes with the functional activity of these organs and is reflected in a compensatory increase in the respiratory rate, which may thus be caused by congestion of the lungs, pneumonia, emphysema, atelectasis or neoplasm.   Any defect in the oxygen-carrying capacity of the blood will require greater respiratory activity—and cardiac activity—to meet the oxygen requirements of the tissues.   Reflex stimulation of the respiratory centre causing an increase in the respiratory rate occurs in acute pain and is particularly noticeable if the pain is located in the extremities or in one of the serous cavities of the body.

The rhythm may vary quite considerably in normal animals.   Pronounced variations in the rhythm are observed in animals that are excited or subjected to any unusual or frightening influence.   It is therefore important to study the respiratory rhythm before disturbing the animal or handling it in any way if it is of an excitable nature.   Gross variations in the respiratory rhythm are commonly observed in dogs in strange surroundings ;   it is frequently necessary to allow a dog to become accustomed to its surroundings before attempting to estimate the respiratory rhythm.   The respiratory rhythm will be disturbed by any obstruction that necessitates an increased effort on either inspiration or expiration, the increased resistance to the passage of air causing either inspiration or expiration to be prolonged.   Thus in chronic alveolar emphysema inspiration is performed normally but expiration is prolonged, due to the increased muscular effort required to expel air from the lungs.   Depression of the respiratory centre occurs in profound toxæmia, coma, narcotic poisoning, and in the toxic stages of anæsthesia ;   in consequence respiration is irregular.

The character or type of respiration may be a considerable diagnostic significance.   In all normal animals respiration is performed by a combined movement of the thoracic and abdominal walls.   Whenever dyspnœa develops, from whatever cause, the muscular efforts of respiration become more forceful.   Exaggeration of either thoracic movements or abdominal movements will alter the character of the respiration.   Gross distension of the abdomen limits the extent to which abdominal movement can assist the respiratory efforts ;   in consequence respiration becomes largely thoracic in character.   This is exemplified by the effect on respiration of pronounced ascites.

A double expiratory movement is characteristic of chronic alveolar emphysema.   Inspiration is performed normally, and after the usual pause at the end of inspiration a normal thoracic expiratory movement takes place. This is insufficient to compress the distended lung, so, in order that the air may be expelled, a secondary movement is made by the abdominal muscles, the contraction of these appearing to raise the abdominal wall. In effect, the expiratory movement is a double one and the second part of it is seen as a " lifting " of the abdominal wall. The recognition of this type of respiration is of diagnostic importance, as a broken-winded horse suffering from pulmonary congestion closely simulates pneumonia, but if the type of respiratory movement is appreciated differential diagnosis will be considerably facilitated.

Limitation of thoracic movement occurs in the early painful stages of pleurisy : a compensatory increase in the movements of the abdominal wall leads to the appearance of a pleuritic line or ridge that is seen on a level with the costo-chondral junctions during each respiratory movement. This pleuritic line is particularly noticeable in horses in the early stages of pleurisy. In pleurisy with effusion the respirations develop a swinging character owing to the great excursion of the abdominal wall necessary to assist the ventilation of lungs surrounded with fluid. This grossly exaggerated abdominal movement is seen in dogs in tuberculous pleurisy with effusion ; to relieve the pressure on the lungs the animal often sits erect on its hind quarters for long periods. Exaggerated " heaving " respirations are produced as a result of intrathoracic pressure on the lungs from other causes as well as fluid ; in diaphragmatic hernia, with invasion of the chest by abdominal organs, the compression of the lung and interference with respiration cause respiratory movements of this type. In extensive bovine tuberculosis the dry nodular pleurisy may cause such extensive fixation between the visceral and parietal pleura that the movements of the lungs are very limited ; the respiratory movements then become very fast. In pneumothorax the respiration remains thoraco-abdominal but the movements are exaggerated ; dyspnoea is proportional to the amount of air or gas that has entered the pleural cavity.

Congestion of the lungs and pneumonia, by interfering with respiratory efficiency of the lungs, cause a fast shallow type of respiration. The ratio between respiratory rate and pulse rate is decreased in congestion of the lungs and pneumonia, and in extensive pneumonia in a heavy horse the ratio may be almost 1 to 1, compared to the normal of 1 to 3.

A peculiar jerky type of breathing occurs during massive migration of helminth larvæ through the lungs ; this is observed chiefly in horses and pigs. A similar type of breathing may develop as a result of pulmonary consolidation arising from causes other than those associated with helminthiasis.

Rupture of the diaphragm permitting organs from the abdominal cavity to pass forward into the thoracic cavity may cause dyspnoea which varies in intensity according to the extent expansion of the lungs is restricted. In small animals, if the fore-end is raised and if the organs fall back into the abdominal cavity the dyspnœa is relieved, whereas, if the hind quarters of the animal are raised, dyspnœa is intensified. It may be observed that the abdominal cavity has an empty appearance that is corrected when the fore-end of the animal is raised. Physical examination of the chest may reveal abnormalities varying according to which organs have passed forward. An X-ray examination may prove helpful in differential diagnosis.

Attention should be paid at this stage to any abnormal sounds arising in the respiratory system and discernible by simply listening to the animal breathing. Snuffling noises are caused by the presence of nasal discharge in such quantities that the air passing up and down the nasal passages has to force its way through the discharge ; exceptionally, snuffling may be due to œdema of the nasal mucous membrane or deformity of the nasal passages caused by chronic inflammatory changes or tumour growth, accompanied by exudation. Snuffling is usually present during both inspiration and expiration, though it may be more pronounced during one than the other.

Snoring or stertorous breathing may be caused by alterations in the contours of the respiratory passages so that obstruction is presented to the free passage of air ; this may be present in the nasal cavities, pharynx, larynx or trachea. If only one side of nasal passages is involved the sound will be stopped by occluding the nostril on that side. Enlarged lymphatic glands pressing on the pharyngeal wall may cause snoring as in tuberculosis of the retropharyngeal lymph gland in cattle. Polypoid growths arising from the mucous membrane of the upper respiratory passages, though uncommon in the domestic animals, may vibrate in the air currents, thus creating stertorous sounds. Ulceration of the respiratory mucosa, especially if in the larynx, causes a whistling or roaring sound that may be heard either on inspiration or expiration. Hunting pointed out that the sudden development of this sound in a horse may be due to glanders ulceration of the laryngeal mucous membrane. The application of the Mallein test (see p. 294) would be necessary for the differential diagnosis in such a case if glanders was suspected. Grunting and groaning is a common symptom of acute respiratory disease involving the lungs in cattle.

The term " grunting " is applied in horses to the sound that may be produced in forced inspiration occurring when a horse is suddenly threatened. It is considered that this sound is evidence of a tardy action of the laryngeal muscles. A considerable proportion of horses that grunt when threatened either are, or subsequently prove to be, " roarers." The term " roarer " is used to describe a horse that, if strenuously exerted, makes a roaring or whistling sound at the end of forced inspiration, due to air entering an abnormally patent lateral laryngeal ventricle and passing over the open entrance to the ventricle. The abnormal patency of the ventricle is due to paralysis of the muscles of one side of the larynx as a result of paralysis of the recurrent laryngeal nerve ; the condition most commonly affects the left side.

Spasm of the diaphragm (hiccup) causes an abrupt sound, varying in volume according to the size of the animal, and also a peculiar jerky movement of the animal's body. In the horse spasm of the diaphragm may superficially resemble cardiac palpitation, but the sound created by cardiac palpitation can be co-related with the heart impulse.

NASAL DISCHARGE.—The presence of nasal discharge would be noticed during the preliminary general examination. The significance of the nasal discharge may now be considered. Nasal discharge may be evidence of inflammatory changes in the nasal mucous membranes alone, but it is also present in cases involving other parts of the respiratory system.

In cattle a few drops of clear watery (serous) fluid are normally present in the nostrils. A thick yellow purulent nasal discharge is present in malignant bovine catarrh and in calf diphtheria. One of the symptoms of rinderpest (cattle plague) is a dirty nasal discharge. Actinobacillosis of the nasal mucous membrane and actinomycosis of the bones of the nasal passages cause at first a thin watery nasal discharge, but later the discharge may become purulent.

A slight watery discharge from a sheep's nostrils is quite common. A purulent nasal discharge may arise in the lower part of the nasal passages from the spread of infection therein from the lesions of orf. Infestation of the nostrils with the larvæ of Œstrus ovis irritates the nasal mucosa, causing some discharge along with sneezing.

In the horse a thin watery nasal discharge may be the first sign of respiratory disease or of general specific disease. Thus a nasal discharge at first serous in character is an early sign of equine influenza, strangles or purpura. In equine influenza the discharge becomes thicker as the disease progresses. In strangles the discharge rapidly becomes purulent in character. In purpura hæmorrhagica the nasal discharge is serous in character and pale pink in colour due to the extravasation of small quantities of blood from petechial hæmorrhages in the nasal mucous membrane. In glanders the nasal discharge is grey in colour and gleety in character. A slightly rusty nasal discharge may be present in acute congestion of the lungs or pneumonia. A dirty rusty nasal discharge with an offensive smell is present in gangrene of the lung. A unilateral nasal discharge is usually evidence of a local condition. This may arise from disease of the nasal passage, infection of the facial sinuses or a diseased tooth causing empyema of the sinus. The nasal discharge in these conditions is purulent in character and if necrosis of bone or tooth is present there is an offensive smell.   The presence of pus in the guttural pouches causes a purulent nasal discharge that is most profuse when the horse's head is lowered.   Clinical examination of the region concerned will reveal the distension of the pouch.

In the pig nasal discharge, often of a purulent character, is a constant symptom of the specific fevers affecting that animal, e.g. swine fever. A serous discharge accompanied by sneezing is often the first symptom observed in piglet influenza.   Nasal discharge of a muco-purulent type is a feature of well developed atrophic rhinitis in pigs.   The discharge may be expelled in the form of plugs after a violent attack of sneezing.   Partial or almost complete occlusion of the nasal passages may compel the pig to breathe through the mouth and deformity of the nose may be noticed.

In the dog a nasal discharge, at first serous but later in some forms becoming purulent, is an important sign of the distemper group of diseases. There may be a conjunctival discharge in association with the nasal discharge.   Nasal discharge is also observed in catarrhal conditions of the respiratory tract due to infections other than distemper virus—e.g. B. bronchisepticus.   Tumour growth involving the nasal region may cause a persistent serous nasal discharge that becomes hæmorrhagic if ulceration takes place.   Nasal discharge with violent sneezing and snorting may be caused by the parasite Linguatula tænoides.   In cats nasal catarrh is commonly a symptom of infectious feline catarrh ; the discharge is serous and the cat sneezes.

COUGH.—The act of coughing is preceded by a deep inspiratory effort, then with the glottis closed an expiratory movement commences which compresses the air in the respiratory system so that when the glottis is opened the air rushes out forcefully and carries with it mucus and exudate from the respiratory mucous membrane.   All coughing in the domestic animals is involuntary and is evidence of abnormality. Coughing may be initiated in various parts of the respiratory system and it is obviously necessary to ascertain the source of the cough.

The first point that requires attention in the investigation of a cough is whether the cough consists of a single act or if paroxysms of coughing occur.   At the onset of catarrh of the respiratory passages in horses and dogs the only symptom noticeable may be single coughs at intervals ; as the disease progresses these become more frequent.   In the early stages of respiratory tuberculosis in cattle the cough is infrequent, but in the later stages of the disease coughing is almost continuous.   In the later stages of any respiratory disease that causes profuse exudation the cough becomes frequent and a series of explosive efforts may be necessary to expel the exudate and clear the respiratory passages for the time being. Paroxysmal coughing occurs in the parasitic respiratory diseases that affect principally cattle and sheep.   In parasitic bronchitis (Hoose) in cattle the animal stands with its neck extended, the head lowered and the tongue protruding. The actual paroxysm of coughing may in severe cases last several minutes and the animal shows quite pronounced dyspnœa at the end of the paroxysm. Parasitic bronchitis and parasitic pneumonia in sheep cause paroxysms of coughing similar to those in cattle. Detailed consideration of the diagnosis of these parasitic conditions is given in the chapter on clinical helminthology. Paroxysmal coughing in the dog, accompanied by relatively little exudate, occurs during pharyngitis and laryngitis. Paroxysmal coughing with marked exudate is a pronounced feature of bronchopneumonia following canine distemper and a persistent harsh cough in the dog may be due to the irritation caused by the presence of the parasite *Filaroides osleri* (formerly *Oslerus osleri*) in small nodules formed in the mucous membrane of the lower part of the trachea and commencement of the bronchial tree. Specimens of sputum or fæces should be examined for the presence of larvae of the casual parasite. Passage of an endoscope under light anæsthesia will permit a visual inspection of the lesions.

Chronic cough is a symptom of certain important infective diseases of the domestic animals and also is characteristic of some non-infective conditions. The principal infective disease characterised by a chronic cough is tuberculosis. In the horse a chronic cough is a constant concomitant of chronic alveolar emphysema (broken wind), and frequently occurs in laryngeal paralysis (roaring). In the pig chronic swine fever, virus pneumonia of pigs, chronic swine erysipelas and the chronic type of piglet influenza all cause a chronic cough. In the dog chronic bronchial catarrh and spasm of the bronchial muscles give rise to a chronic cough.

The cough is dry, harsh and painful in the early stages of acute inflammation of the respiratory mucous membrane. The cough becomes moist and soft when exudation occurs, which may be due to catarrhal diseases or may be due to the later exudative stages of croupous conditions. The cough may be deep and powerful in character when much exudate requires to be expelled.

The cough tends to be short and ineffective either when the animal is too exhausted to make the necessary respiratory effort or when the deep inspiration that precedes the act of coughing is painful and the animal checks inspiration before the lungs are fully expanded. A short or suppressed cough is present in the early painful stages of acute inflammation of the respiratory mucous membrane and of pleurisy. If extensive consolidation of the lungs has occurred the animal is unable to create the necessary respiratory pressure required to produce a powerful cough. In advanced thoracic tuberculosis of cattle with fixation of the visceral and parietal pleura the cough, though chronic and persistent, is of a short suppressed type. In acute terminal miliary tuberculosis of the lungs in horses and cattle the cough is short and suppressed. In thoracic tuberculosis in the dog coughing may be frequent in the early stages, but if pleurisy with voluminous exudation occurs, leading to compression of the lung, the cough may practically cease.

The tone of the cough may be of some assistance in diagnosis. The cough of a broken-winded horse is prolonged, deep and hollow. In the dog a barking type of cough occurs in chronic bronchitis. In pulmonary or mediastinal tumour formation the cough at first resembles that of bronchitis, later it may develop a peculiar resonant brassy tone.

While coughing principally arises in connection with the respiratory system, it may be a symptom of disease elsewhere. Choking gives rise to powerful expiratory efforts directed towards expelling the foreign body. Cardiac disease, if it has reached a stage when the heart is unable to sustain the needs of exertion, may result in passive congestion of the lungs, evidenced by respiratory distress and coughing. Over-exertion of unfit horses or dogs or over-driving of fat cattle or sheep may also result in acute congestion of the lungs, which in addition to marked dyspnœa causes much coughing. Coughing may arise from peripheral irritation of the abdominal viscera, acting in the same way as a reflex expectorant, but before accepting this as the cause of the cough, particular care should be taken to make certain that there is no disease located in the respiratory system that is the real cause of the cough. Thus many cattle affected with tuberculosis show lack of appetite with other evidence of digestive disturbance, and a cough is present. At first it may seem that the cough is reflex in origin from the digestive system, but a more critical examination will reveal clinical signs of tuberculosis of the respiratory system.

LYMPHATIC GLANDS.—Examination of the respiratory system should always include inspection and palpation of the superficial lymphatic glands of the head and neck. The glands most commonly involved are those of the pharyngeal region. The submaxillary glands are frequently involved. The retropharyngeal, the subparotid and the submaxillary are commonly involved in bovine tuberculosis. Tumour formation involving lymphatic tissue of the head and neck is seen principally in the dog. It appears that many of these tumours arise from the tonsillar tissue. Their presence may create a syndrome resembling that of sub-acute pharyngitis, but manual examination of the region will reveal the enlargement and deformity of the tissues concerned.

PHYSICAL EXAMINATION OF THE CHEST

Physical examination of the chest consists of palpation, percussion and auscultation. Inspection of the chest has already been described.

PALPATION

Palpation provides relatively little direct information regarding the state of the thoracic organs, but may provide some useful indirect information. Palpation reveals abnormal sensitivity of the thoracic wall and the intercostal spaces. It is sometimes difficult to distinguish between the flinching of sensitive highly-strung animals and manifestations of pain. The general behaviour of the animal in response to approach and handling will be a guide to the type of animal that is being examined. Abnormal sensitivity of the thoracic wall and intercostal space is most pronounced in inflammatory conditions affecting the pleura ; it is rather less pronounced when the lungs and bronchi only are involved. Extensive pneumonia will be accompanied by at least some measure of pleurisy.

Œdema of the chest wall is found by palpation. Œdema develops first between the forelegs and along the region of the sternum. If extensive the lower part of the neck may be involved and the œdema may encroach on the abdominal wall. Œdema of the chest wall results from any condition causing venous stasis, and may thus occur in any respiratory disease responsible for pressure on the great veins as is the case in pleurisy with effusion. Œdema of the chest wall is also a symptom of venous stasis resulting from cardiac disease.

Friction between the visceral and parietal pleura can seldom be appreciated by palpation, except in tuberculosis of cattle with extensive development of granular lesions. It is rarely possible to feel by palpation the impulse of waves in pleuritic fluid caused by the respiratory movements.

PERCUSSION

The lungs and heart do not occupy the whole of the cavity enclosed by the spine, ribs and sternum. The convexity of the diaphragm is projected into the thoracic cavity and the postero-lateral limits of the chest cavity are determined by the costal attachment of the diaphragm. Dorsally the bodies of the vertebræ, the spinous processes and the muscular masses filling the triangular space between the spinous processes, the vertebræ and the ribs form a solid mass that precludes percussion of the thoracic organs in this region. Anteriorly the scapula, the humerus and the heavy mass of the muscle filling the triangular area between them shield the chest wall from percussion. Movement of the fore-limb alters the position of anterior limit of the area of the chest wall that is available for percussion. Except in the dog and cat, the most anterior part of the chest is not available to physical examination even if the limb is drawn forward as far as possible. Bearing these anatomical points in mind it will be realised that a triangular area of percussion may

H

be mapped out. The superior limit is marked by the anterior portion of a line joining the posterior angle of the scapula to the coxal tuber of the ilium. The anterior limit is formed by a line joining the olecranon process of the ulna to the posterior angle of the scapula. The third side of the triangle is formed—except in the pig—by a line connecting the olecranon to the superior limit at the second last intercostal space. In the horse this line forms a curve that is concave in a dorso-anterior direction ; the line passes over the costo-chondral junction of the 7th rib and the middle of the 12th rib. In cattle the posterior limit, formed by the line joining the olecranon to the second last intercostal space, is practically a straight line. In the dog the posterior limit forms a gentle curve with its concavity facing anteriorly and dorsally. In the pig the posterior limit is formed by a straight line running from the olecranon to the third or fourth last intercostal space. It will be realised that the posterior limit is subject to variation in position during respiratory movement. The positions described are those occupied by the border of the lung midway between complete expiration and full inspiration. It must not be forgotten that the area of percussion is modified by the presence of other organs, particularly those of the digestive system. Dorsally on the right side at the posterior end of the area, the mass of the liver tends to cause an abrupt termination to pulmonary resonance compared to the left side. On the left side a tympanitic stomach or in cattle and sheep a tympanitic rumen gives an exaggerated resonance to the posterior area of percussion. Impaction of the stomach or rumen will give a corresponding reduction in resonance on percussion in this area. In the lower anterior part of the left side a dull area is present; this corresponds to the area of the heart and is known as the area of cardiac dullness.

Percussion entails the production of vibrations in the chest wall that are reflected by the underlying tissues. The texture of the chest wall has therefore a considerable influence on the success attending percussion and the information that can be obtained by it. In heavy draught horses in good bodily condition the thoracic wall is so thick that the clinical value of percussion is necessarily limited. In thin-skinned light horses, such as thoroughbreds, the chest wall is not sufficiently dense to mitigate against successful percussion. Similarly in fat cattle of the beef breeds and in bulls the value of percussion is definitely limited, but in cows of the dairy breeds accurate percussion is quite practicable. In pigs percussion is seldom possible. In dogs the breed and bodily condition determine the extent to which clinical information can be elicited by percussion. In all animals the state of the coat has an effect on percussion, a thick coat acting as an acoustic damper. To some extent the damping effect of the coat can be overcome by separating the hair or wool so that the fingers applied to the chest wall come as nearly in contact with the skin as possible. The force used in percussion must be varied to suit the thickness of the chest wall and the depth of the underlying tissues in the different animal species. Thus fairly vigorous percussion is necessary in any of the larger animals and quite appreciable force is necessary in heavy horses. On the other hand, in the small animals light percussion is essential if any measure of accuracy is to be obtained. The need for light percussion is particularly marked in cats. Very often it is found necessary to compare the corresponding area on either side of the same animal. When this is being done it is of obvious importance that the same degree of force should be used when each side is percussed. It will be found most satisfactory if in percussion the most resonant part is percussed first and percussion is continued from the resonant to the less resonant areas.

Percussion may be employed to determine the position occupied by the borders of the lung in so far as this is possible in the domestic animals. The dorsal border is fixed by the dense structures limiting percussion. The anterior limit is determined not by the condition of the underlying thoracic tissues but by the position of the fore-limb in relation to the chest wall. The posterior border does, however, vary in position according to the state of the thoracic organs. The posterior border is displaced backwards in well-marked alveolar emphysema ; this displacement can be demonstrated by percussion in horses with chronic alveolar emphysema. The posterior border may also be displaced backwards in pneumothorax. Displacement of the posterior border in a forward direction is appreciated in any condition limiting full expansion of the lungs. This may be intrathoracic in origin and arise from disease of the lungs or pleura. In cattle acute tympany of the rumen, by diaphragmatic pressure, may limit expansion of the lungs, and therefore the posterior border of the area of percussion appears to be further forward than in the normal animal, but the degree of tympany necessary to produce this is such that its presence is obvious on inspection of the animal.

The area of percussion on each side may be divided into upper, middle and lower thirds. In the horse on the left side the upper third is resonant in the anterior part ; resonance gradually diminishes as percussion proceeds from the thicker portion of the lung to the thin border. In the middle third resonance is pronounced in the anterior part but diminishes more rapidly than in the upper third as percussion is carried backwards. In the lower third the anterior two-thirds are mainly occupied by the area of cardiac dullness ; the remaining posterior part contains insufficient lung tissue to give any degree of resonance to percussion. On the right side, resonance in the upper third terminates abruptly, due to the interposition of the dullness due to the liver. In the middle third, resonance is the same as in the middle third of the left side. In the lower third the cardiac dullness is not so marked and slight resonance may be elicited from the underlying lung tissue.   In cattle the antero-posterior dimensions of the area of percussion are much less than in the horse.   On the left side the resonance from the lung in the upper third merges with that of the upper part of the rumen that normally contains no food material.   In the middle third resonance ends abruptly owing to the solid mass of foodstuff in the rumen.   The lower third is similar to that in the horse.   The right side presents comparable regions to those described in the horse.   In dogs and cats the upper and middle thirds do not differ materially, except in regard to size, from the same areas in the horse.   In the lower third clear resonance can be demonstrated with the exception of the area of cardiac dullness.   In the pig the heavy chest wall limits percussion.

Assiduous practice in the different species and breeds of animal is necessary if the student is to achieve success in the use of percussion as a means of physical examination of the chest.   It will often be found helpful to compare the percussion note obtained in an apparently normal animal of the same species, breed and bodily condition as that of the patient being examined.   Such a comparison may be found of great assistance when dealing with cattle and horses.

The changes in resonance demonstrable by percussion fall into two main categories ; firstly the resonance may be increased ; secondly the resonance may be diminished.   Increase in resonance may be due to either pronounced emphysema or to pneumothorax.   In extensive alveolar emphysema the characteristic expiratory effort will be noticeable, but in pneumothorax both inspiratory and expiratory efforts are exaggerated.

. Reduction of resonance may be general or it may be confined to a particular area of which the borders can be defined ; the area may be fixed or it may be found to be movable according to the position assumed by the animal.   Reduction in resonance of a general character is demonstrable in any widespread disease of the lung causing a reduction in the amount of air contained in the lung.   The reduction of resonance may be difficult to appreciate in animals with a thick chest wall, even when comparisons are made between both sides of the chest and a comparison is made with the chest of a normal animal.   Acute congestion of the lungs causes some reduction in resonance.   This may be widespread or may be confined to the lower parts of the lung.   Congestion of the dependent parts of the lung is often encountered as a complication of equine influenza ; hypostatic congestion may occur in the lower lung during lateral recumbency.   Consolidation of the lung, due to confluent broncho-pneumonia, causes a marked reduction of resonance on percussion.   If extensive and including the greater part of the area of percussion it may not be possible to define the area, which then appears to cause a general dullness.   If the area is smaller it may be possible to define its borders by percussion. Accurate definition of the edges of the area may not be possible in large fat animals ; in the smaller animals, especially in the toy breeds of dogs and in cats, the small size of the whole area of percussion mitigates against a precise definition of an area of dullness. In interstitial pneumonia, as seen in the so-called hard pad form of distemper, a reduction in resonance may be appreciated in the upper third of the area of percussion, that is to say, the area overlying the thicker part of the lung. A general reduction in resonance may be demonstrated in miliary tuberculosis of the lungs. Thickening of the pleura, as it occurs in bovine tuberculosis, causes some reduction in resonance. An extensive granulomatous lesion in the chest producing fixation of the visceral and parietal pleura may occur in advanced bovine tuberculosis ; the area involved in such a lesion produces a dull wooden note on percussion.

Dullness in the lower part of the chest with a horizontal upper limit above which resonance is clear and almost tympanitic is indicative of fluid in the pleural cavity. If the position of the animal can be altered so that the long axis of the body is no longer parallel to the ground the position of the upper limit to the area of dullness will still be found to be horizontal but will have altered in relation to the chest wall. In small animals, if they are turned on their backs, the area of dullness and the area of resonance will be found to have changed places. Acute dyspnœa may be caused in an animal with extensive pleuritic fluid if it is placed on its back, as the pressure of the fluid is brought to bear on the thicker and more vital parts of the lung, whereas in the former position the pressure was mainly exerted on the thin lower border of the lung. If such dyspnœa is caused the examination should be as brief as possible. Pleuritic fluid in the horse is found on both sides of the chest and the two sides are usually involved to nearly the same extent owing to the communication that exists in the horse between the left and right sides of the pleural cavity. In many cases in other animals both sides are involved but not necessarily to the same extent. Pleuritic effusion is present in tuberculosis of the chest in both the dog and cat and in actinomycosis of the chest in the dog, while in cattle tuberculosis of the chest is almost invariably of the dry granulomatous type. A voluminous pleuritic exudate is present in contagious bovine pleuropneumonia and in bovine pasteurellosis (hæmorrhagic septicæmia). Hydrothorax—a noninflammatory transudate in the pleural cavity—gives rise to a similar type of dullness to percussion ; hydrothorax is frequently a sequel to circulatory defects.

Thoracic tumours, if sufficiently large, may give dull areas on percussion. A pulmonary tumour may give a well-defined area of dullness that is found on examination at a later date to have increased in size. Tumours arising in the mediastinum attain considerable dimensions before causing appreciable alteration in resonance on percussion.

AUSCULTATION

From the beginning the student should always use a stethoscope when auscultating the chest, for it is only by using a stethoscope that accurate results can be obtained.   The chest piece of the binaural stethoscope should be sufficiently firmly applied to the chest to prevent movement between it and the surface of the chest wall during respiration.   If the coat is short and smooth the chest piece is applied without any preliminary preparation.   If the hairs of the coat are erect it is desirable that they should be smoothed down with the hand.   If the coat is very long it will be necessary to separate the hair or wool at the point of application of the chest piece so that a pad of wool or hair does not form a layer that is impenetrable to sound.   When the stethoscope is applied to a particular point on the chest wall, it should be retained there until at least one complete respiratory movement has been performed by the patient. The chest should be methodically explored, moving the stethoscope from place to place so that when the examination is completed every part of the lung available for examination has been auscultated.   Different parts of the same lung may require to be compared one with another;   it may also be found necessary to compare corresponding portions of the lung on both sides.   The areas of auscultation are the same as those of percussion.

The object of auscultation is to determine the character of the respiratory sounds and the presence of abnormal sounds.   In the domestic animals it is not possible to obtain any co-operation from the patient during the clinical examination of the chest, so the clinician must adapt his examination to the patient, as alterations in the character and depth of the respiration cannot be obtained at will to facilitate the examination. The act of coughing may be provoked by pinching the larynx and the first two or three rings of the trachea or the lower cervical part of the trachea immediately before it enters the chest.   The normal respiratory sounds consist of the vesicular sound and bronchial sounds.   The vesicular sound, as the name implies, is the sound caused by air entering and leaving the alveoli ;   it therefore consists of an inspiratory sound and an expiratory sound.   It is the inspiratory sound that possesses the characteristics by which the vesicular murmur can be recognised.   In a normal chest the inspiratory sound may be described as soft and rustling ;   it may be compared to the sound produced if the letter " f " is whispered softly.   In the large animals at rest with the breathing quiescent it may be difficult to detect the vesicular sound.   In the horse it will be found that the sound can be detected if the horse is trotted a few yards by an assistant, and is halted beside the examiner, who immediately auscultates the chest.   It is frequently almost impossible clearly to hear the vesicular sound in the normal chest of a pig.   In dogs and cats the sound is clearly audible. In young animals of all species the vesicular sound is harsher than the corresponding sound in the adult. The expiratory sound follows the inspiratory sound without any appreciable interval ; it is much less intense than the inspiratory sound. It is practically imperceptible in horses and cattle, but it is quite distinct in dogs and cats. The expiratory sound is of shorter duration than the inspiratory sound.

Bronchial sounds are blowing in character ; they commence and end abruptly. The inspiratory sound and the expiratory sound are of approximately the same duration. The expiratory sound is separated from the inspiratory sound by a short but distinct pause. This appears to be due to the bronchial inspiratory sound terminating shortly before the end of inspiration. The bronchial expiratory sound is prolonged to the end of expiration. The bronchial sounds are heard in the normal lung only in those areas of the chest where the larger bronchi are relatively near to the chest wall, that is to say principally in the anterior part of the middle third of the area of auscultation. The student will find it of assistance in recognising the bronchial sounds if he listens over the lower end of the trachea with his stethoscope and then listens to the chest for the bronchial sound, bearing in mind that the bronchial sound, though similar in character, is much less in volume and intensity than the sound heard in the trachea. The bronchial sound is not conducted any distance by the normal lung tissue, so in the larger animals it is only heard over a limited area in the chest. In the dog, particularly in the small breeds, and in the cat, the bronchial sounds are heard over a considerable part of the area of auscultation. If the breathing is accelerated for any reason such as fear or fever, even if not associated with any abnormality in the lung, the bronchial sounds may be audible throughout the area of auscultation in the dog. This may be very marked in young dogs and puppies.

A number of important alterations in the vesicular sound may be detected on auscultation. The sound may be exaggerated and harsh in character, resembling that in a young animal if the respiratory effort is increased. A sound of this type can be heard if the chest is auscultated immediately after active exertion ; it is also heard when the respiratory movements are increased in fever or reflexly stimulated by pain, as is well illustrated by the respiratory disturbance present in the early acutely painful stages of lymphangitis in the horse. The increased respiratory efforts associated with interstitial pneumonia increase the volume of the vesicular sound but do not create any adventitious sounds. Harsh vesicular sounds are heard in emphysema, whether acute alveolar emphysema as a concomitant of pneumonia, or chronic alveolar emphysema as in broken wind of the horse. Such sounds are also heard in interstitial emphysema as for instance in acute pulmonary œdema in cattle (Fog Fever).

Jerky interrupted respiration, sometimes known as " cog-wheel " respiration, may occur in animals as a result of fear, and is heard all over the area of auscultation and will affect both sides equally. Interrupted vesicular sounds localised to particular areas indicate an irregular expansion of portions of the lung ; this is believed to be due to a lack of elasticity of the lung tissue, and it commonly indicates fibrosis of a part of the lung. Barely audible or inaudible vesicular sounds, in an animal showing symptoms of respiratory disease involving the lung, are indicative of defective expansion of the lung. In pleurisy, if the exudate is voluminous, the vesicular sound will be completely inaudible below the upper level of the fluid, while above the level of the fluid the vesicular sounds are clearly audible and tend to be increased in volume and rather harsh in character. Consolidation of the lung due to confluent bronchopneumonia, so that air is no longer able to enter the alveoli, will lead to a complete absence of vesicular sound from the affected portions of the lung. The area involved in the consolidation must be of considerable dimensions in relation to the size of the area of auscultation before the complete absence of sound can be appreciated owing to sounds from adjacent areas being picked up by the stethoscope. Loss of vesicular sound is present in an area of lung invaded by a tumour causing consolidation thereof. It may be possible to appreciate prolongation and duplication of the expiratory sound in chronic alveolar emphysema in the horse. It is important that the student should distinguish between subdued but normal vesicular sounds and the absence of vesicular sound due to disease. As a general rule respiratory disease involving the lung is associated with disturbance of the respiratory rate, rhythm or character.

Extension of the bronchial sound into those parts of the lung where normally only the vesicular sound should be heard, occurs if for any reason the lung contains less air than normally, and in consequence the conduction of sound by the lung tissue is enhanced. Thus consolidation of the lung produces an extension of the bronchial sound. If the consolidation only involves part of the area under examination the bronchial sounds will be superimposed on the vesicular sound. If consolidation is complete the bronchial sound only will be heard and owing to more perfect conduction will be correspondingly louder. A sound similar to that produced by blowing across the open mouth of a tube is known as an amphoric sound. This sound is heard if there is a direct communication between a bronchus and a lung cavity, but cavitation, sufficiently extensive to produce this sound, is comparatively rare in the domestic animals.

Adventitious sounds are definitely abnormal sounds arising from disease of the bronchi, lungs or pleura, as distinct from modifications or alterations of the normal respiratory sounds. These adventitious sounds fall into four main categories—Rhonchi or Dry Sounds, Moist Sounds, Crepitations and Friction Sounds.

Rhonchi or Dry Sounds are produced at a partial obstruction of the bronchial tubes, owing to the air being forced through an irregular or constricted tube. These sounds vary in pitch according to the size of the tube in which they are produced. In the larger bronchi the sound is low pitched and snoring and is known as a sonorous sound, and in the smaller bronchi the sound is higher in pitch and is known as a sibilant sound. The partial obstruction of the bronchi may be due to inflammatory swelling of the mucosa as in acute bronchitis, or to thick tenacious exudate firmly adherent to the mucous membrane, or to distortion of the bronchi by pressure as in tuberculosis and tumour formation, or to constriction of the bronchial muscle.

Moist sounds may be produced in the bronchi, bronchioles or alveoli. These moist sounds, sometimes known as moist râles or mucous râles, are caused by air passing through or forcing aside fluid material, whether secretion or exudate, and are of a bubbling character. They are modified by coughing, since that act will move the fluid from the point where the sound was heard prior to coughing. Moist sounds are always recognisable in catarrhal inflammation and are thus an important clinical sign of bronchitis and bronchopneumonia (lobular pneumonia). These moist sounds may be further classified into fine and coarse sounds, the fine sounds being those produced in the smaller bronchioles and the alveoli, while the coarse sounds are produced in the larger bronchioles and bronchi.

Crepitations are crackling or very fine sharp sounds heard only during inspiration and usually towards the end of inspiration. The sound is very similar to that produced by separating the moistened forefinger and thumb; this requires to be done quite close to the ear for the sound to be appreciated. Crepitation is caused by the sudden separation of the walls of alveoli that have become adherent on account of the presence of exudate. The separation of the walls only takes place when sufficient negative pressure has been created by the inspiratory movement to draw apart the walls of the alveoli, hence the sound tends to occur chiefly towards the end of inspiration. Friction between the chest piece of the stethoscope and the stiff hair of an animal's coat produces a sound similar to crepitation, but it is of a harsher nature. If the chest piece of the stethoscope is fitted with a rubber cushion and is held firmly to the chest wall, sounds due to friction with the hair can largely be eliminated. If doubt exists as to the origin of the sound the coat may be damped and laid flat when any sound arising from the hair should cease. The student should make himself familiar with the sounds produced by the hair of the coat, as these may prove confusing if the animal's coat is stiff and harsh.

Crepitation is recognised as one of the cardinal signs of the first stage of pneumonia; it disappears from any portion of the lung that has undergone consolidation. Crepitation is usually appreciable on the periphery of an area of consolidation if that area is surrounded by a zone wherein the pneumonic process has not advanced to the stage of consolidation. During the stage of resolution crepitation reappears when air again enters the affected part of the lung. Crepitation is present in miliary tuberculosis in those areas where the disease has not advanced sufficiently to prevent the entrance of air. Similarly crepitation is heard in glanders of the lung, the so-called glanders pneumonia. Crepitation is occasionally heard during the onset of œdema of the lung, and at this stage definite bubbling sounds may also be heard.

Emphysema produces a harsh crackling sound ; this to some extent resembles that produced by crushing a piece of newspaper. The sound in emphysema is continuous during the whole of inspiration and is also to a lesser extent in evidence during expiration. Attention has already been drawn to the characteristic double expiratory effort in chronic alveolar emphysema, this leading to a prolongation of expiration.

The sounds in the lung may be dull and toneless if a sodden condition prevails in the lung ; this may be due to thickening of the pleura, or it may be that sufficient exudate is present between the visceral and parietal pleura to act as an acoustic damper. Metallic or tinkling sounds in the area of auscultation arise either in conjunction with amphoric breathing or in pneumothorax. These metallic sounds must be distinguished from the tinkling sounds present in some cases of pericarditis with extensive exudation into the pericardial sac ; a similar sound is sometimes heard in hydropericardium.

Friction sounds are of a creaking or rubbing character and have been compared to the sound produced by rubbing together two pieces of unpolished leather ; perhaps a better simile is that of the sound produced by leather saddlery when either the horse or rider moves. Friction sounds are produced by the inflamed roughened visceral and parietal layers of the pleura rubbing together when there is not sufficient exudate to separate the two layers ; they are therefore characteristic of the early stages of pleurisy. Though synchronous with the respiratory movements the sounds are not necessarily continuous, as they only occur when the roughened areas of the pleura rub against each other ; the sounds are usually heard best during inspiration. Friction sounds are not altered by coughing. The inflammatory process that causes a friction sound necessarily causes pain during the respiratory movements, so the respiratory character is altered, being principally abdominal with the appearance of the pleuritic line ; in the horse symptoms of subacute colic may also be present. Pressure on the chest wall may increase the pain but it is only in the dog and cat that pressure on the chest wall with the stethoscope may increase the intensity of the friction sound, owing to the increased resistance offered to the movement of the inflamed pleural surfaces.

Friction sounds disappear as soon as sufficient exudate is formed to separate the inflamed pleural layers. It should be appreciated that pleurisy may be a concomitant of pneumonia ; therefore friction sounds may accompany other abnormal lung sounds.

EXPLORATORY PUNCTURE OF THE CHEST

Exploratory puncture of the chest is justified if the presence of fluid in the pleural cavity is suspected. The operation should be performed with due regard to asepsis. In the large animals a needle $3\frac{1}{2}$ to 4 inches long and 2·5 to 3 mm. in diameter is used, alternatively a small trocar and cannula may be used ; in the smaller breeds of dogs and in cats a needle 1 inch long and 0·9 mm. in diameter is used ; in very large dogs a needle $1\frac{1}{2}$ inches long and 1·4 mm. in diameter may be required. The site of the puncture is the seventh or eighth intercostal space in the lower third. The needle should be introduced as close as possible to the anterior border of the rib to avoid the intercostal nerve, artery and vein. The site of the puncture may be rendered insensitive by infiltration with a local anæsthetic solution.

RADIOLOGICAL EXAMINATION OF THE CHEST

A radiological examination of the chest is only practicable in the dog and cat. In these animals it provides useful assistance in diagnosis of certain types of respiratory disease. Examination of the chest by means of the fluoroscopic screen makes it possible to inspect the movements of both the ribs and diaphragm and any abnormality of the respiratory movements can be appreciated.

In some cases of foreign body in the thoracic œsophagus, causing perforation and septic mediastinitis, the symptoms and clinical signs may rather indicate the presence of a septic pleurisy without any indication of the original cause. Radiological examination of the chest will reveal the true nature of the case.

Confirmation of a tentative diagnosis of pulmonary or mediastinal tumour is made possible by a radiological examination ; in order to define the form of the tumour, films should be taken giving a dorso-ventral and a lateral view of the chest. Interpretation of the radiographs is facilitated if the relative position of the various organs in the chest is studied. Thus a tumour in the left lung will push the heart over to the right side of the chest. The trachea may be displaced to either the right or left, and both it and the œsophagus may be compressed between the tumour mass and the roof of the chest.

In pleurisy with exudation, or in hydrothorax, the fluid compresses the lung so that a space exists between the chest wall and margin of the lung. This fluid is sufficiently opaque to X-rays to show up by contrast with the lung tissue that offers relatively little resistance to the passage of the ray. When there is a great amount of fluid present in the pleural cavity the shadow of the lung is completely obliterated and the chest on that side presents a homogeneous opaque appearance. Introduction of an opaque substance such as iodised poppy-seed oil into the bronchial tree by means of an intratracheal injection will show up the collapsed lung very clearly. Such opaque substances may also be used to show up bronchiectasis and pulmonary cavitation. In pneumothorax the lung is separated from the chest wall by a zone that offers less resistance to X-rays than the lung tissue, and so appears to be sharply delineated. Furthermore, the greatly exaggerated respiratory movements can be studied by means of the fluoroscopic screen.

In diaphragmatic hernia the smooth contour of the diaphragm may be broken ; the tissues that have passed from the abdomen into the chest may be opaque to X-rays, *e.g.* the liver, or if not opaque, can be rendered visible by the administration of a meal containing an opaque substance such as bismuth carbonate or barium sulphate.

ANALYSIS OF THE SYMPTOMS AND CLINICAL SIGNS OF THE CHIEF RESPIRATORY DISEASES

In order to assist the student in the co-relation of the symptoms and signs presented by the chief respiratory diseases, a brief analysis of these is now given. (See Table IV, p. 126.)

NASAL CATARRH.—The leading symptom in nasal catarrh is the presence of nasal discharge. The discharge at first is serous in character, but, as the disease progresses, becomes either mucoid or purulent. There may be a slight febrile reaction and the associated lymphatic glands may show signs of a defensive reaction. Symptoms and clinical signs suggesting involvement of other parts of the respiratory system are absent. Simple nasal catarrh is a benign condition, but in all animals nasal catarrh may be a symptom of specific infections or contagious disease, as in equine influenza, equine strangles, cattle plague, malignant bovine catarrh, swine fever, canine distemper and infectious feline catarrh. In the earliest stages of these diseases nasal catarrh may be the only leading symptom, but very soon other symptoms and clinical signs become manifest.

PHARYNGITIS.—In the majority of cases the first symptom is a dry painful cough ; this later becomes less painful and more moist in character. There is some nasal discharge. Difficulty in swallowing is present and may be so marked as to cause complete refusal of food. In the horse, attempts at swallowing may cause an attack of coughing and some food material may be expelled through the nose. In the dog and cat attacks of coughing may terminate with retching and vomiting. There is tenderness of the pharyngeal region ; the associated lymphatic glands may be swollen and painful. In those animals in which the pharynx can be inspected the mucous membrane will be seen to be inflamed. A febrile reaction is present ; this may be quite severe in character. As in nasal catarrh, pharyngitis may be a symptom of a specific fever.

LARYNGITIS.—Laryngitis seldom if ever occurs without a corresponding degree of inflammation of the pharyngeal mucous membrane. Frequently laryngitis is a complication by extension of a pre-existent pharyngitis. The onset of laryngitis is evidenced by a painful paroxysmal cough that is harsh and distressing. Changes in the vocal tone are only appreciable in the dog when the bark becomes hoarse and sometimes barely audible. Involvement of the larynx in an inflammatory process renders the larynx very sensitive to external manipulation which provokes an attack of coughing. Inspection of the larynx, which is only practicable in the dog and cat, will reveal the inflammatory process.

ACUTE BRONCHITIS.—Febrile symptoms are present in acute bronchitis. There is a varying amount of dyspnœa, and coughing is always marked. The cough is at first dry, hard and painful ; after a spasm of coughing the dyspnœa will be more pronounced. The cough soon becomes moister and less painful, due to exudation. Later the expectorate consists of considerable quantities of muco-purulent or purulent matter. Percussion of the chest reveals no alteration in resonance. Auscultation in the early stages demonstrates sonorous and sibilant rhonchi, these being replaced by moist bubbling sounds caused by the presence of exudate. Bronchitis is a common complication of specific disease, e.g. canine distemper. Parasitic bronchitis is discussed further in the chapter dealing with clinical helminthology.

CHRONIC BRONCHITIS.—It is only in the dog that chronic bronchitis is of clinical importance. The leading symptom is a persistent cough that may be paroxysmal in character. There is no febrile reaction and the dog may be in good bodily condition. Though at rest respiration is normal, any sudden or violent exertion provokes an attack of coughing and dyspnœa develops, the latter being out of all proportion to the amount of exertion. Percussion of the chest shows resonance to be normal. Sibilant and sonorous rhonchi with slight mucous sounds will be heard on auscultation. There may be evidence of secondary emphysema. Cardiac disturbances are frequently present in these cases.

BRONCHOPNEUMONIA : Lobular or Catarrhal Pneumonia.—This is the common form of pneumonia encountered in the domestic animals. The patient is febrile, breathless and coughing. Copious exudate is rapidly formed and the expulsion of this may cause the patient much distress. A general reduction of resonance on percussion may be demonstrable ; if the involvement of an area of the lung is extensive

TABLE IV

	Nasal Catarrh	Pharyngitis	Bronchitis	Lobular Pneumonia	Interstitial Pneumonia	Chronic Alveolar Emphysema	Pleurisy	
							1st Stage	2nd Stage
Nasal discharge	1. Serous 2. Mucoid 3. Purulent	May be mucoid or purulent	May be mucoid or purulent	May be mucoid or purulent	—	—	—	—
Swallowing	—	May be difficult	—	—	—	—	—	—
Cough	Absent	1. Dry and harsh 2. Moist and soft	1. Dry and harsh 2. Moist and soft. May be paroxysms	Copious expectorate. Cough may be very frequent	—	Deep hollow cough	—	—
Respirations	Normal	Normal	Dyspnoea may be severe	Dyspnoea may be severe	Rapid Shallow	Double expiratory effort. Dyspnoea on exertion	Mainly abdominal. Pleuritic line	Dyspnoea if exudate voluminous
Fever	Usually only slight	May be marked	May be marked	May be marked	Slight	Absent	Present	Present
Regional (throat) lymphatic glands	May be swollen	May be swollen	—	—	—	—	—	—
CHEST. Vesicular sounds	—	—	May be exaggerated	May be exaggerated	Exaggerated	Increased in volume. Crackling noises	—	—
Bronchial sounds	—	—	Sonorous and sibilant rhonchi	Sonorous and sibilant rhonchi	Loud	—	—	—
Moist sounds	—	—	Present	Present	—	—	—	—
Crepitation	—	—	—	Present	May be crackling due to alveolar emphysema	No true crepitation	—	—
Friction sounds	—	—	—	—	—	—	Present	Absent
Percussion	—	—	Normal	General reduction in resonance. May be dull areas due to confluence	Loss of resonance develops in upper third	May be an increase in resonance and size of area	Normal	Dull area in lower part of chest

and the individual zones of consolidation have become confluent an area of dullness may be delinated by percussion. On auscultation there will be found rhonchi, mucous sounds, crepitation and areas, if these are sufficiently large, devoid of all sounds ; the vesicular sounds in the healthy lung tissues are increased in intensity.

Lobar pneumonia, as understood by the pathologist, is remarkably rare in the domestic animals. A pneumonia that appears to be lobar in distribution is not uncommon, but the lesion does not possess the homogeneous character of a genuine lobar pneumonia, being a lobular pneumonia in which the affected lobules are contiguous. Massive bacterial invasion of the lung tissue may occur in equine influenza and in acute congestion of lungs in an unfit horse following excessive exertion. The onset may be sudden and the patient is acutely ill with a sharp febrile reaction. Dyspnœa is marked, being roughly proportional to the extent of the pulmonary involvement. The mucous membranes are congested and in severe cases show some degree of cyanosis. There is a rusty nasal discharge, which in pulmonary gangrene has an offensive smell. The incidence of pulmonary gangrene in the horse has been markedly reduced by the early use of antibiotic therapy.

INTERSTITIAL PNEUMONIA.—An interstitial pneumonia occurs in paradistemper, the so-called hard-pad type of distemper of dogs. It is characterised by dyspnœa with very little coughing. Percussion may reveal some reduction in resonance in the upper third of the chest but auscultation fails to reveal anything beyond some increase in volume of the normal respiratory sounds.

EMPHYSEMA.—Acute alveolar emphysema occurs as a concomitant of, or sequel to, other acute respiratory disease. It is recognised by the development of fine crackling sounds audible on auscultation.

Chronic alveolar emphysema is only of clinical importance in horses ; in these animals it is the cause of broken wind. The animal has a low respiratory efficiency and dyspnœa develops on exertion. A prolonged deep hollow cough is present ; this can be provoked by pinching the lower end of the trachea at the entrance to the chest. The expiratory effort is duplicated, giving the characteristic abdominal " lift," and in consequence of the double expiratory effort the time occupied by expiration is prolonged. Percussion may show an increase in resonance and the posterior border of the area of percussion may be found to be displaced backwards and downwards. Auscultation shows increased vesicular sounds and crackling sounds may be heard.

Acute interstitial emphysema occurs in cows affected with septic metritis or septic mastitis, when as a result of the local sepsis a general septicæmia has developed. There is a marked febrile reaction ; the respiratory rate is increased and on auscultation of the chest crackling sounds are heard. The importance of noting the condition of the udder and uterus in relation to the differential diagnosis of the case will be readily appreciated.

Acute interstitial emphysema is frequently present in cases of acute pulmonary œdema of cattle—so-called " Fog-Fever." The signs of this condition are those of intense dyspnœa ; auscultation of the chest reveals loud harsh crackling sounds. Rupture of the emphysematous interstitial tissue of the lung into the mediastinum may allow air to pass forward in the fascial planes to reach the subcutaneous tissue of the neck whence it spreads along the back.

PLEURISY.—In the early painful stages horses show symptoms of subacute colic, cattle grunt and dogs flinch if the chest wall is palpated. The respiratory movement is largely abdominal, producing the pleuritic line. Some fever is present ; the pulse is accelerated and hard. Auscultation shows friction sounds.

If exudation occurs the pain abates, friction sounds disappear and the pulse becomes softer. If the exudate is voluminous, the respiratory movements become exaggerated and dyspnœa may be pronounced. Percussion shows dullness in the lower part of the chest, the upper margin of the dull area being horizontal. No respiratory sounds are heard in the dull areas on auscultation, but in the upper part of the chest the normal vesicular sounds are heard ; these may be exaggerated. Exploratory puncture of the chest will confirm the presence of fluid.

PNEUMOTHORAX.—Except when arising from trauma to the chest wall, pneumothorax is rare in the domestic animals. In cases due to trauma the nature of the injuries will be such as will suggest the possibility of pneumothorax developing. In cattle perforation of the thoracic œsophagus and consequent passage of gas from the rumen may cause a form of pneumothorax if the pleura is punctured. The gas may pass along fascial planes to reach the subcutaneous tissue of the neck and chest.

Occasionally in the dog, and very rarely in the horse, pneumothorax occurs as a result of the rupture of a portion of lung tissue so that air is forced into the pleural cavity. The movement of the affected lung is restricted and sudden dyspnœa develops. If unilateral it may be appreciated that the affected side of the chest appears distended and does not complete the expiratory movement made by the normal side. Percussion reveals increased resonance on the affected side ; if sufficient air be present the chest may be tympanitic. If the lung on the affected side is extensively collapsed neither vesicular nor bronchial sounds will be heard on that side. If the lung is only partially collapsed the sounds will be faint and apparently remote. In small animals a radiological examination may assist differential diagnosis.

TUBERCULOSIS

CATTLE.—Tuberculous pleurisy in cattle is, with very rare exceptions, a dry granular inflammation leading to the development of grape-like lesions on both the visceral and parietal pleura. These lesions cause friction sounds detectable on auscultation. Percussion will only reveal dullness if the grape lesions have attained a sufficient size to produce a definite zone of consolidation within the chest wall. Tuberculous pleurisy may be present in cattle without any symptoms being observed, and its presence may only be realised if the chest is subjected to a careful physical examination. Frequently the animal is in good bodily condition, and it is only on examination of the carcase in the abattoir that the disease is discovered.

Tuberculosis of the lungs is first evidenced by a cough that to begin with is abrupt and harsh; later it becomes softer and a considerable quantity of exudate is expectorated. As the disease progresses loss of condition becomes obvious, the coat is dry and harsh and the skin is hidebound. If the animal is a cow in milk there is a reduction in the milk yield. The appetite becomes capricious and rumination is performed irregularly. The temperature will be found to be elevated in the later part of the day and subnormal in the early morning. Any unusual strain, such as passage through a market or the act of parturition, may lower the animal's powers of resistance, so that the disease enters on an acute terminal phase. If the involvement of the lungs is extensive the respiration is rapid and shallow; any exertion produces dyspnœa and the act of coughing is followed by a period of dyspnœa. In the early stages the lesions are too small to be detected by physical examination of the chest. It is only when there is extensive consolidation of the lung that a definite area of dullness can be mapped out by percussion. Similarly the disease process must be fairly well advanced before auscultation shows marked abnormality of the respiratory sounds, the vesicular sound is increased, bronchial breathing is evident over considerable areas; sibilant and sonorous rhonchi, mucous sounds and crepitations may all be heard. There may be clinical signs of tuberculosis in other parts of the body, e.g. enlargement of lymphatic glands and tuberculous mastitis. A diagnosis of tuberculosis of the lungs is only justified if the symptoms and clinical signs are very pronounced; in the majority of cases diagnosis must be confirmed by a bacteriological demonstration of tubercle bacilli in the sputum. The early detection of tuberculous infection must depend on use of the tuberculin test.

PIG.—Pulmonary tuberculosis in the pig frequently runs a very rapid course. The pig soon becomes emaciated, the skin is dry and harsh, looking rather like parchment paper. Respiratory distress is pronounced and coughing is almost continuous. Diagnosis may be assisted by a

I

bacteriological examination or a tuberculin test, but it is often found more satisfactory to destroy the animal, so that the diagnosis can be confirmed by post-mortem examination. If the suspected animal is one of a number of pigs kept under similar conditions, its destruction with a view to post-mortem diagnosis is advisable in the interest of the herd as a whole.

HORSE.—Pulmonary tuberculosis in the horse is nearly always secondary to abdominal lesions and often takes the form of an acute miliary tuberculosis. The horse is acutely ill with a marked febrile disturbance. The respirations are fast and shallow. Though it is possible that some reduction in resonance may be demonstrable on percussion, it will be found that the information obtained by percussion is of somewhat limited value. Auscultation shows marked abnormality of the respiratory sounds similar to those described in cattle. Diagnosis will depend on the recognition of clinical signs of tuberculosis in other parts of the body.

DOG AND CAT.—Thoracic tuberculosis in the dog and cat frequently takes the form of pleurisy with great exudation. There may be a history of a cough that has persisted for some time. The animal may have presented the symptoms and clinical signs associated with pneumonia, but the illness followed an indefinite course. In a considerable proportion of cases the illness commences acutely with the sudden onset of intense respiratory distress. The animal is found to be in poor bodily condition and the mucous membranes are pale and anæmic. There are exaggerated abdominal respiratory movements in addition to the maximum possible costal movement. The animal prefers to sit in an upright position, and if it is placed on its back severe dyspnœa ensues. Physical examination of the chest reveals the presence of fluid. A sample of the fluid can be withdrawn and submitted to a bacteriological and, if necessary, a biological examination. The organisms may be very scanty and even after prolonged centrifugalisation cannot be demonstrated microscopically in the deposits. If the fluid is of a clear straw colour the organisms are usually not numerous, but if the fluid is turbid or blood-stained the organisms are commonly present in sufficient quantity to be found by microscopic examination of stained smears made from the deposit obtained by centrifugalisation. So large a proportion of cases of pleurisy with exudation in the dog and cat are of tuberculous origin that a provisional diagnosis of tuberculosis is justified if no other adequate explanation of the cause of the pleuritic fluid is obtained by a clinical examination, e.g. hydrothorax due to defective heart action.

TUMOUR

Thoracic tumours are rarely encountered in the domestic animals except in the dog. Carcinoma of the lung, and lympho-sarcoma of the mediastinal lymph glands are encountered in this animal as also are heart-base tumours. The development of the tumour causes first a harsh cough that resembles that associated with chronic bronchitis ; the brassy character of the cough may be appreciated. With the increase in size of the tumour the respiratory efficiency of the lungs is impaired and dyspnœa is easily provoked on exertion. An area of consolidation may be delineated by percussion and auscultation and this area will be found to be slowly increasing in size. Radiographic examination of the chest is of great assistance in diagnosis. Mediastinal tumours, by pressing on the œsophagus, interfere with swallowing, and attempts to ingest solid food may result in the regurgitation of the foodstuff.

CHAPTER V
CIRCULATORY SYSTEM

Regional Anatomy :—Horse—Cattle—Dog
Cardiac Cycle and Cardiac Sounds
Clinical Examination :—Pulse—Abnormalities—Heart—Sounds—Rhythm
—Murmurs—Pericardial Sounds—Venous System—Posture and
Gait. Examination of Blood
Electrocardiograph—Radiological Examination
Analysis of the Symptoms and Clinical Signs of the Chief Diseases of
the Circulation

CARDIAC disturbance may occur reflexly as a result of disease in another part of the body, as for instance, reflex acceleration of the heart in spasmodic colic. A more serious form of circulatory disturbance follows any disease that imposes a severe strain on the heart ; thus pneumonia inevitably causes cardiac disturbance due to the increased resistance opposed by the lung to the flow of blood from the right heart, but in addition the heart muscle is affected by the relative anoxæmia. Toxæmia and septicæmia may not only involve the heart muscle, but may also involve the blood vessels and the vasomotor centre. Anæmia has an inevitable effect on the heart. Cardiac disease not associated with identifiable lesions is termed functional disease of the heart, but if lesions be present the condition is termed organic disease of the heart. In some cases it may appear that cardiac disease alone is responsible for the symptoms and signs shown by the animal. In the horse this type of cardiac disease is very frequently functional ; organic disease of the heart is only rarely encountered in the horse. In the dog both functional and organic disease of the heart are commonly encountered. In cattle the most common forms of cardiac disease are traumatic pericarditis, endocarditis and tuberculous pericarditis. In pigs verrucose endocarditis caused by chronic swine erysipelas is the form of cardiac disease most frequently encountered. In sheep cardiac disease is rare except as a complication of severe systemic illness. Outbreaks of endocarditis in sheep caused by *Erysipelothrin rhusioparhiæ* are sometimes encountered. Frequently in such outbreaks a proportion of the sheep show lameness due to fibrosis of joints and tendon sheaths.

REGIONAL ANATOMY

In all the domestic animals the chest is flattened laterally and the heart lies in the lower two-thirds of the thoracic cavity. The apex of the heart lies practically in the middle line and it is the side of the ventricle that comes in contact with the chest wall.

HORSE.—The left ventricle is in contact with the chest wall in an area extending from the 3rd to the 6th rib ; this area extends nearly to the upper margin of the lower third of the area of auscultation and percussion described under the respiratory system. A small area of the right ventricle comes nearly into contact with the chest wall from the

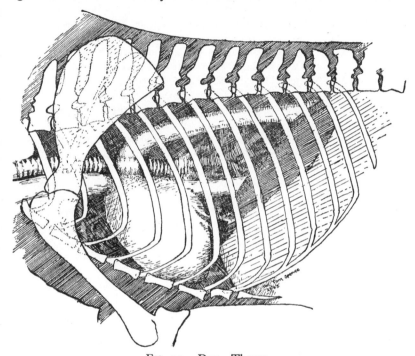

FIG. 12.—Dog. Thorax.
Drawn from Radiographs. One-third actual size.

4th to the 6th rib, but owing to the small size of the cardiac notch in the right lung in the normal animal auscultation and percussion of the heart on the right side gives no positive information (see Figs. 1 and 2, pp. 42 and 43). If of normal size approximately two-thirds of the heart lie to the left of the median plane. Enlargement of the heart will cause an increased proportion of the heart to extend to the right of the median plane and in gross cardiac enlargement contact between the heart and the chest wall on the right side may extend to a considerable area. The long axis of the heart lies obliquely in the chest, forming an acute angle with the long axis of the sternum. The base of the heart is fixed by the great vessels entering and arising from it. The right atrioventricular opening, guarded by the tricuspid valve, lies opposite the fourth intercostal space in the lower third of the cardiac area. The pulmonary orifice lies opposite the third intercostal space slightly above the right atrioventricular opening. The left atrioventricular opening, guarded by the bicuspid or mitral valve, is opposite the fifth intercostal space and midway between the level of the right atrioventricular opening and the pulmonary orifice. The aortic orifice lies opposite the fourth intercostal space and occupies the most dorsal position of the four cardiac openings, being on the level of the lower border of the upper third of the heart. Accurate location of the positions of the valvular orifices by auscultation is very difficult and where the heart is enlarged may be quite impossible.

CATTLE.—The heart is only separated by the thickness of the diaphragm from the reticulum which occupies the lower anterior part of the abdominal cavity formed by the curve of the diaphragm. This close approximation of the reticulum to the heart makes it possible for penetrant foreign bodies to enter the pericardial sac and impinge on the cardiac muscle (see Fig. 3, p. 61).

DOG.—The heart is placed more obliquely in the chest than in the horse, so that the base of the heart faces in a more anterior direction than in the horse, in which the base of the heart faces mainly in a dorsal direction. The contact of the wall of the ventricle with the left side of the chest wall extends from the 3rd rib to the 6th rib.

CARDIAC CYCLE AND CARDIAC SOUNDS

When relaxation of the ventricles is just commencing, both atria will have filled from the great veins entering them (*i.e.* the cranial and caudal venæ cavæ on the right side and the pulmonary veins on the left side). The cycle of contraction commences in the atria, their contraction being sufficient to pass blood into the ventricles, thereby assisting the latter to fill. The ventricles then contract, and simultaneously with their contraction the chordæ tendinæ are tensed and the atrioventricular valves close, thus preventing the return of blood into the atria. The contraction of the ventricle and closure of the atrioventricular valves in association with tension on the chorda tendinæ produce the first heart sound that is commonly described as resembling the phonetic sound " lub." This first sound, corresponding as it does to the early part of the phase of contraction or systole in the cardiac cycle, is sometimes referred to as the systolic sound. The contraction of the ventricles forces the blood along the pulmonary artery to the lungs and along the aorta through the arteries to the systemic circulation. During the later part of ventricular contraction the atria relax and fill with blood from the great veins ; and when the contraction is completed the ventricles relax. Immediately the ventricles commence to relax the pressure exerted by the heart on the column of blood in the large vessels is reduced and the blood pressure in the great vessels is sufficient to close the valves in the aorta and pulmonary artery. The closure of these valves produces the second heart sound ; this is commonly described as resembling the phonetic sound " dup." The second heart sound is synchronous with the onset of ventricular relaxation or diastole, and so the second sound is sometimes referred to as the diastolic sound. The intensity of the second heart sound is dependent on the blood pressure in the great arteries at the onset of diastole.

CLINICAL EXAMINATION

The clinical examination of the circulatory system falls into the main categories : (1) taking the pulse, (2) examining the heart, (3) examining the venous system, and (4) if necessary examining the circulating fluid.

PULSE

The method of taking the pulse has been described under the preliminary general examination of the patient. The importance of the information that can be obtained by taking the pulse in the domestic animals is emphasised by the fact that this is the principal clinical method available for the estimation of the cardiac efficiency. As it is not possible to utilise the sphygmograph in the domestic animals no visual record of the pulse can be obtained. Though by experimental methods the arterial blood pressure may be estimated, no form of sphygmomanometer has been devised that permits the estimation of the blood pressure of animals in clinical veterinary practice. The clinician has, therefore, to depend on the acuity of his digital perception to estimate not only the rate and rhythm of the pulse but also the character of the pressure wave in the artery. These points are exemplified by consideration of the following types of pulse.

Rapid Pulse.—Acceleration of the pulse may be due to cardiac disease, or it may be caused by the reflex stimulation of pain or may result from diseases such as the infective fevers, debility or anæmia.

Slow Pulse.—A slow or infrequent pulse may be a natural condition in an animal that is accustomed to strenuous muscular exertion, when the animal has been resting for some hours. Thus in seasoned hunters, after a night's rest in the stable, the pulse may be as slow as 36 per minute. In some comatose conditions the pulse is very slow. In cardiac disease an extremely slow pulse will probably indicate heart-block.

Soft Pulse.—A soft pulse with a poorly developed wave may be due to the depressing effect of focal sepsis. Fatigue or depression of the heart muscle may also be responsible for the production of a soft pulse.

Strong Pulse.—A strong bounding pulse is indicative of increased blood pressure. Such a pulse is sometimes, though inaccurately, referred to as a " full " pulse, the implication in the term " full " being that the artery is abnormally distended with each pulsation.

Wiry Pulse.—A wiry pulse occurs when the heart-beat is reasonably strong and rapid and there is some degree of vaso-constriction. A wiry pulse is present in acute pleurisy and in acute peritonitis. It also results from acute irritation of the endocardium and is present in the early stages of acute pericarditis.

Thready Pulse.—In this form of pulse the pulsation of the artery feels like a piece of thread being rendered tense under the fingers. A thready pulse is indicative of weakness of the heart's action. It may precede a fatal termination of disease.

Running-down Pulse.—If repeated examination shows that the heart action is becoming increasingly weak and fast and that there is a lack of vessel tone, the pulse is spoken of as having a " running down " character.

Small Pulse.—A small pulse may be due to lack of force in the ventricular contraction. It may, however, be due to atrioventricular incompetence or aortic stenosis or mitral stenosis.

Water-hammer Pulse.—The water-hammer or Corrigan's pulse consists of a sharp increase of pressure followed by a rapid collapse of the pressure in the vessel. This type of pulse is characteristic of aortic incompetence, the defective valves being unable to sustain the pressure in the great vessels when the ventricles relax.

When abnormalities of the pulse are encountered these should be co-related with the cardiac action. In order to achieve this the examination of the heart and vessels, now to be described, should be carried out.

EXAMINATION OF THE HEART

INSPECTION

Inspection of the heart in the domestic animals can only provide information of very restricted value. This is due partly to the configuration of the chest, as in the normal animal only part of the wall of the left ventricle comes in contact with the chest wall, and in many animals it is also due to the thickness of the chest wall being sufficient to occlude any visual evidence of the heart's action. Except in those animals in which the chest wall is thin and the coat comparatively short, distinct signs of cardiac activity visible on the chest wall of an animal at rest may be regarded as evidence of abnormality. This abnormality is not necessarily indicative of serious cardiac disease. In highly strung excitable animals, handling by strangers, restraint and unusual surroundings quite often cause the pulsation of the heart to become so vigorous that its beating against the side of the chest wall is clearly visible. The preliminary clinical examination of the animal will already have made clear to the clinician that his patient is of this excitable type. As the animal becomes accustomed to its surroundings and ceases to be excited the heart action will become more normal and the beating of the heart against the chest wall will no longer be evident. If an animal is compelled to perform vigorous muscular activities that tax its strength the heart's action may become tumultuous and the beating of the heart is obvious on the side of the chest wall ; thus in a horse that has just finished a gallop, or in a cow that has been chased, the beating of the heart may be seen.

When the action of the heart is tumultuous, as in palpitation, the efforts of the heart can in many animals be discerned quite clearly on inspection of the chest wall. Gross increase in the size of the heart brings it into more intimate and more extensive contact with the chest wall, so that even if the heart's action is not abnormally vigorous the pulsations are perceived with greater facility than is normal. But it commonly occurs that the cause of the increase in the size of the heart also induces an increased effort on the part of the heart muscle so that the impact against the chest wall is increased in force as well as in area. It will be appreciated that increase in the size of the heart will cause the area of contact with the right side of the chest to be larger and pulsation of the heart may become visible on the right as well as on the left side. The presence of a substantial quantity of fluid on one side of the chest may displace the heart to the opposite side, so that the closer contact made between the heart and the chest wall renders the movement of the heart more obvious on inspection. In the same manner displacement of the heart may originate from the presence of a tumour in the thoracic cavity.

If the pulsations of the heart can be seen it may be possible for the clinician to notice the nature of the heart's action. Any observations of this type are necessarily of a rather vague and general character, and they should only be interpreted in conjunction with other symptoms and clinical signs that may indicate the nature of the circulatory disturbance.

PALPATION

It will usually be found convenient to combine palpation with inspection, as the conjoint interpretation of inspection and palpation may be of some assistance in diagnosis. Palpation of the chest wall may indicate that the impulse of the heart is appreciable over a larger area than is normal. Some information as to the force of the heart impulse may be obtained by palpation, if due allowance is made for the deadening effect of the chest wall. There are many abnormalities in the character of the beat that cannot be determined by palpation. Palpation of both sides of the chest wall may reveal increased contact between the heart and both the right and left sides of the chest. It is very doubtful if pericardial friction could be determined by palpation. Palpation of the heart may well be regarded as a minor method of examination that may on occasion provide some useful confirmatory clinical signs.

PERCUSSION

The limitations of percussion as a method of clinical examination of organs in the thoracic cavity of the domestic animals have already been discussed. These limitations should be kept in mind when considering the value of percussion in the investigation of cardiac disease in animals. Exact definition of the periphery of the heart is rendered difficult by the insinuation of the edge of the lung between the heart and the chest wall. In animals with a thick chest wall and a substantial layer of subcutaneous fat it will be found impossible to map out the borders of the area of cardiac dullness, and percussion of the heart may be found an impracticable procedure. But in animals of a less substantial build with a relatively thin chest wall and not too heavy a coat, percussion will be found to give results that are of considerable assistance in diagnosis.

The object of percussion is to determine the size of the heart and the extent to which the heart is in contact with the chest wall. Percussion should be performed in order to contrast the resonant with the less resonant, commencing over the lung and progressing towards the area occupied by the heart. The force employed in percussion must be adapted to suit the size of the individual animal and the configuration of the chest wall; if, as has been indicated, the lung is percussed first the optimum force can be determined by a few blows of varying force. In general, it may be said that the larger the animal the greater the force necessary for the purpose of percussion; in very small animals the force of percussion will require to be light and the distance separating the point of impact of successive strokes must also be correspondingly small. Reduction in the area of cardiac dullness, due to changes in the heart, is unknown. Emphysema, by causing the insinuation of abnormally resonant lung tissue between the heart and the chest wall, may create an apparent reduction in the area of cardiac dullness. The presence of fluid in the lower part of the chest cavity, if sufficient in volume, will render definition of the cardiac area impossible, as the resonance of the lung tissue surrounding the heart is obliterated by the pressure of the fluid.

Owing to the position of the heart and its anatomical relations, an increase in the size of the area of cardiac dullness always leads to a displacement of the peripheral limit of the area in an upward and backward direction. In the larger animals this displacement may extend to as much as from two to three inches, but in the smaller animals the displacement may only be a fraction of an inch. Increase in the area of cardiac dullness is caused either by dilatation of the pericardial sac with fluid or by an increase in the size of the heart. Enlargement of the heart may be due to either dilatation or hypertrophy; in either case the heart sounds are distinct though they may be abnormal in character. Fluid in the pericardial sac may be a transudate as in hydropericardium, or an exudate as in pericarditis. Pericarditis in cattle is not infrequently the result of infection with anaerobic gas-forming organisms; in this case the pericardial sac contains both fluid and gas, when it may be possible to demonstrate by percussion that the posterior border of the cardiac area is displaced backwards, but apparently the upper border is not displaced owing to the resonance produced in the pericardial sac by gas that has accumulated in its upper spaces. The infection with gas-forming organisms in traumatic pericarditis in cattle is due to the penetration of a foreign body from the reticulum, carrying with it infection from the contents of that organ. Difficulty may be experienced in distinguishing between fluid in the pericardial sac and fluid in the lower part of the pleural cavity. If the fluid is in the pericardial sac its position is restricted by the fact that it is contained within a limiting membrane, so alterations in the position of the animal do not materially alter the position of the area of dullness. If the fluid is in the pleural cavity only the dorsal limit can be determined and whatever the position of the animal the fluid occupies the lowest part of the chest cavity and the upper limit to the area of dullness caused by the fluid is always horizontal.

AUSCULTATION

The purpose of auscultation is first to determine the volume or intensity of the heart sounds, their rhythm and the character or quality of the sounds, and secondly, the existence of abnormal sounds arising from, or associated with, the heart-beat; these abnormal sounds may be endocardial in origin or they may arise from the pericardium. It is essential that the student should make himself familiar with the normal heart sounds as they occur in the differing species and types of domestic animals. Not only do the sounds vary according to the species and size of the animal, but great variations occur in the extent to which the sounds are deadened by the chest wall; for instance, in a fat bullock the heart sounds may appear to be remote and not at all distinct. The approximate position of the valves of the heart in relation to the chest wall has been referred to in the description of the regional anatomy of the heart. It is seldom, if ever, possible to decide by topographical means alone if a particular valve is involved in a disease process.

The co-relation of the heart sounds with the movement of the heart will be facilitated if the cardiac impulse can be felt through the chest wall. If the impact of the heart is sufficiently powerful the chest piece of the stethoscope may be felt to jerk with each beat of the heart ; if the force is insufficient to produce this effect the impact may be felt by palpation of the chest wall over the region of the heart. It should be realised that a distinct lag occurs between the commencement of the contraction of the ventricles—thereby producing the first heart sound—and the pulsation of the median, facial or femoral artery, owing to the time necessary for the propagation of the pressure wave along the aorta and arteries. As has already been explained the first sound corresponds with the commencement of ventricular systole and the second sound with the commencement of ventricular diastole, the sounds being essentially connected with the closure of the appropriate valves. In the normal animal the valves close completely and the sounds are distinct and the terminations of the first and second sound are quite clearly defined. This definite termination to the sound is important clinical evidence of the complete closure of the valves.

The heart sounds may be reduced in volume if the action of the heart is weakened by the effect of illness. This need not necessarily be associated with organic disease of the heart ; it may be the effect of acute febrile disease, septicæmia or toxæmia. Reduction in the volume of the heart sound may be an indication of cardiac failure ; in severe illness this diminution of volume may occur very rapidly and is then a clinical sign with an ominous significance. The heart sounds may appear weaker if they are muffled by fluid in the pericardial sac.

An increase in the volume of the heart sound is evidence of greater muscular activity. Thus in hypertrophy of the heart associated with increased peripheral resistance the sound is loud, rather prolonged and of a thudding character. The increased muscular activity does not necessarily indicate cardiac efficiency and a loud tumultuous heart beat may be associated with a weak pulse, indicating that the cardiac output is poor in spite of the apparently vigorous action. This seemingly para-doxical state of affairs is exemplified by the loud heart sound present in palpitation of the heart caused by anæmia, when the pulse may be found to be almost imperceptible. If the heart is enlarged it may be appreciated that the sounds are heard clearly over a larger area on the left side. Since enlargement of the heart also causes it to make greater contact with the chest wall on the right side, the heart sounds on the right side may be unusually distinct and audible over an area appreciably larger than normal.

A comparison may be made between the volume of the two heart sounds. The volume of the first sound is related to the force of ventri-cular contraction, the volume of the second sound is dependent on the pressure in the great vessels at the time ventricular diastole commences. If, therefore, circumstances exist that alter the factors producing these sounds, their relative volume may be altered. Obstruction to the passage of blood through the lungs will cause an increase in the pressure in the pulmonary arteries and the volume of the sound caused by the closure of the pulmonary valves is increased ; but the force of the ventricle may increase in order to overcome the increased resistance, and so the volume of the first sound may also increase. While theoretically there should follow a further increase in the volume of the second sound, it will often be found difficult to appreciate a true difference in volume and the distinction may be more apparent than real.

Reduplication of the heart sound may involve the first or the second sound. Reduplication of the first sound may be heard in healthy animals if the blood pressure is high. A lesion of one branch of the bundle of His delaying the conduction of impulses will cause the ventricles to contract asynchronously, thus producing a double first sound. It may be possible to confirm the suspected existence of such a lesion by means of an electrocardiogram. It is important that reduplication of the first sound be distinguished from a pre-systolic murmur ; this distinction may be made possible by clinical signs revealed during the further examination of the patient. Reduplication of the second sound is most likely to occur when there is an increase in the pressure on the pulmonary artery causing an early closure of the pulmonary valves. This increase of pressure may be due to an increased resistance to the flow of blood through the lung caused by pulmonary disease or to stenosis of the mitral valve which causes damming back of the blood through the lung. Alterations in the synchrony of the contraction of the ventricles may cause reduplication of the second sound.

Alterations in the cardiac rhythm may have been detected when the pulse was taken. It is often found that slight deviations from the normal cardiac rhythm are more easily detected by auscultation of the heart sounds than by taking the pulse ; similarly the accurate study of serious disturbances of rhythm is facilitated by listening to the cardiac sounds over a reasonable period of time—say one minute. The greater value of auscultation in this respect is due to the aural appreciation of rhythm being, in most people, more acute than the tactile sense located in the finger tips. The normal cardiac rhythm of both horses and cattle is very regular, and though exertion may produce a great increase in the rate the rhythm does not alter. In the dog irregularities of the rhythm may be normal ; these irregularities tend to follow the respiratory movement ; they are not excessive in character. The student will find that, after examining the hearts of a number of normal dogs, he will have little difficulty in identifying the normal canine cardiac rhythm, and he will find it possible to distinguish it from an abnormal rhythm arising from cardiac disease or dysfunction. In a horse at rest and after a period of rest a regular dropping of one beat may be found on auscultation ; for instance, every fifth or every seventh beat may not be audible. If the horse's heart is normal the dropped beat is restored after exertion, when the normal cardiac rhythm asserts itself and may remain regular and without intermission for some considerable time. If, however, the disturbance of rhythm is evidence of cardiac abnormality, exercise will have the effect of accentuating the disturbance of rhythm. In addition to revealing the significance of any disturbance of rhythm, exertion will cause the heart to accelerate. Following acceleration due to such exercise the heart, if free from disease, should rapidly return to its normal rate. In cattle an alteration of rhythm of this type is unknown and it is sufficient to auscultate the heart with the animal at rest. In the normal dog exertion tends to cause a smoothing out of the irregularities of the cardiac rhythm so that the beat becomes more regular though faster than in the animal at rest. If the irregularity of rhythm is greater than in a normal dog and is evidence of cardiac disease, exertion will have the effect of causing an increase in the degree of irregularity, and the acceleration of the heart will be very much more than would be expected in a normal animal that had undergone a comparable amount of exertion.

Abnormalities in the cardiac rhythm may involve the rate, the spacing and the volume of the heart sounds. The rate may be found to vary in different ways ; thus there may be a period of increasing rate followed by a pause that is succeeded by a few powerful rhythmic beats leading to another period of increasing rate. In other cases the rate may show great fluctuations in any given unit of time, but the fluctuations do not appear to follow any regular sequence. Disturbances of rate, if pronounced, must be regarded as evidence of grave disturbance of the nervous control of the heart; they may occur at the end of an acute exhausting disease extra-cardiac in origin, or they may be evidence of severe cardiac disease. Disturbances of rate and rhythm are not uncommon in excitable dogs. The fact that the animal is excitable and restless will have been noticed during the general clinical examination. Well-established alterations in the spacing of the heart beats may indicate interference with conduction between the sino-auricular node and the ventricles, being in fact evidence of heart-block. In the horse the significance of these alterations in spacing may be investigated more fully by means of the electrocardiogram. If the force of the ventricular contraction is not constant the volume of both the first and second sounds will be found to vary. This may also be evidence of interference with or delay in conduction within the intrinsic nerve mechanism of the heart. In cardiac disease the heart sounds often lose their normal characteristics and the two sounds are almost identical in nature ; such sounds may, for instance, be described as resembling the syllables " clack-clack," and may well be compared to the sound made by a paddle wheel striking still water.

ADVENTITIOUS SOUNDS

Adventitious sounds may have their origin in the endocardium or the pericardium.

ENDOCARDIAL SOUNDS.—If endocardial in origin they are called murmurs, and may be caused by valvular lesions ; but endocardial murmurs may be evidence of functional disturbances of the heart that interfere with the free flow of blood through the cavities of the heart and the vessels in the immediate proximity of the heart. Thus palpitation of the heart is often observed in cases of acute anæmia especially after exertion. Under stress the heart action may become quite tumultuous producing a variety of endocardial sounds. In the normal heart the flow of blood through the chambers of the heart and its passage into the great vessels produces no sound, the only sounds heard on auscultation being those associated with the commencement of systole and diastole and the closure of the atrioventricular valves and the aortic and pulmonary valves. If the valvular orifices are altered in contour and their lumen restricted, the blood must be forced through a narrow irregular orifice before it escapes into a wider cavity ; the passage of the blood in these circumstances produces a murmur that is recognised as clinical evidence of stenosis of the valvular orifice. If the valves fail to close completely, blood is forced back through the valvular orifice into the part of the heart that is guarded by the defective valve. This return flow of blood produces a murmur that is evidence of regurgitation of blood and is indicative of incompetence of the valve concerned. When a murmur has been heard on auscultation, certain points concerning its occurrence should be investigated.

(1) The location of the murmur in the cardiac cycle may be determined by its relation to the normal heart sounds. In the horse with a comparatively slow heart-beat no great difficulty may be experienced in the co-relation of the murmur to the heart sounds, but if the heart rate is fast, as in a small dog with a pulse of 100 beats or more to the minute, it may be difficult, if not impossible, to establish this relationship. Some assistance may be obtained by palpating the beat of the heart against the chest wall and simultaneously auscultating the heart. Owing to the time taken for the pressure wave to extend from the heart to the site of pulse, simultaneous auscultation of the heart and pulse-taking may not be of assistance in the identification of the position in the cardiac cycle occupied by a murmur.

(2) Murmurs vary in character, and a knowledge of their different characters may be of help in deciding the site and type of a valvular

lesion.   The murmur due to stenosis tends to have a rough harsh ragged tone.   The murmur caused by regurgitation has a softer blowing or purring character.   The murmur produced by a disorderly tumultuous action of the heart, such as occurs in anæmic palpitation, has a humming character.   The volume of a murmur is not necessarily an indication of the severity of the valvular lesion, since the volume is dependent on the pressure and volume of fluid passing throug'a the orifice and on the form of the projections in the valve that are causing disturbances of the flow.   Thus a valve may be the site of serious incompetence, but if the heart's action is weak and the edges of the valvular lesion relatively smooth, comparatively little volume of sound is produced and the murmur has a soft blowing character.

(3) It may be possible to establish a point on the chest wall where the murmur is loudest and the anatomical relationship of this point to the position of the cardiac valves may be considered.   But, as has already been indicated, it is improbable that diagnosis of a lesion in a particular valve can be achieved by topographical means, but the position of the maximum sound may prove of some assistance in differential diagnosis if considered along with other symptoms and clinical signs.

(4) As has already been indicated, the type of pulse may give some indication of the type of valvular disturbance present in the heart, *e.g.* small pulse and water-hammer pulse.

(5) The state of the venous system may indicate damming back of the blood stream or regurgitation.   Thus the jugular veins may be distended or a jugular pulse synchronous with the heart-beat may be present.   Further details of the examination of the venous system are given later.

If an accurate diagnosis of the nature of cardiac disease is to be achieved the site of a cardiac murmur must be determined.   Prognosis is dependent on diagnosis and is of economic importance, as it may not be desirable to attempt treatment if there is no prospect of restoring the animal to a reasonable measure of efficiency.   The choice of treatment must obviously be influenced by a knowledge of the nature of the cardiac disease.

Murmurs may be described according to the time of their occurrence in the cardiac cycle as presystolic, systolic and diastolic.

PRESYSTOLIC MURMUR.—A presystolic murmur immediately precedes the systolic sound (the first heart sound).   The sounds originating in the heart then consist of *brr—lub—dup, brr—lub—dup*.   A presystolic murmur is an indication of stenosis either of the tricuspid valve (right atrioventricular valve) or of the mitral valve (left atrioventricular valve).   If the tricuspid valve is the site of stenosis there will be signs of venous congestion ; this will involve the superficial veins which can be seen to be distended ; some subcutaneous œdema and ascites may be present. If the mitral valve is the site of stenosis a retrograde pressure on the pulmonary circulation is produced, and passive congestion of the lungs ensues. After a period of rest, if the stenosis is not too far advanced there will be little disturbance of the respiratory rate. Exertion is followed by an increase in the respiratory rate and, if the stenosis is severe, intense dyspnœa may develop. Due to mitral stenosis there is an increase in the pressure on the pulmonary artery, and that part of the second heart sound, produced by closure of the valves guarding the pulmonary artery, is loud and distinct ; and as the increased pressure in the pulmonary artery may lead to early closure of the pulmonary valves, reduplication of the second heart sound may result.

SYSTOLIC MURMUR.—A systolic murmur succeeds the systolic sound (first heart sound). The sounds originating in the heart depend in character and tone on whether the systolic murmur is due to stenosis or incompetence. If the cause is stenosis the murmur is harsher than if due to incompetence. So in the case of incompetence the sounds consist of *lub—pss—dup, lub—pss—dup* ; in the case of stenosis the sounds are *lub—brr—dup, lub—brr—dup*. The systolic murmur may be due to tricuspid incompetence, mitral incompetence, pulmonary stenosis or aortic stenosis.

In tricuspid incompetence when the ventricle contracts there is a regurgitation of blood from the right ventricle into the right atrium ; this forces blood back into the venous system, causing venous congestion and in many cases a venous pulse. Owing to the leakage through the valve the heart is lacking in efficiency ; the heart can compensate for minor valvular incompetence, but when the valvular inefficiency is advanced the output of the heart suffers and the pulse loses strength ; alterations in rate and rhythm of the pulse may follow failure of compensation. Tricuspid incompetence may be due to valvular lesions (organic disease). Or it may be due to dilatation of the ventricle and the tricuspid orifice, so that the valves are not able to close the dilated orifice. Some of the murmurs encountered in anæmic palpitation may be due to dilatation of the heart that has resulted from the heart muscle being weakened in consequence of defective nutrition of its musculature. Owing to the reduction in the oxygen-carrying capacity of the blood in anæmia, a greater volume of blood must be passed through the lungs in order that an adequate supply of oxygen may be obtained ; this need places an increased strain on the right side of the heart.

Mitral incompetence allows regurgitation of blood into the left atrium when the left ventricle contracts. This regurgitation will cause some back pressure in the pulmonary veins and so passive congestion of the lungs may follow with its concomitant effect on respiration and the second heart sound. The incompetence may be due to organic lesions

K

or to dilatation of the orifice, but dilatation of the left ventricle is less commonly associated with anæmia than is dilatation of the right ventricle.

A systolic murmur may be caused by pulmonary stenosis, but except as a congenital condition pulmonary stenosis does not occur. In pulmonary stenosis the murmur is prolonged and harsh in character ; the second heart sound is poorly defined ; cyanosis accompanies pulmonary stenosis. The pulse is small and the wave develops slowly. Aortic stenosis is only rarely encountered in the domestic animals.

DIASTOLIC MURMUR.—A diastolic murmur immediately follows the diastolic sound (second heart sound). Diastolic murmurs can be distinguished from presystolic murmurs in that they are practically continuous with the second heart sound and are separated from the succeeding first sound by a definite pause. Diastolic murmurs are always due to incompetence of the valves. The sounds originating in the heart consist of *lub—dup—bss, lub—dup—bss.* Incompetence of the pulmonary valves is exceedingly rare and no further description of it will be given. Aortic incompetence permits the regurgitation of blood from the aorta into the left ventricle immediately ventricle diastole commences. The volume of the murmur, as well as the volume of the second heart sound, will be dependent on the pressure in the aorta at the time diastole commences. The murmur of aortic incompetence is propagated along the course of the large arteries, and if the regurgitation is marked an abnormal sound may be detected in the large animals on auscultation of the carotid arteries where they emerge from the chest.

MIXED AND MULTIPLE MURMURS.—In cardiac disease it not infrequently happens that the defect in the valve is not confined to one site. If this is the case more than one murmur will be heard on auscultation. It may be possible to establish the position occupied by each murmur in relation to the cardiac cycle and the two heart sounds. Frequently it will only be possible to decide the source of the murmurs by considering the symptoms and clinical signs arising from the effects of the cardiac disturbance on the general circulation. Multiple cardiac murmurs may be due to organic lesions of more than one valve in the heart, or they may be due to dilatation affecting both ventricles and the valvular orifices of both atrioventricular openings.

SIGNIFICANCE OF CARDIAC MURMURS.—The following points, in relation to cardiac disease in the domestic animals, will be found of assistance in considering the significance of a cardiac murmur. Organic disease, producing definite lesions on or in the neighbourhood of the cardiac valves is rare in the horse. Acute endocarditis causing murmurs may be encountered in serious cases of septicæmia. Dilatation and hypertrophy of the heart is comparatively common in the horse. Dilatation of the heart may develop in race horses and hunters as a result of unduly strenuous "training," and is a not uncommon cause of break-down in this class of animal. Dilatation of the heart may also follow a debilitating illness, or acute pulmonary disease, such as pneumonia. Chronic pulmonary disease may also have secondary effects on the heart. Cardiac arrhythmia, functional irregularity of the heart, or disorderly action of the heart may, if pronounced, give rise to cardiac murmurs. These may be absent at rest but in evidence after exertion ; it is seldom possible to co-relate the murmur with any particular cardiac valve. In cattle and sheep acute septicæmic conditions giving rise to acute endo-carditis may in the later stages be associated with endocardial murmurs. In cattle valvular lesions of endocardial origin are more common than was at one time thought; the diagnosis of these lesions in the living animal is dependent on detecting an endocardial murmur by auscultation. In the pig the only cardiac condition of clinical importance is the verrucose endocarditis that is an almost constant feature of chronic swine erysipelas. Organic lesions involving the cardiac valves and the endocardium in the neighbourhood of the valves are very common in the dog. In many dogs the heart is able to compensate for the defect caused by a valvular lesion and the animal appears normal and is able to sustain exertion without distress. Such an animal may survive to a substantial age without showing any outward evidence of cardiac difficulty. The existence of the valvular defect can be detected by auscultation (see p. 143). It is only when cardiac compensation fails that the animal shows evidence of circulatory failure. Acute endocarditis arising from septicæmia occurs in the dog as in other animals. Dilatation and hypertrophy are frequently encoun-tered in sporting and racing dogs that have been subjected to abnormal strain. Dilatation of the heart may follow a debilitating illness or acute pulmonary disease, e.g. extensive pneumonia.

PERICARDIAL SOUNDS.—The movement of the heart within the smooth pericardial sac creates no sound. In the early stages of pericarditis the roughened pericardial surfaces rubbing together produce a friction sound. This friction sound is not very loud, and in animals with a substantial chest wall the sound may not be audible ; furthermore, quite early in the course of the disease sufficient exudation may take place to separate the two layers of the pericardium and so the friction is obliterated. Very distinct pericardial friction sounds may be heard in tuberculous pericarditis in cattle.

Pericardial friction sounds do not necessarily correspond with any particular part of the cardiac cycle. The sound may be continuous, but more often it is intermittent and only occurs when two rough areas come in contact with one another. The sound may be present only during diastole or only during systole ; in some cases the sound occurs both during systole and diastole. If the sound is intermittent it may be possible to determine that the sound corresponds to the heart-beat, thereby co-relating it with the heart. It may be easier first to establish that the friction sounds are not connected with the respiratory movements and then they may be co-related with the cardiac function.

Not only does pericardial fluid obliterate all friction sound, but once sufficient fluid has been poured out the heart sounds become faint and muffled. Invasion of the pericardial sac with gas-forming organisms will result in the pericardial sac containing both fluid and gas. When that occurs a very distinct tinkling sound can sometimes be heard on auscultation ; this sound has been compared to that produced when a glass tumbler is lightly struck with a silver fork. Except in traumatic pericarditis in cattle caused by a foreign body passing forward from the reticulum, invasion of the pericardium by gas-forming organisms is exceptional. The presence of the tinkling sound, in addition to other symptoms and clinical signs, can be of material assistance in diagnosis of traumatic pericarditis in cattle. It should be realised that pleurisy and pericarditis may be present in the same case if both serous cavities are infected by the same causal agent.

EXAMINATION OF THE VENOUS SYSTEM

The state of the venous system may be of appreciable significance in differential diagnosis. In cattle, with the exception of the mammary vein in the cow, the veins lying immediately under the skin are not usually visible on inspection ; but in cattle with short coats in warm surroundings the superficial veins may be so engorged that they become visible. In thin-skinned horses with short coats, such as thoroughbreds and hunters, the veins of the face and limbs may be clearly visible for a short time after active exercise ; if the animal's circulation is functioning normally this temporary venous congestion soon disappears. In sheep and pigs subcutaneous veins are very rarely visible. In dogs with short coats the small saphenous vein can be seen as it curves round the lower end of the lateral aspect of the tibia. Persistent dilatation of superficial veins is an indication of venous congestion. It is in horses and cattle that such venous congestion can readily be appreciated. The veins of the face and limbs being easily seen provide the most suitable places for inspection of the venous system.

Prominent distension of the jugular veins, so that they become visible as thick cords running down the neck, is an important symptom of venous congestion. Slight pulsation in the jugular vein that cannot be appreciated by inspection, but may be felt by palpation, is present in many animals. This is due to conduction through the jugular vein of the pulsation of the carotid artery that lies beneath the jugular vein ; this type of jugular pulsation is sometimes referred to as a false jugular pulse. True pulsation in the jugular vein, originating from the heart and extending back up the vein, is a clinical sign of abnormality of the heart ; in addition to pulsation it is usually seen that the vein is markedly distended. Jugular pulsation may be due to the pressure of pericardial fluid on the thin-walled atrium ; a jugular pulse arising in this way is a clinical sign that is commonly encountered in traumatic pericarditis in cattle. Jugular pulsation also occurs in advanced tricuspid incompetence ; thus in the horse pronounced jugular pulsation synchronous with the arterial pulse may be found to arise from dilatation of the right ventricle and the atrioventricular orifice. Though tricuspid incompetence is not uncommon in dogs, the presence of jugular pulsation is not easily seen unless the dog is laid in a position so that its neck is fully extended. Fine fast pulsation of the jugular vein is seen in horses suffering from atrial flutter, the contractions of the first chamber of the right heart having adopted a rhythm independent of the ventricular contraction ; in these cases a jugular pulse of 120 or more per minute may be present when the arterial pulse is 80, 60 or less.

Distension of the venous system may result from disease not directly connected with the circulatory system. Acute distension of the stomach, marked tympany or any other cause of increased abdominal pressure may cause dilatation of the superficial veins. Chronic alveolar emphysema in the horse is frequently accompanied by distension of the venous system that becomes exceedingly prominent on and after exertion.

In addition to inspection of the superficial veins, inspection of the conjunctiva will be of assistance in assessing the state of the venous system. In venous congestion the small vessels of the conjunctiva are seen to be distended and stand out prominently under the mucous membrane. Cyanosis in the case of animals with pigmented skins can only be seen if the visible mucous membranes are inspected. Cyanosis is clinical evidence of defective oxygenation of the blood, it may be a sign of cardiac defect, but may be due to respiratory disease.

POSTURE AND GAIT IN RELATION TO CIRCULATORY DISEASE

In some forms of circulatory disease the animal adopts a posture that reduces the pressure by the fore-limbs on the lower part of the chest. To do this the elbows are abducted, and when the animal is viewed from behind the presence of a space between the elbow and the chest wall is very noticeable. Any acute cardiac condition that is painful may necessitate the adoption of this posture, but it is most characteristic of traumatic pericarditis in cattle. Dogs may achieve a measure of relief from cardiac pain by sitting upright with the elbows abducted as far as possible from the chest wall. Animals with painful cardiac conditions frequently show disinclination to move, and if forced to do so may emit a groan. When turning they do not flex the body but tend to keep the spine rigid in a straight line, so requiring a larger circle than normal in which to turn. Dogs frequently refuse to go up or down stairs.

EXAMINATION OF THE BLOOD

Alterations in the composition of the blood inevitably affect the function of the heart. In the investigation of circulatory disease it is important that such alterations should be determined. Any disease that is accompanied by dehydration will cause an increased viscosity of the blood that increases the work the heart must perform.

Anæmia is the most important abnormality of the blood that produces clinical signs of cardiac disturbance. The principal symptoms and clinical signs of anæmia are conveniently discussed at this point as the diagnosis of anæmia may be an essential preliminary in the interpretation of an apparent circulatory disease. Anæmia may be due to blood loss or it may be due to failure of production. Blood loss may be a result of hæmolysis as it occurs in babesiasis in cattle or in post-parturient hæmoglobinuria in cows. Blood loss may be due to hæmorrhage whether severe and recent or less acute but more chronic. Hæmorrhage may be a result of trauma or in pigs and dogs as a result of ingesting an anticoagulant such as warfarin rat poison. On the other hand hæmorrhage may result from the continued loss of small quantities of blood from any system of the body. Blood-sucking intestinal helminths can thus cause anæmia, while other helminths can cause ulceration of the mucosa leading to hæmorrhage.

Anæmia due to failure of production may be nutritional in origin. It is seen in gross malnutrition which practically amounts to starvation, but is often associated with trace element deficiencies such as cobalt or copper deficiency.

The anæmia that accompanies heavy fluke infestations in cattle and sheep results from disturbance of intermediate metabolism in the liver.

Hypoplasia and aplasia of the bone marrow causes anæmia by depressing or stopping the production of red blood cells. Such changes in the bone marrow can be caused by some toxic substances, by irradiation and by neoplasia of the bone marrow.

Animals suffering from anæmia show general symptoms of debility; the coat or fleece is harsh and lacks lustre, the animal is easily fatigued and any strenuous exertion causes dyspnœa, the animal being unable to sustain the effort for anything more than a short period. Frequently the animal is thin and may even be emaciated. Ascites may be so marked that the animal has a large pendulous abdomen and the flanks on both sides below the lumbar transverse processes appear hollow. Accumulations of fluid may be present in the pleural cavity and pericardial sac. Œdema of the limbs, of the substernal region and of the lower part of the abdominal wall may be present. The visible mucous membranes are pale and watery in appearance; owing to pigmentation of the skin this pallor is not noticed until the mucous membranes are inspected, and owners are frequently unaware of the presence of anæmia and the time of its development. The pulse is fast and weak. On auscultation the heart-beat is loud and tumultuous, the volume of sound being out of all proportion to the strength of the pulse. Following exertion the heart's efforts are increased and the beating of the heart may be heard at a distance of several feet from the animal. In severe anæmia due to the rapid destruction of red blood cells, as occurs in bovine piroplasmosis, the loud palpitating action of the heart may be heard at some distance from the animal even when it is at rest and recumbent.

Further investigation of a case of anæmia entails an analysis of the history and clinical evidence supplemented by examination of the blood for hæmoglobin content, red cell count, with examination of the red cells for abnormalities, and white cell count with a differential cell count. Details of these examinations are given in Chapter XVIII. If parasitism is suspected fæces and other suitable material should be examined for eggs and larvae ; details of the techniques are given in Chapter XVII.

THE ELECTROCARDIOGRAPH

The electrocardiograph is an instrument that provides a permanent visual record of the very small electric currents generated in the heart muscle during the various phases of its muscular activity.

It cannot be too strongly emphasised that the electrocardiograph is an aid to diagnosis and that a complete clinical investigation must precede the use of the electrocardiograph.

The electrocardiograph record must always be interpreted in conjunction with the clinical findings. Any attempt to use the electrocardiograph as a short-cut to diagnosis will inevitably lead to confusion and errors in diagnosis. There are abnormalities of the heart that are not revealed by the electrocardiograph and there are deviations in electrocardiograph records that are of no clinical significance. Clinical examination of the circulation, particularly careful assessment of the pulse and auscultation of the heart, will in many cases provide more information than can be obtained by means of an electrocardiograph, and there are cases in which the clinical examination reveals cardiac defects not recorded by the electrocardiograph.

In suitable cases the electrocardiograph provides a very useful method for the careful study of cardiac disease. The selection of cases for study by means of the electrocardiograph must depend on a clear appreciation of what can be demonstrated by the electrocardiograph, and this in turn depends on a knowledge of the principles involved in electrocardiography.

In the horse the electrocardiograph has proved useful in the investigation of cases of cardiac disease. In this animal the student will find that the electrocardiograph, by providing a visual record of the heart action, may be of considerable assistance in understanding the nature of some forms of cardiac disease. In cattle, sheep and pigs little need has been found for the use of the electrocardiograph in the investigation of cardiac disease. In the dog, when careful analysis of the findings by clinical examination indicate that the nature of the case is such that the electrocardiograph could be expected to provide additional information, a greater degree of accuracy in diagnosis may be achieved. In the dog, however, non-specific electrocardiograph deviations from the normal are common.

The principle underlying the electrocardiograph is that when a portion of muscle is stimulated to contract, a difference in electrical potential is created between the active contracting part and the inactive part. When the wave of contraction has extended to involve the whole of the muscle there is no difference in electrical potential between the two parts—*i.e.* iso-electric state. If the contraction ceases at the point where it first commenced but persists in the part of the muscle to which the excitation process spread, a difference of electrical potential between the two portions of muscle will again be present, but when recorded will be found to be in the reverse direction to that of the original difference in potential. If these differences in electrical potential are recorded on paper moving at a constant speed it will be found that they take the form of a curve consisting of deflections either above or below the iso-electric line. The rhythmic contraction of the heart spreading through its muscular tissues produces comparable differences in electrical potential and it is these that are recorded by the electrocardiograph. The technical principles involved in constructing an electrocardiograph are that the very small currents generated by the heart muscle are picked up by electrodes applied to suitable parts of the body and are passed through a very sensitive measuring and recording apparatus. The form of measuring instrument used in the original apparatus was the Einthoven string galvanometer ; the deviations of the string being recorded on sensitised photograph film or paper by means of a beam of light projected across the string and focussed by means of a system of lenses.

In order to obtain satisfactory records it is essential that the animal remains still during the recording. In the case of horses this means that the animal may require to be rested after a journey or exercise until its breathing has settled down and the animal if excited has calmed down. In dogs the procedure is to lay the dog on its right side ; with gentle handling they generally lie quietly ; though a sedative may be given, it is better avoided.

The most satisfactory form of electrocardiograph in clinical veterinary practice is the direct writing electronic electrocardiograph operated by alternating current from the electricity supply mains. This instrument has the advantage that the records are available for inspection as they are being made and adjustments can be made on the instrument as may be required during the actual recording.

Various methods of applying the electrodes have been described and quite naturally there is room for difference of opinion as to what may be the best method. It is, however, necessary if consistent results are to be obtained, to adhere to the method adopted. The method described here is that used consistently in the Department of Veterinary Medicine in the Royal (Dick) School of Veterinary Studies of Edinburgh University. It has been found most convenient to use sites just above the carpus and tarsus selecting sites where muscle underlies the skin. The areas on each limb, to which the non-polarisable metal electrodes are applied, are clipped ; the skin of the areas is then rubbed with an electrode jelly to ensure efficient electrical contact. The electrodes lightly smeared with electrode jelly are held in place with broad elastic bands which should be just sufficiently tight to keep the electrode in position without causing undue constriction. The three active electrodes are applied to the right and left forelimbs and the left hind limb ; a fourth electrode applied to the right hind limb is connected to earth through the machine. In making connections between the electrocardiograph and a horse it has been found useful to employ extension leads fitted with quick release sockets into which the normal terminals are fitted. This procession safeguards the machine from a sudden jerk should the horse make a rapid movement. Careful checks have shown that these extension leads do not reduce the quality of recording. A switch on the electrocardiograph enables the operator to select a combination of electrodes from which to obtain a recording ; these combinations are known as leads and are shown in the table below :

LEAD	CONNECTION AND POLARITY	
	+	−
Simple Leads		
I	Left foreleg	Right foreleg
II	Left leg	Right foreleg
III	Left leg	Left foreleg
Augmented Leads		
AVr	Right foreleg	Left foreleg, left leg connected together
AVl	Left foreleg	Right foreleg and left leg connected together
AVf	Left leg	Right foreleg and left foreleg connected together

It will be realised that the use of these leads makes it possible to record the currents derived from six positions of the electrical axis relative to the anatomical axis of the heart. In this way the maximum possible information can be obtained from the electrocardiograph. In addition to these leads it is possible to obtain recordings in which the three limb leads are connected together through 5000 ohms resistance in each lead to form the negative pole while the right arm, left arm and left leg are used as a single lead for the positive pole. A further combination is to use a suction electrode in the chest wall over the heart to form the positive pole with the right arm forming the negative pole.

As a bare minimum the three simple leads I, II and III should always be recorded, but as a general rule it is desirable also to record the augmented leads AVr, AVl and AVf.

The paper used in the electrocardiograph is provided with a time scale, the smaller horizontal divisions representing $\frac{1}{25}$ second and the larger divisions $\frac{1}{5}$ second. Before using, the apparatus is adjusted so that an impulse of 1 millivolt raises the writing point through two of the larger vertical divisions (*i.e.* 1 cm.).

Before reviewing in detail the information obtainable from an electrocardiograph it is useful to consider the salient features of what can be seen in a recording. The rate of the heart can be counted accurately. The rhythm of the heart can be studied. The rate of conduction of impulses forming the cardiac cycle can be measured. Defects in conduction can be seen. Deviations in the normal curves can be appreciated and corelated to such changes as preponderance of one ventricle.

There are certain conditions that can only be diagnosed with certainty by means of the electrocardiograph. These include heart block, disassociation between atria and ventricles as represented by atrial flutter and atrial fibrillation. On the other hand the electrocardiograph will give visual confirmation of conditions such as disturbances of cardiac rhythm that have been recognised by ordinary clinical methods. The electrocardiograph cannot indicate the presence of a leaking atrioventricular valve ; it may record preponderance of the ventricle concerned before failure of compensation and the low voltage of an exhausted heart muscle when compensation has failed.

The letters P, Q, R, S, T are used to describe the components of the cardiac cycle as recorded by the electrocardiograph. The first upward curve P corresponds to the period of contraction of the atria. In the horse this may have a pointed or rounded summit but in many normal horses there is a slight saddle-shaped bifurcation ; the duration of the P-wave is about 0·12 second. Following P is an iso-electric period lasting about 0·16 second. The ventricular complex that follows consists of four components labelled Q, R, S, and T. Q is normally a small downward deflection, that is absent from many records. This is followed by a pronounced upward deflection R and a downward deflection S ; the S-wave is frequently not very pronounced and may be absent. The duration of Q, R, S is about 0·08 second and represents the period of ventricular contraction. Following Q, R, S is an iso-electric period lasting about 0·34 second. The final deflection T lasts about 0·10 second.

The T-wave in the conventional diagram of an electrocardiograph is represented as being in an upward direction, but in many apparently normal horses the T-wave is a downward direction and is then described as being inverted. The T-wave, sometimes termed the terminal deflection of the ventricular complex, is the electrical effect of ventricular de-activation *i.e.* depolarisation of the muscle.

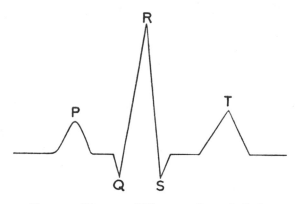

FIG. 13.—Diagram of Electrocardiograph Cycle.

The P-R interval is considered to represent the conduction time of the bundle of His and is therefore a measure of the conductivity of the intrinsic nerve mechanism of the heart. A series of records from normal horses showed that the P-R interval was very consistent at 0·32 second.

In dogs the heart rate is at least double that of a normal horse in consequence the duration of each cardiac cycle is less than that in the horse. Q and S waves are usually well marked and the excursion of the R-wave is usually pronounced.

USE AND INTERPRETATION OF ELECTROCARDIOGRAPHS

HORSE.—Though it is frequently possible to count a horse's pulse with accuracy there are those cases in which the pulse is irregular and the horse restless and it is in these cases that the electrocardiograph makes it possible to achieve an accurate estimate of the pulse rate. At the same time the record will show the type of irregularity and may give an indication of the cause of the irregularity.

The rate of conduction of the impulses forming the cardiac cycle can be measured and in this connection the P-R interval is of particular importance. Thus in a case of incomplete heart block the P-R interval was never less than 0·48 second compared with the normal of 0·32 second,

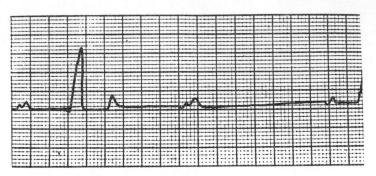

LEAD II

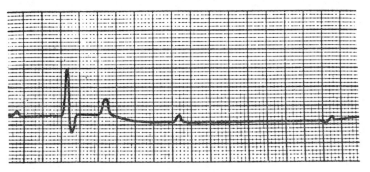

LEAD III

FIG. 14. — Electrocardiographs.   Horse.   11 year old Thoroughbred Mare.   Notched P-wave.   Prolonged P-R interval.   Irregular and unpredictable failure of ventricles to contract following atrial contraction. Incomplete heart-block.

the P-R interval at times exceeding 0·48 second immediately before the cardiac cycle in which the ventricles failed to contract following an atrial contraction.   It follows that the electrocardiograph is an invaluable means of diagnosing incomplete heart block.   In a case of incomplete heart block failure of the ventricle to contract in association with the atrial contraction may only occur at irregular intervals in a horse after a period of rest, but suspicions may be aroused by the lengthened P-R interval. If the horse is exerted and as soon as it has settled sufficiently another record is taken the presence of heart block may be picked up more quickly. In complete heart block there is complete disassociation of the atria and ventricles. As a general rule the atria are beating at a greater rate than the ventricles. In consequence the number of P-waves exceeds those

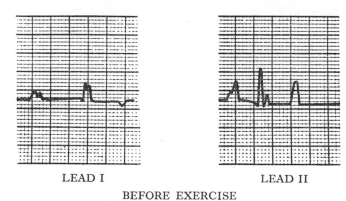

LEAD I   LEAD II

BEFORE EXERCISE

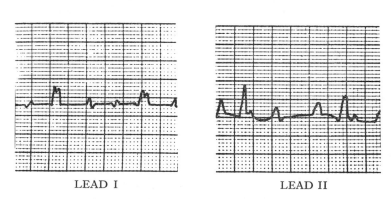

LEAD I   LEAD II

AFTER EXERCISE

Fig. 15. — Electrocardiographs.   Horse.   6 year old Thoroughbred Gelding.   Increasing dyspnœa on exertion.

Lead I   Splitting of P-wave and notching of R-wave.
Lead II   Similar.

Excessive preponderance of left ventricle.   Branch bundle block.

formed by the Q, R, S, T complex.   The P-waves may be fairly regular, but the Q, R, S, T complexes are frequently irregular.   In atrial flutter the P-waves are numerous and close together but identifiable as P-waves. In atrial fibrillation the atria are not contracting effectively and P-waves are absent.   In their place there is a very rapid continuous series of small elevations of the writing point ; these may be as frequent as 300 per minute. Imposed on this are frequent but irregular records of the ventricular contractions which are frequently of small extent, the electrocardiograph of the ventricular activity being found to correspond to the fast weak irregular pulse.

Heart block does not always equally involve both branches of the bundle of His. If conduction in one branch is more impaired than in the other there will be delay in the excitation process extending to the ventricle supplied through the branch involved in the greater impairment. If complete block of one branch is present there will be a considerable delay in the spread of the excitation wave to that ventricle. These delays in the spread of the excitation process are reflected in the record of the ventricular complex. Thus the apex of the R-wave may be bifurcated, or the down stroke of the R-wave may have an obvious notch on it. The leads in which these changes can be seen depends on the relationship of the electrical axis of the lead concerned to the anatomical axis of the heart, and that in turn depends on whether any hypertrophy of the heart has preceded the development of branch blunder block. Thus the electrocardiograph of branch bundle block in a horse breaking down in training with gross cardiac hypertrophy will be different from that in a horse showing severe cardiac irregularity after an attack of *purpura hæmorrhagica*.

Preponderance of one ventricle in the horse is usually related to hypertrophy and most often involves the left ventricle. Preponderance of the right ventricle is usually a sequel to some respiratory difficulty that will have been depicted during the general clinical examination. Thus a horse with chronic alveolar emphysema develops some degree of hypertrophy of the right ventricle.

In ventricular hypertrophy the R-wave is increased in amplitude, owing to the longer time required for the excitation process to spread through the increased muscle mass the Q, R, S complex is increased in width, giving the R-wave a broader base than normal. Quite frequently the S, T segment is depressed, that is to say, instead of S, T following the iso-electric line it drifts downwards into the T-wave, a return to the iso-electric line only following the T-wave and that sometimes only by a gradual drift. Distinction between right and left ventricular hypertrophy in electrocardiographic evidence alone may be difficult if not impossible. In any case some compensatory hypertrophy of the second ventricle is usually present. If the electrocardiograph is considered in relation to the clinical evidence, which has shown that the cardiac difficulties are sequel to respiratory difficulty it may be possible to establish a right-sided preponderance. In the absence of antecedent respiratory difficulty, electrocardiographic evidence of ventricular hypertrophy is most likely to relate to the left ventricle in a fast moving horse. A certain degree of electrocardiographic evidence of ventricular hypertrophy is almost always seen in records from horses used for fast work and is a normal condition related to the physiological response to training.

In horses with a disorderly heart action with other electrocardiographic evidence of heart block, the P-wave has the appearance of being split into two sharp peaks. This indicates a measure of disassociation of the contraction of the atria which are no longer contracting simultaneously In horses with very weak pulse and faint heart sounds it will be found that the excursion of the R-wave is much reduced thus confirming the clinical opinion of myocardial weakness.

Dog.—The most common cardiac disease in the dog is chronic valvular endocarditis followed by failure of compensation. This form of cardiac disease is essentially one in which diagnosis is based on the result of a clinical examination. The electrocardiograph cannot contribute to diagnosis of this disease.

In the dog irregularities of cardiac rhythm are a normal feature. These can readily be seen on electrocardiograph records and it is necessary to appreciate that great variations in these irregularities occur as between individual healthy dogs. Paroxysmal tachycardia is not uncommon in dogs when clinical investigation of the case may be difficult because of the extreme speed of the heart. In these cases electrocardiograph studies may assist interpretation of the cardiac disorder. The normal rhythmic irregularities disappear in these cases ; the entire complex is reduced in time and the Q, R, S, and T waves are increased in amplitude, the increase in the R-wave being very marked.

Atrial flutter, atrial fibrillation and cardiac hypertrophy are encountered in the dog. The electrocardiographic changes are comparable to those seen in the horse bearing in mind the greater rate of the normal heart in the dog.

Cattle.—Very satisfactory electrocardiographs can be obtained from normal cattle. There does not appear to be any clinical applications of electrocardiography in cattle.

Radiological Examination of the Heart

Radiological examination of the heart is only possible in the smaller domestic animals, and its use is practically confined to the dog. A radiological examination may furnish additional information regarding the size, shape and position of the heart. It should be clearly appreciated that the information thus obtained is of little value by itself, but if taken in conjunction with the symptoms and clinical signs may be of value. The radiographs should be taken in two planes, namely lateral and ventrodorsal. If the ventro-dorsal film is to be of any value it must be taken with the dog held with its sternum directly above the spine so that the film presents a symmetrical view of the chest. Increase in size of the heart can only be determined with certainty on an X-ray film when the increase is of substantial proportions and the X-ray picture may be of assistance in supporting the clinical findings. The fluid in hydropericardium is of practically the same density to X-rays as heart muscle and therefore an X-ray film in hydropericardium shows an enlarged heart shadow ; the distinction between enlarged heart and hydropericardium must then be based on the clinical findings.

Analysis of the Symptoms and Clinical Signs of the Chief Diseases of the Circulation

I. General

ACUTE MYOCARDITIS AND ENDOCARDITIS.—Acute myocarditis is usually secondary to severe infectious disease or septicæmic states. There is marked evidence of depression and weakness ; a phase of acute fever may terminate with a rapid fall of the temperature to below normal immediately before death. The pulse is fast, weak and irregular. The heart sounds are feeble and may appear indistinct. The condition is responsible for a high mortality, the course being short. Acute myocarditis will very frequently be associated with acute endocarditis. The presence of acute endocarditis can only be diagnosed with certainty if an endocardial murmur is detectable on auscultation. In very many cases death occurs before the lesions on the endocardium have attained a character that will produce such a murmur. A differential white cell count may show a marked neutrophilia with an increase in the proportion of non-lobulated neutrophils.

ACUTE PERICARDITIS.—Acute pericarditis is also a secondary condition. There is a febrile reaction and a small fast pulse. In the early stages a pericardial friction rub may be detected. Once a sufficient volume of exudate is present the friction disappears and the heart sounds become muffled. An increase in the area of cardiac dullness may be detected on percussion. The course and termination depend on the cause, but in many cases the course is short and the termination fatal.

HYDROPERICARDIUM.—Hydropericardium may be present to a small extent in debilitated and anæmic animals, especially those suffering from the effects of gross parasitic infestations. If severe the condition is usually due to defective heart action ; the symptoms and clinical signs are partly attributable to the causal disease. The animal shows severe dyspnœa on exertion and may stagger if the effort has been unduly strenuous. Many cases are afebrile ; if fever is present it is due to the causal condition, not to hydropericardium. There will be signs of venous congestion and pulsation of the jugular vein may be seen. The pulse is rather small and accelerated. The heart sounds are muffled and an increase in the area of cardiac dullness may be discerned.

II. AFFECTING INDIVIDUAL SPECIES

(1) HORSE

CARDIAC ARRHYTHMIA.—In a moderate degree of cardiac arrhythmia no symptoms may be in evidence ; it is only when the circulation is examined that the arrhythmia is detected. If the disturbance of rhythm is severe, the heart is unable to respond to demands made on it, and exertion produces symptoms of respiratory distress, inability to continue the exertion and possibly staggering. The pulse is found to be irregular in rate, rhythm and character. Further investigation of cardiac arrhythmia in the horse with a view to determining its nature is facilitated by the electrocardiograph.

EXTRA-SYSTOLE.—Extra-systole or premature contraction is not a common condition in the domesticated animals ; it is occasionally encountered in the horse and rarely in the dog. Occurrence of premature contraction appears to be an indication of irritability of the myocardium and endocardium. As a result of this irritability the ventricles irregularly contract independently of the cardiac rhythm. If this premature contraction or extra-systole occurs when the ventricle is partly filled, a pulse wave is propagated and both atrio-ventricular and aortic valves close. The pulse wave may be recognised as being less than normal. Following premature contraction the heart rests in diastole filling completely and producing after an appreciable pause a pulse wave and heart sounds that are stronger than normal.

If premature contraction occurs when the ventricle is relatively empty, the atrio-ventricular valves close producing a weak first sound but neither pulse wave nor second heart sound are produced. After a pause the ventricles contract forcibly after filling completely. Though the presence of extra-systole or premature contraction may be suspected as a result of a clinical examination, confirmation of its presence is dependent on electrocardiograph evidence.

DILATATION.—Dilatation of the heart may be present for a considerable time without any symptoms being shown. When the dilatation of the heart attains dimensions that render closure of the valves no longer possible, symptoms of valvular insufficiency appear. Exertion will cause severe dyspnœa due to pulmonary congestion. The venous system is engorged and there may be jugular pulsation. The arterial pulse is rapid and irregular in rhythm and force. A blowing systolic murmur is heard on auscultation ; this becomes very loud on exertion. An increase in the area of cardiac dullness may be discerned by percussion. The horse tends to lose bodily condition. Death may occur suddenly.

HYPERTROPHY.—A certain degree of cardiac hypertrophy is a physiological response to the continued graded exercise that constitutes the

L

process of training. If kept within normal physiological limits no symptoms will be evident. If hypertrophy becomes excessive the atrio-ventricular orifices become sufficiently enlarged to render the valves guarding them incapable of completely closing the orifices during systole. For a time the heart will compensate for the valvular insufficiency, but as soon as compensation fails symptoms and clinical signs similar to those of cardiac dilatation appear.

PALPITATION.—Cardiac palpitation is a violent tumultuous beating of the heart that may be a symptom of other disease. Cardiac palpitation is observed in highly strung nervous horses and also in young horses when these are first subjected to handling. Cardiac palpitation is a constant concomitant of acute anæmia. It may be due to a diseased condition of the heart. The characteristic feature of cardiac palpitation is the loud tumultuous disorderly beating of the heart, the sound being readily heard some distance from the animal. The sound is found to be related to the cardiac impulse. In spite of the violent efforts of the heart the pulse is weak. The horse is excited and may show signs of distress. Other symptoms and clinical signs will depend on the causal condition.

(2) CATTLE

TRAUMATIC PERICARDITIS.—There may be a history of digestive disturbance that has persisted for a length of time varying from a day or so to as much as five and a half months. The animal tends to remain standing with its head poked out and the elbows abducted. If lying it is unwilling to rise. There may be some œdema of the dewlap extending back between the forelegs. The jugular veins are corded and pulsation may be seen in them. If made to move the animal turns with the body held rigidly and does not flex the spine ; the gait is stiff. The pulse is rapid and rather wiry in character. The temperature is variable. Extensive exudation into the pericardial sac rapidly takes place, and it is unlikely that the animal will be examined sufficiently early in the illness for pericardial friction to be detected. Once exudation has occurred the heart sound is muffled and appears far away. An increase in the area of cardiac dullness can only be detected in thin animals whose chest wall is not too substantial. If gas as well as fluid is present in the peri-cardial sac a tinkling sound may be heard on auscultation. The act of parturition causing a great increase in intra-abdominal pressure may precipitate a fatal conclusion by forcing the foreign body further forward until it actually impinges on the heart muscle. Exertion of any kind may also lead to a fatality.

TUBERCULOUS PERICARDITIS.—Many cases of tuberculous pericarditis are only found in the abattoir or post-mortem room. Tuberculous peri-carditis may be part of a generalised tuberculosis. Not infrequently it is found without extensive involvement of the thoracic organs though the lymph glands in various parts of the body may be affected. Tuberculous pericarditis by itself may give rise to symptoms of cardiac disturbance. In cattle the lesion is dry in character and no increase in the area of cardiac dullness is likely to be detected. Pericardial friction sound may be heard on auscultation, but these sounds are not always sufficiently distinct to be recognised. Diagnosis is necessarily difficult and a post-mortem examination may be necessary before a diagnosis of tuberculous pericarditis can be established.

ENDOCARDITIS.—Acute endocarditis occurs in the course of septicæmic disease, the clinical picture is one of a febrile reaction with depression of the circulation, if the animal survives long enough for lesions on the valves of the heart to cause insufficiency an endocardial murmur can be detected. In chronic endocarditis the lesion is found to be involving an atrio-ventricular valve. The clinical picture is one of malaise with dyspnœa on exertion, possibly some inco-ordination of gait. The pulse is accelerated and lacks volume ; auscultation reveals a blowing endocardial murmur.

PALPITATION.—Pronounced cardiac palpitation is common in bovine piroplasmosis (bovine hæmoglobinuria) and in post-parturient hæmoglobinuria. The symptoms and clinical signs of cardiac palpitation in cattle are similar to those described as occurring in the horse.

(3) PIG

VERRUCOSE ENDOCARDITIS.—Verrucose endocarditis is an important lesion of swine erysipelas and is present in practically every case of chronic swine erysipelas. In some cases no symptoms are seen, the pig being found dead ; in others there may be symptoms of cyanosis and acute respiratory distress. Auscultation may show that the normal heart sounds are practically obliterated by the harsh murmurs caused by the large vegetative growths arising from the atrioventricular valves. These may be so extensive as practically to fill the cavity of the ventricle. Death almost invariably results and the presence of verrucose endocarditis may be confirmed by a post-mortem examination.

PIGLET ANÆMIA.—In young pigs suffering from nutritional anæmia (iron deficiency) there is great dilatation of the heart, which on postmortem examination may be so large as to appear to fill the chest cavity. In these cases cardiac palpitation is pronounced.

(4) DOG

ACUTE ENDOCARDITIS.—Acute endocarditis may occur as a complication of infective fever or septicæmia; it is probable that a certain amount of myocarditis is also present in such cases. In the earlier stages acute endocarditis is manifested by acceleration of the pulse and reduction in the cardiac output. It is only in the later stages when definite valvular lesions have caused a murmur that the existence of endocarditis can be determined with certainty.

In the dog a disease resembling rheumatic fever of man is encountered. There is a sharp febrile reaction with marked prostration ; the dog is unwilling to move and shows pain when handled or lifted, but careful manipulation will fail to show any point of maximum intensity of pain. The pulse is fast and wiry and very often a distinct thrill is felt running through the pulse. In a matter of a few days a distinct endocardial murmur can be heard. The course usually extends to about three weeks ; the mortality is low but chronic endocardial lesions persist.

CHRONIC ENDOCARDITIS.—In a small proportion of cases a history is obtained of a previous illness corresponding to that described under acute endocarditis, but in the majority of cases no relevant history of antecedent illnesses is obtainable. So long as the heart is able to compensate for the valvular defects caused by chronic endocarditis no symptoms will be manifested. Physical examination of the heart will reveal the presence of an endocardial murmur and this may be localised to an individual valve. When compensation fails and the heart is no longer capable of making good the valvular defects, symptoms of cardiac deficiency become manifest. Failure of compensation may take place gradually, but quite often there is a sudden acute failure of compensation.

At rest the animal may appear to be quite normal, but very slight exertion causes a marked increase in the respiratory rate. Strenuous efforts will cause severe dyspnœa and the animal may stagger and collapse. Temporary rigidity of the skeletal muscles may exist for a few minutes after the animal has collapsed. The pulse is fast, weak and very irregular ; in not a few cases it may be found to be almost imperceptible. There may be evidence of venous congestion. Physical examination of the heart will reveal a pronounced endocardial murmur. In a considerable proportion of cases the tricuspid (right atrioventricular) is the valve principally involved. The size of the heart may be found to be considerably increased, the sounds being clear and distinct on the right side as well as the left side of the chest.

HYDROPERICARDIUM.—As a result of cardiac defects hydropericardium is encountered in association with hydrothorax and ascites. The pulse is weak and the heart sounds muffled by the fluid in the chest. The electrocardiograph shows evidence of myocardial weakness.

TUBERCULOUS PERICARDITIS.—In the dog tuberculous pericarditis is of a wet type and is characterised by considerable exudation into the pericardial sac. Symptoms are not shown until exudation has taken place, when dyspnœa, after even slight exertion, attracts attention to the animal. The pulse is small and fast. Auscultation of the heart shows that the sounds are muffled and are nearly as audible on the right as on the left side. Percussion shows an increased area of cardiac dullness that must be distinguished from the dullness caused by fluid in the pleural cavity. It will be necessary to obtain fluid from the pericardial sac in order that the presence of tuberculosis may be demonstrated by microscopic, and if necessary, biological methods.

HYPERTROPHY.—Cardiac hypertrophy may occur in sporting dogs in circumstances similar to these described as occurring in the horse. Cardiac hypertrophy is also encountered in the dog, when there is an increase in the peripheral resistance of the circulation, as occurs in chronic interstitial nephritis ; in these cases the pulse is strong and the cardiac sounds loud. It may be possible to demonstrate an increase in the area of cardiac dullness.

TACHYCARDIA.—A paroxysmal tachycardia is met with chiefly in excitable animals. The pulse is excessively fast and weak ; the heart sounds though distinct are rather weak. The electrocardiograph will confirm that the cardiac abnormality is one of tachycardia.

HEART-BLOCK, ATRIAL FLUTTER AND ATRIAL FIBRILLATION.— These are conditions associated with a fast weak irregular pulse. An electro-cardiograph investigation is necessary to establish the nature of the cardiac defect.

PALPITATION AND DILATATION.—The symptoms and clinical signs of cardiac palpitation and dilatation are similar to those described as occurring in these conditions in the horse.

URINARY SYSTEM

CLINICALLY recognisable diseases of the urinary system are not very commonly encountered in horses, cattle, sheep and pigs ; though in some areas the incidence of calculi in kidney, bladder and urethra is sufficiently high to render the condition one of importance. In the dog and cat diseases of the urinary system are of frequent occurrence. In the dog chronic interstitial nephritis and the presence of urinary calculi are of considerable clinical importance. In the adult castrated male cat cystitis, due to retention of the urine following obstruction of the urethra with sabulous material, is common.

Symptoms and clinical signs suggestive of disease of the urinary system may be sufficient to justify a tentative diagnosis, but in many cases before a diagnosis can be established analysis of a specimen of urine is necessary. It should be realised that the symptoms, that may lead to professional advice being sought, do not necessarily suggest that the disease is located in the urinary system. Inefficient renal function may lead to symptoms and clinical signs usually associated with organs remote from the kidney ; thus vomiting may be evidence of chronic interstitial nephritis in the dog. Examination of the urine in cases of indefinite illness may reveal unsuspected disease of the urinary system or a pre-renal condition.

REGIONAL ANATOMY

HORSE.—The left kidney lies under cover of the last rib and the transverse processes of the first two or three lumbar vertebræ. The right kidney lies under cover of the last three ribs and the transverse process of the first lumbar vertebra (see Figs. 1 and 2, pp. 42 and 43). The kidneys in the horse cannot be palpated through the abdominal wall. If the animal is not too large the left kidney may be palpated *per rectum*. It is only in very small animals that both kidneys can be palpated on making a rectal examination. The bladder when empty lies on the anterior part of the floor of the pelvis ; as the bladder becomes distended with urine it extends forward to reach the abdominal floor. In the male the bladder is directly in contact with the ventral surface of the rectum ; in the female the body of the uterus and vagina lie between the bladder and the rectum. The male urethra terminates in the urethral process, a small free part of the membranous tube extending into the fossa of the glans penis. The female urethra terminates at the external urethral orifice in the floor of the vagina at a point four or five inches in front of the ventral commissure of the vulva. The female urethra is capable of considerable dilatation, and with care a finger can be introduced through the external urethral orifice.

CATTLE.—The kidneys are lobulated. The left kidney lies under cover of the third, fourth and fifth lumbar vertebræ. The left kidney is only loosely attached to the sublumbar region, and its position in relation to the median plane depends on the degree of repletion of the rumen. If the rumen is relatively empty the left kidney lies partly to the left of the median plane, but if the rumen is full the left kidney is entirely on the right of the median plane. The right kidney lies under cover of the last rib and the transverse processes of the first two or three lumbar vertebræ (see Fig. 4, p. 62). The kidneys cannot be palpated through the abdominal wall in adult cattle. On making a rectal examination the left kidney can be palpated in all except very large animals. The bladder extends farther forward on the abdominal floor than in the horse. Its relations in the two sexes are similar to those in the horse. The male urethra follows the course of the penis, which forms a sigmoid flexure just behind the scrotum ; the external urethral orifice is small. The female urethra terminates about four or five inches anterior to the ventral commissure of the vulva. Immediately posterior to the external urethral orifice is the suburethral diverticulum ; this is about an inch in length and is sufficiently capacious to permit the entry of the finger.

SHEEP.—The kidneys are not lobulated. The male urethra terminates in the processus urethræ, a twisted tube projecting about an inch and a half beyond the glans penis.

PIG.—The kidneys may lie symmetrically beneath the transverse processes of the first four lumbar vertebræ, but the left kidney is in some animals slightly more anterior than the right. The bladder is large. In the boar the sigmoid flexure of the penis lies in front of the scrotum. In the sow the posterior part of the urethra is fused with the floor of the vagina forming an elevation surrounding the external urethral orifice.

DOG.—The left kidney is somewhat loosely attached and in consequence its position is variable ; it usually lies under the transverse processes of the second, third and fourth lumbar vertebræ, but the anterior pole may lie under the transverse process of the first lumbar vertebra (see Fig. 9, p. 87). The right kidney lies under the transverse processes of the first three lumbar vertebræ ; occasionally the anterior pole may lie under the last rib (see Fig. 11, p. 104). The kidneys cannot be palpated through the abdominal wall in all dogs. The bladder when empty lies within the pelvic cavity ; if very full it may reach as far forward as the umbilicus. The prostate is large and surrounds the neck of the bladder and the commencement of the urethra. The male urethra passes through a groove in the ventral part of the *os penis*, and in this part of the urethra dilatation is restricted by the rigidity of the bone. On either side of the external urethral opening in the bitch there is a depression in the vaginal mucous membrane.

CAT.—The kidneys are loosely attached to the sublumbar region and if the abdomen is empty they may hang down into the abdominal cavity. The male urethra has a very small lumen where it passes through the penis.

CLINICAL EXAMINATION

The symptoms and clinical signs arising from diseases of the urinary system may be described as falling into three categories. First, there are those associated with the act of micturition ; they include frequency, abnormal posture and evidence of pain. Secondly, there are those signs that can be determined by the physical examination of the urinary system. Thirdly, there are those symptoms and signs remote from the urinary system that are caused by the defects in excretion, metabolic disturbances and toxæmia that ensue from urinary diseases ; these symptoms and signs emanate chiefly from the cardiovascular system, the digestive system and the nervous system. The interpretation of the symptoms and clinical signs occurring in these three categories is facilitated by the consideration of them in relation to any abnormalities found by urine analysis.

MICTURITION

Horses as a rule urinate only at rest and frequently do so when the straw bed is laid down or when placed in their stall or box. A horse does not normally urinate when moving. The posture normally adopted by both horses and mares is that the hind-legs are separated and the animal appears to press forward slightly and exert pressure by contracting the abdominal wall. Very often the horse will emit a grunt or groan while urinating. It is found that horses living a regular life conforming to a time-table urinate at remarkably constant times. Cows adopt a posture in the same manner as horses—the tail is elevated and the urine passed fairly rapidly. In male cattle the act of urination might well be described as a dribbling process, the urine being passed frequently in comparatively small amounts. This is done while the animal is walking as well as when it is standing still and the animal does not stop feeding.

Sows pass urine in the same way as mares and cows. Boars and castrated male pigs pass the urine in a series of jets giving an appearance as if the urine was being ejaculated.

Bitches adopt a squatting posture and the urine flows freely and rapidly from the bladder. The male dog raises one of the hind-legs and as a rule directs the stream of urine against some object.

FREQUENCY.—An increase in the frequency of urination may be due to a greater volume of urine. This occurs in equine diabetes insipidus (polyuria), in diabetes mellitus, in chronic interstitial nephritis in dogs, and may be due to a greater fluid intake or to the action of diuretics ; it also occurs in cold weather. Increased frequency of urination may be due to irritation of the urethra, when alterations in the character of the urine render it irritant to the mucous membrane of the urethra ; such alterations occur in acute nephritis and cystitis. If the bladder is not completely emptied the residuum of urine may undergo decomposition and so become highly irritant. If only a small quantity of urine is voided from a distended bladder, tension persists and stimulation of the micturition reflex soon recurs. Vesical calculi by irritating the mucous membrane of the bladder stimulate the wall of the bladder to exert sufficient pressure to extrude urine and initiate the micturition reflex. Inability to adopt the normal posture for urination may prevent emptying of the bladder until the pressure of urine in the bladder is sufficient to overcome the sphincter, when the urine is passed more or less passively in small amount at frequent intervals. Any disease associated with paraplegia may lead to this type of interference with the act of urination.

Infrequent urination may be due to a reduction in the amount of urine ; this will occur if there is dehydration from any cause or if the blood pressure shows a marked fall. Difficulties in micturition may first lead to retention of the urine with apparent reduction of frequency, and then when the bladder is acutely distended and the sphincter overcome by the pressure on the urine incontinence occurs with an apparent increase in frequency.

POSTURE.—Any alteration in the posture adopted for the act of urination must be regarded as evidence of abnormality. It is only very rarely that the altered posture is an aberration on the part of the animal, and then it is usually found that the animal has habitually adopted the abnormal posture. The adoption of an abnormal posture for the act of micturition may be due to some interference with muscular control ; thus a paraplegic dog may be unable to balance on three legs and voids the urine while in the normal standing position. On the other hand the reason for the adoption of the abnormal posture may lie in the urinary system ; thus male dogs with acute cystitis very often pass urine in the squatting position usually adopted by bitches.

PAIN.—Pain on micturition may arise when it is necessary to overcome any obstruction in the urethra ; it is evidenced by groaning and tensing of the abdominal muscles. The pain may be due to stimulation of the urethral mucosa caused by urine that is so altered as to be irritant, *e.g.* concentrated and highly acid urine. Irritation of the urethral mucosa arising in this way will be shown by straining after urination and other evidence of discomfort ; increased frequency also results.

STRAINING.—Straining may be due to the animal having to exert sufficient pressure to overcome a urethral obstruction, when the straining is seen to precede and accompany the passage of urine ; unless the obstruction is completely overcome only a small amount of urine will be passed, but the effort may be repeated again after a short pause. Straining from discomfort following the passage of urine can usually be recognised by the gradual abatement of the straining, which reappears immediately after urine has again been passed. Straining and frequent apparent attempts at micturition due to colic in the horse must be distinguished from a genuine urinary condition. This is nearly always rendered possible by the presence of symptoms and clinical signs arising from the digestive system.

PHYSICAL EXAMINATION OF URINARY SYSTEM

KIDNEYS.—Though lumbar pain may be present in acute renal disease, it is not infrequently found on post-mortem examination that substantial acute renal damage has occurred without sufficient outward evidence of pain to attract the attention of anyone in attendance on the animal. Chronic kidney disease is characterised by an almost complete absence of pain or discomfort arising in the kidney. Renal colic is most commonly due to obstruction of the ureter by a calculus that has entered the ureter from the pelvis of the kidney. The pain thus created is of a most acute character, and in the horse the symptoms will very closely resemble those of acute colic of alimentary origin.

As palpation of the kidneys in horses and cattle is virtually impossible, the posterior thoracic and lumbar regions of the horse may be palpated with a view to eliciting evidence of pain. It will, however, be found that seldom, if ever, is any dependable information obtained by this method. In smaller animals, such as some dogs and most cats, deep palpation of the abdomen should enable the presence of pain in the kidneys to be accurately assessed. The only dependable method of determining the presence of abnormalities in the kidneys is the examination of samples of urine.

BLADDER.—Disease conditions of the bladder are manifested by increased frequency of urination, evidence of discomfort during or after micturition, changes in the urine and the signs determined by physical examination.

In the large animals it is possible to palpate the bladder *per rectum,* when the clinician should be able to determine the degree of distension and the existence of pain in the bladder when it is manipulated. It may also be possible to assess thickening of the bladder wall due to inflammatory process. If the bladder is empty vesical calculi can be palpated. In smaller animals the bladder must be examined by palpation through the abdominal wall. If the animal is small this may be done with one hand, but it will usually be found more convenient to place a hand on either side of the abdomen and by gentle pressure the fingers are brought together over the bladder. Occasionally it may be found of assistance if, with the forefinger of one hand in the rectum, the bladder is grasped between the forefinger and thumb of the other hand through the abdominal wall so that the bladder can be pushed back into contact with the tip of the finger in the rectum. This procedure is sometimes useful in small dogs in determining the presence of a calculus in the bladder. In cats the pyriform mass of a distended bladder is usually determined with little difficulty on palpation through the abdominal wall.

URETHRA.—Obstruction of the urethra will, as soon as the bladder becomes sufficiently distended, give rise to frequent repeated attempts at micturition. Inflammation of the urethra maintains by irritation a constant succession of stimuli to the micturition reflex resulting in the frequent passage of small quantities of urine. Palpation of the urethra is of rather limited value in any animal ; it may be possible in the horse or dog to palpate a calculus in the urethra. Palpation is, of course, of value in determining gross abnormalities such as a tumour involving the urethra or the neighbouring tissues. In the horse and dog the passage of a sound or catheter is the only satisfactory method of investigating the patency of the urethra. In cattle and pigs the sound can only be passed as far as the sigmoid flexure, and very frequently the obstruction is immediately behind the flexure and therefore beyond the point to which a sound can be passed. In examining the urethra in the male an inspection of the prepuce and penis should always be made. Obstruction of the preputial opening, phimosis and paraphimosis prevent the passage of urine ; such conditions are immediately recognised on inspection of the parts.

In the female the short dilatable urethra is seldom obstructed, but may be the site of inflammatory changes that not infrequently involve, or may originate from, the vaginal wall in the immediate neighbourhood of the external urethral openings. The presence of inflammatory changes involving the external urethral opening can only be ascertained by inspection. In the smaller animals such vaginal inspection may only be possible if a suitable speculum is employed ; in the larger animals the lips of the vulva may be separated manually or a speculum may be employed.

INTERPRETATION OF URINE ANALYSIS IN RELATION TO URINARY DISEASE

The details of the technique employed in urine analysis are given in Chapter XV. Abnormalities that would point to urinary disease are the presence of protein, blood and deposits in the urine, in addition changes in specific gravity and reaction may be noted. The results of urine analysis must always be interpreted in conjunction with the history and clinical picture of the case ; when that is done urine analysis will be found to be of great assistance in diagnosis and differential diagnosis.

With the exception of urine containing sufficient quantity of blood or blood pigment to give a definite colour, any opinion founded solely on the appearance of a sample of urine is notoriously unreliable and will in all probability be seriously misleading. As hæmoglobinuria as distinct from hæmaturia is the result a pre-renal condition and hæmaturia is a result of a renal or post-renal condition, the distinction between hæmaturia and hæmoglobinuria is of vital importance.

SPECIFIC GRAVITY.—With perhaps one exception estimation of the specific gravity of an isolated random sample of urine is of little help in diagnosis of urinary disease, since there are so many factors known and unknown that may have influenced the volume and specific gravity of such a sample. The exception is the very low specific gravity of any sample of urine obtained from a dog suffering from advanced chronic interstitial nephritis.

REACTION.—While quite substantial variations in the pH of urine take place in cases of urinary disease these are not necessarily of specific diagnostic significance ; thus a strongly alkaline sample of dog's urine may be related to acute bacterial cystitis, but the mere existence of alkaline urine does not justify a diagnosis of cystitis.

PROTEIN.—Though the presence of protein in urine is one of the earliest and most easily recognised signs of renal disease, the presence of protein does not necessarily indicate the existence of renal disease. Transient proteinuria is encountered in acute febrile disease and may indicate nothing more than cloudy swelling of kidney cells associated with the general systemic infection. Protein in urine may be post-renal in origin ; thus in cystitis the products of the inflammatory process are voided in the urine, and these contain protein. In acute nephritis, in addition to the cells of the kidney becoming permeable to colloids, the inflammatory process contributes to the amount of protein in the urine and the quantity may be considerable. In chronic interstitial nephritis the amount of protein in the urine tends to decrease as the disease progresses, until in the later stages only traces of protein may be present.

When protein is found in urine, an examination for deposits should be made. A consideration of the clinical findings along with the evidence obtained by examining the deposits will enable the clinician to decide on the source and significance of proteinuria.

BLOOD.—The normal routine in testing urine is to use a test for blood pigment ; if that is positive the next step is to decide whether the condition is one of hæmoglobinuria or hæmaturia. Hæmoglobinuria indicates a pre-renal condition ; hæmaturia indicates a renal or post-renal condition. Hæmaturia may be renal in origin when the deposits will show evidence of the source. Hæmaturia occurs in acute cystitis, in damage to the bladder mucosa caused by calculi, in cases of tumour formation in the bladder wall and in cases of chronic cystic hæmaturia in cattle associated with papillomatous growths protruding from the bladder mucosa.

DEPOSITS.—As the deposits in urine are of significance in the differential diagnosis of diseases of the urinary system a description of their characteristics is given here (see also p. 316). The deposits obtained from samples of urine fall into two main categories, the unorganised deposits consisting of various salts and other substances that have settled out of the urine and the organised deposits consisting of tissue elements such as red blood cells, white blood corpuscles, epithelial cells and casts. In addition to these two main categories the deposits from urine may contain large numbers of organisms.

The unorganised deposits vary according to the reaction of the urine. If the urine is acid in reaction, deposits of uric acid and urates are commonly present ; these are seen as small granular particles that may be described as amorphous deposits. Deposits of calcium oxalate are comparatively rare in the domestic animals; they take two principal forms, either a dumb-bell form, or a form rather like the back of a square envelope, the square being crossed by two diagonals. If the urine is alkaline in reaction phosphates and carbonates may be deposited. Phosphates occur most commonly as an amorphous deposit of white granular material that settles to the bottom of the urine, and, unlike urate deposits in acid urine, is not pigmented. A deposit of phosphate in the form of stellar crystals is rather uncommon. Carbonates are deposited as granular particles that resemble amorphous phosphates, but are soluble in acetic acid with the liberation of carbon dioxide. Phosphates are not soluble in acetic acid and no gas is evolved. Examination of the deposits will show the presence of the fine sabulous material that is present in the urine in cases where very numerous extremely small calculi are present in the urinary tract—a condition sometimes spoken of as " gravel."

The organised deposits occur in urine irrespective of its reaction. Red blood cells may be recognised in unstained smears made from the deposits obtained from fresh urine, but it is more satisfactory, especially when the specimen of urine has stood for some time, if the smear be stained with a suitable blood stain. The presence of red blood cells necessarily indicates a break in the continuity of the urinary tissue with the extravasation of blood. The presence of leucocytes and pus cells indicates an inflammatory reaction of a suppurative character ;

this may be situated in any part of the urinary tract. The identification of epithelial cells may indicate the site of the inflammatory reaction that has led to their appearance in the urine. Unfortunately, as a result of the inflammatory process that led to their separation, the cells may have been so damaged that the recognition of their source is rendered difficult : even prolonged exposure of the cells to the macerating effects of urine will produce much change in their morphology. Renal epithelial cells are polygonal, or columnar if coming from the tubules ; they are rather larger than a leucocyte and have a large nucleus. Epithelial cells from the pelvis of the kidney, ureter, bladder and urethra are squamous in character and can usually be distinguished from those originating in the kidney tissue, but it may be found impossible to decide from which part of the urinary passage the cells have originated. It may be thought that larger cells will have been detached from the bladder wall, but the relative size is more dependent on the depth to which the inflammatory process has extended into the mucous membrane than on the exact position in the urinary tract.

Casts, as the term implies, are models of the tubule from which they originated, and their presence in urine undoubtedly indicates an inflammatory condition of the kidneys. Casts containing a high proportion of cellular elements are indicative of an acute inflammatory condition of the kidney. Blood casts consist of a clot to the surface of which are attached large numbers of red blood cells. Epithelial casts may result from the complete separation of a cylindrical mass of cells from the wall of the tubule, or the epithelial cells may have become detached individually and subsequently been moulded on to colloid material extravasated into the tubules during the inflammatory process. The epithelial cells may be at various stages of disintegration. Granular casts are probably the remains of disintegrated epithelial casts ; they therefore occur in older standing cases. Hyaline casts are homogeneous, only slightly refractile and nearly transparent ; they consist of protein. Their presence is usually indicative of renal disease that has existed for some considerable time. Other types of cast, such as amyloid casts, waxy casts and lipoid casts, are not very commonly encountered.

UREA CONCENTRATION.—There are substantial variations in the concentration of urea in the urine passed at different times of the day. In dairy cows the percentage of urea is normally very low, while in horses it is usually high. It is uncommon for a healthy dog to pass urine with a urea content of less than 1·5 per cent. ; but if the fluid intake has been large the urea content may be considerably reduced. The most satisfactory test in regard to the excretory efficiency of the kidney in relation to products of nitrogen metabolism is an estimation of the blood urea.

Estimation of the amount of urea in an isolated sample of urine is of little value, but a substantial increase in the blood urea may be an indication of renal insufficiency (see p. 369).

RADIOLOGICAL EXAMINATION

Radiological examination of the urinary system is limited to the small animals. It is principally employed to demonstrate calculi. Intravenous pyelography has a very limited application. Retrograde pyelography is only possible in the bitch and is very rarely practised.

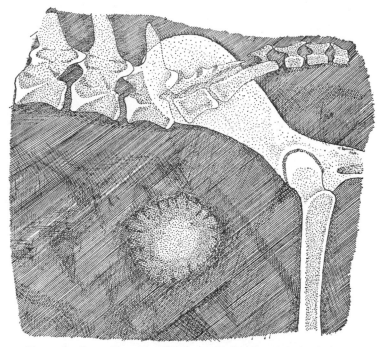

FIG. 16.—Dog. Drawing of radiograph showing vesical calculus.
One-third actual size.

ANALYSIS OF THE SYMPTOMS AND CLINICAL SIGNS OF DISEASE OF THE URINARY SYSTEM

ACUTE PARENCHYMATOUS NEPHRITIS.—The onset of symptoms is frequently sudden; there is a sharp febrile reaction with all the concomitant symptoms of fever. The animal stands with its back arched; it resents attempts being made to cause it to move and if forced to do so the gait is stiff. In the dog vomiting nearly always occurs. Though the pulse is accelerated there is no definite increase of pressure. Attempts at micturition are frequent and the passage of urine may cause considerable discomfort. Following a transient increase in the amount of urine there is a reduction in the volume that is related to the severity of the disease process in the kidneys. The amount of blood in the urine varies from just sufficient to give it a smoky appearance to a quantity that forms a flocculent reddish-brown precipitate immediately the urine is allowed to stand. The specific gravity of the urine is increased, the reaction is acid and the urine is usually heavily loaded with protein. Microscopic examination of the deposits shows the presence of blood, blood casts and epithelial casts in the first stages ; in the later stages granular casts may appear. Hyaline casts will only be found in longer-standing cases. The presence of micro-organisms and pus cells in the urinary deposits is not a feature of acute parenchymatous nephritis and would suggest the existence of pyæmic nephritis, pyelonephritis or pyelitis.

Acute parenchymatous nephritis causes a degree of toxæmia proportional to its severity. In the dog the tongue, gums and teeth are coated with an evil-smelling brown scum, and necrosis of the oral mucous membrane may occur. While the symptoms and clinical signs may suggest the possibility of acute nephritis, a definite diagnosis must depend on the examination of a specimen of urine.

ACUTE INTERSTITIAL NEPHRITIS.—In the dog acute interstitial nephritis is a feature of infection with *Leptospira canicola*. McIntyre and Stuart (1949) describe this phase of the illness as that of primary renal damage. It follows about one or two weeks after the invasive stage. The affected animals appear to have lost condition and are depressed. The breath is unpleasant and the teeth, gums and tongue may be coated with a reddish-brown scum. The pulse is increased in rate and force. Protein is present in the urine and casts can be demonstrated in the deposits. Leptospiræ can be found in the urine in a high proportion of cases. The blood urea varies from 40 to 200 mgs. or more per 100 ml. The agglutination titre for *Leptospira canicola* is either high (say 1 in 10,000) or shows a distinct rise between successive samples at a week's interval.

CHRONIC INTERSTITIAL NEPHRITIS.—Two forms of chronic interstitial nephritis are recognised in dogs. The first occurs within weeks or at the most a few months after an attack of leptospirosis and can be regarded as the clinical manifestation of secondary renal damage resulting from that illness. The second form occurs later in life and co-relation of it with an earlier attack of leptospirosis may or may not be possible.

The first form occurs in both young or old dogs. The dog has become thin and is very thirsty. Its appetite is impaired. The breath is often unpleasant and the pulse is full and bounding. There may also be a history of occasional vomiting. The urine is passed in increasing quantities, its specific gravity is low, traces of protein are found, the deposits contain hyaline casts and epithelial cells, and the urea content is low. The blood urea is increased in severe cases to 150 mgs. per 100 ml. or more. Co-relation with leptospirosis depends on the demonstration of an abnormal agglutination titre, the figure varying from 1 in 30 to 1 in 3000.

The second form is encountered most frequently in dogs from six or seven years and upwards. This form may be the sequel to a leptospirosis infection earlier in life but it may also result from other causes.

Very frequently there is obtained a history of irregular vomiting extending over a period varying from a few weeks to one or two years. This vomiting may have been attributed to some indefinite gastric disorder. Recently the attacks of vomiting have become more frequent and more severe and at the same time a great increase in the animal's thirst has been noticed. Thirst is associated with polyuria and nocturnal incontinence. Loss of condition, at first gradual, becomes accentuated and the animal in the final phase of the disease may be very emaciated. Catarrhal conjunctivitis is frequently present ; opacity of the lens and in some cases subretinal hæmorrhages may be seen on examination of the eyes. The skin is dirty and has an unpleasant smell. A characteristic feature of the disease is the arterial hypertension causing a strong bounding pulse that may be difficult to compress. Physical examination of the chest will reveal an increase in the size of the heart. The urine is pale and limpid in appearance. The specific gravity is very low—e.g. 1·003. The reaction is acid or amphoteric to litmus. Protein is present in small amounts and proteinuria tends to decrease as the disease progresses until in later stages only traces of protein are present ; but small quantities of protein are invariably present. The deposits are very scanty ; hyaline and granular casts may be found ; recognisable epithelial cells are very rarely seen. The percentage of urea in the urine is low and becomes progressively lower as the kidneys lose their power to concentrate urine, in consequence there is an increase in the blood urea. The history symptoms and clinical signs may be very strongly suggestive, but diagnosis must be confirmed by an examination of a specimen of urine. Estimation of the urea content of blood enables the clinician to assess the degree of renal insufficiency.

REFERENCE

McIntyre, W. I. M., and Stuart, R. D. (1949). " Canine Leptospirosis." Vet. Record, vol. lxi, pp. 411-414.

Pyæmic Nephritis.—Pyæmic nephritis is always a secondary condition, and in the majority of cases the predominant symptoms are those of the primary disease. The symptoms attributable to the renal condition resemble those of acute nephritis. Demonstration of pus in the urine is necessary before the nature of the renal condition can be determined. Since the infection reaches the kidneys through the blood stream the initial site of the lesions is in the glomerular tufts ; the urine does not

M

contain pus until, as a result of the inflammatory process, pus can pass into the collecting tubule. The animal may succumb to the causal pyæmia before pus appears in the urine.

PYELONEPHRITIS AND PYELITIS.—Pyelonephritis and pyelitis commonly affect one kidney only. Various organisms have been associated with pyelitis and pyelonephritis ; in cattle perhaps the most common is *Corynebacterium renale*. In the majority of cases there is some measure of febrile reaction, though this may not be very pronounced. Other symptoms may be of a very indefinite character. In dairy cattle colicky pain is often observed. Palpation of the affected kidney, if possible, will reveal the presence of pain. The ureter on the affected side is often substantially thickened and can be detected by rectal palpation. The urine may be cloudy and if allowed to stand the deposits, if sufficient, will produce a definite layer in the bottom of the vessel. The reaction is acid, and the urine contains protein ; blood is only irregularly present. The deposits are found to contain pus and epithelial cells. Diagnosis depends on the demonstration of pus cells and organisms. Pyelitis may be distinguished from pyelonephritis by the demonstration of columnar epithelial cells from the renal tubules, these being absent if the condition is one of pyelitis alone.

CYSTITIS.—Usually the first symptom noticed is frequent painful micturition. Horses and cattle show colicky pains. Male dogs adopt the posture of a bitch when urinating. The gait tends to be straddled, due to abduction of the hind-legs. Cats adopt a squatting position and are very disinclined to move. Constipation is nearly always present and in dogs and cats in advanced cases vomiting may occur. The pulse is reflexly accelerated, but elevation of temperature is not constant. Palpation of the bladder will show it to be painful, thickening of the bladder wall may be appreciated if the bladder is relatively empty. Retention of urine may occur in some cases. The urine in many cases has a most offensive smell; it is turbid and a heavy deposit rapidly settles out. The reaction tends to become alkaline and in a proportion of cases the degree of alkalinity is marked. The specific gravity is increased and both protein and blood are present. The deposits consist of red blood cells, blood clots, epithelial debris, pus cells and numerous bacteria. Though the symptoms and clinical signs point to involvement of the bladder, examination of a specimen of urine is necessary before the diagnosis can be confirmed.

PROSTATITIS.—It is only in the male dog that inflammation of the prostate is of clinical importance. The majority of cases are chronic in nature and develop insidiously in old dogs ; occasionally acute cases are encountered in both young and old dogs. Interference with the passage of urine is not common. The enlarged prostate does, however, interfere with the movement of the fæcal mass through the rectum ; in consequence the animal becomes very constipated. In acute cases the pain is intense and the animal strains continuously and may howl with pain. Violent straining may lead to local tissue damage when blood is passed. Some ataxia of the gait may be observed. Rectal examination will reveal the state of the gland. Diagnosis is dependent on the findings of a rectal examination.

URETHRITIS.—Urethritis in the domestic animals, except as a result of trauma or irritation of the urethra by urine that is abnormal in character, is very rare.

URINARY CALCULI.—Renal calculi are frequently found on post-mortem examination in animals that have shown no symptoms during life. Sometimes the whole of the tissue of one kidney has been destroyed and the capsule of the kidney contains one large calculus that conforms to the original shape of the kidney. It appears that a unilateral renal calculus may cause only subjective symptoms that are not discernible to the clinician. If renal calculi are bilateral the damage to the kidney tissue may be sufficient to cause renal inefficiency that is manifested by signs of uræmia. Calculi in the pelvis of the kidney may, by irritation, cause pyelitis ; this later, by invasion of micro-organisms, may become suppurative. One of the earliest recognisable signs of irritation of the pelvis of the kidney is the appearance of blood in the urine ; if, in addition, the urinary deposits are sabulous in character, the clinical evidence is reasonably conclusive. Calculi in the pelvis of the kidney may give rise to no serious symptoms until they move into the ureter, when, if too large to pass along its narrow lumen, an obstruction of the ureter occurs, causing acute renal colic. Determination of the cause of the renal colic is only possible in the large animals if the calculus can be palpated *per rectum*, but if lying in the anterior part of the ureter it will be beyond the reach of the clinician ; if the animal is fat the course of the ureter cannot be traced. In the smaller domestic animals a radiological examination should be carried out with a view to demonstrating the calculus, but as the calculus is relatively small it may be difficult to do so.

Vesical calculi, by irritation of the bladder wall, cause increased frequency of micturition with straining subsequent to the passage of urine ; as a result of the straining some drops of blood are passed. The continuous irritation of the bladder wall inevitably causes cystitis. The calculus or calculi in the bladder may be palpated *per rectum* in the larger animals and through the abdominal wall in the smaller animals. In dogs the painful condition of the bladder results in tensing of the abdominal wall, rendering accurate palpation impossible in these cases ; the demonstration of the calculus by radiological examination is desirable.

Urethral calculi cause retention of urine by obstruction of the urethra. Constant frequent attempts to pass urine result in only a few drops of blood-stained urine being expelled. The passage of a catheter or sound in the horse or dog will reveal the presence and situation of the urethral obstruction. In the male dog the obstruction is most commonly located at the posterior end of the os penis. In cattle, sheep and pigs the obstruction is usually found posterior to the sigmoid flexure in the urethra, a point to which the catheter cannot be passed. In the male cat the distended bladder can be felt through the abdominal wall and examination of the penis will show that the urethra is impacted with sabulous material. Obstruction of the urethra in the female by a calculus is very rare owing to the great dilatation that can take place.

URÆMIA.—The term uræmia is applied to the state of toxæmia that follows renal insufficiency. This may be due to primary disease of the kidneys, or it may result from secondary damage to the kidneys caused by continued back pressure, as occurs in a complete urethral obstruction. The condition is essentially toxic in character, the severity varying in proportion to the degree of renal insufficiency. Uræmia develops in acute nephritis : even in the less severe cases a certain degree of uræmia is inevitably present, but in very severe cases with marked suppression of urine secretion uræmia is profound. Similarly, in complete urethral obstruction, uræmia develops as the function of the kidney diminishes under the influence of the retrograde pressure of urine ; in old-standing cases the final acute phase of the illness is due to the complete failure of renal function.

The symptoms and clinical signs of uræmia, occurring as a sequel to acute nephritis or failure of renal function due to retrograde pressure, are those of profound depression, terminating in coma. A proportion of cases exhibit symptoms of a convulsive phase before the onset of coma. The mucous membranes are dull and injected, the breath is offensive, the mouth is dirty and the mucous membranes may show necrotic changes. Vomiting occurs in the dog and cat. The pulse is soft and weak. The temperature is variable, but in the later stages, marked by coma, becomes subnormal. Diagnosis of the nature of the toxæmia is dependent on the realisation that the origin lies in a urinary condition.

Uræmia in the dog, occurring as a result of interstitial nephritis, may present itself in three forms. The most common is the gastro-intestinal form, characterised by vomiting and loss of condition ; changes in the conjunctiva and opacity of the lens are seen ; the skin is dirty and evil-smelling ; coma gradually develops, sometimes the period of coma lasts for a day or two before death occurs. The respiratory form is less common and is characterised by recurrent attacks of respiratory distress. If the presence of renal insufficiency is not realised a diagnosis of asthma may be made. The cerebral form is comparatively rare ; it is characterised by convulsions and coma. The cause of the nervous symptoms can only be demonstrated by the examination of a specimen of urine, but the suspicions of the clinician should have been aroused by the strength of the pulse, as marked arterial hypertension is characteristic of chronic interstitial nephritis.

CHAPTER VII
NERVOUS SYSTEM

Introductory :—Regional Anatomy
Clinical Examination :—General Details—Cranial Nerves—Autonomic
    Nervous System—Peripheral Nerves—Motor Nerves—Sensory
    Nerves
Reflexes :—Superficial—Deep—Organic
Interpretation of Symptoms and Signs

MANY general diseases, by extension, ultimately involve the nervous system in the disease process ; others, by interfering with the nutrition of the nervous system, cause disturbance of its function. Lesions in the nervous system may indicate the reaction of the tissues to the access of infection. Normally the vasculo-meningeal barrier affords considerable resistance to the penetration of infection into the central nervous system, but the protection thus afforded is reduced by a number of factors, perhaps the most important of these being a sustained febrile reaction. Tuberculosis produces organic changes in the brain, spinal cord and its coverings. Louping-ill in sheep and other animals is characterised by a meningo-encephalomyelitis. Rabies in any animal causes definite lesions in certain parts of the brain, and confirmation of a diagnosis of rabies is dependent on the demonstration of these lesions. Similarly, the symptoms and clinical signs of tetanus are entirely due to the invasion of the nervous tissue by the toxin elaborated by *Cl. tetani* at the site of the wound. Lesions of the central nervous system also occur in the form of neoplasms. Such new growths may be located in either the brain or the spinal cord. The damage caused to the nervous tissue may be due to direct involvement of the tissues by the tumour, or the tumour may be so located that it exerts pressure on veins causing a local circulatory stasis and consequent anoxæmia of the nerve tissues drained by these veins. The presence of cysts within the cranial cavity inflict damage on the brain by pressure. *Cœnurus cerebralis*, the cystic stage of the tapeworm *T. multiceps* (*T. cœnurus*), whose normal host is the dog, causes a disease in cattle and sheep known as " sturdy " or " gid " that is manifested principally by locomotor disturbances. Certain poisons produce degenerative changes in nerve tissue, causing either local paralysis or general symptoms arising from the central nervous system. For example, lead poisoning may cause local paralysis of a limb, paraplegia, or general convulsive symptoms. Degenerative changes of unknown ætiology may cause ataxia or paraplegia, as for instance swayback in lambs associated with demyelination of the cerebral white matter.

Disease of the nervous system in which no lesion is demonstrable is often referred to as functional disturbance, but probably in many of these diseases an unrecognised lesion is present. " Megrims " in the horse, a condition characterised by irregularly recurrent attacks of loss of equilibrium, is an example of functional disturbance of the nervous system. Some forms of canine hysteria are also examples of this form of nervous disease. Canine chorea has been regarded as a functional disturbance of the nervous system, but though histo-pathologists have failed to demonstrate constant lesions, there can be little doubt that the majority of cases of chorea in the dog result from the invasion of the central nervous system by the virus of distemper, chorea being a symptom of the reaction of the central nervous tissue to the invasion of the virus.

Apart from these conditions that can conveniently be classified as either organic disease or functional disturbance of the central nervous system, the clinician is constantly encountering cases that present symptoms apparently arising from the central nervous system. These nervous symptoms are clinical manifestations of either a general or local condition that may be remote from the central nervous system. Symptoms of this type, arising from a general condition, are exemplified by the nervous manifestations of milk fever in cows. In this disease there is a precipitate reduction of the blood calcium, the relative lack of calcium being the immediate cause of the nervous symptoms. Muscular tetany occurs in young animals whose calcium intake is below that required to maintain the normal blood concentration, pathological changes in the bones may be observed in these cases. Similarly a severe reduction in the blood magnesium causes intense nervous symptoms ; such a state prevails in grass tetany in adult cattle ; magnesium deficiency in calves results in nervous signs manifested by muscular tremors or convulsive seizures. So-called " Mad-Staggers " of horses is an acute anaphylactic reaction manifested by icterus, urticaria and violent convulsive symptoms. Nervous disease in dogs may arise from dietetic deficiencies such as lack of vitamin B. Convulsions in calves may arise from a vitamin E deficiency in the diet.

Nervous symptoms are frequently reflex in origin. Thus intense local pain causes a reflex stimulation of the central nervous system that causes, in addition to acceleration of the pulse and increase in the respiratory rate, restlessness and excitement. Foreign bodies in the alimentary canal on occasion give rise to nervous symptoms ; for example, a hair ball or mass of binder twine lodged in the pylorus of a calf may cause acute convulsive symptoms that often rapidly terminate in death, but many calves harbour foreign bodies in the abomasum that do not appear to cause any harm. While foreign bodies in the abomasum in lambs may cause convulsive symptoms, it has to be borne in mind that frequently the cause of the disease is an enterotoxæmia due to *Cl. welchii*, and the presence of a foreign body in the abomasum does not represent the real cause of the lamb's illness and death ; if the true nature of the disease is not appreciated, appropriate steps cannot be taken to control the spread of the disease in the flock. Heavy helminth infestations, especially in young animals, cause symptoms attributable to the central nervous system. In yearling colts generalised stiffness, simulating the symptoms of tetanus, is frequently found to be due to a massive infestation of the alimentary tract with helminths. Piglets and puppies, if suffering from a heavy intestinal infestation with ascarids, often exhibit convulsive symptoms amounting to a series of " fits." Severe cutaneous irritation, such as occurs in heavy infestations of lice, may cause reflex nervous symptoms of restlessness ; in the dog excitement and convulsive seizures arising from the same cause are sometimes observed. Persistent irritation of the external auditory meatus in many cases results in nervous symptoms. In the dog an apparently minor local irritation often causes such a degree of frenzy in an excitable animal that, at first sight, it appears as though the dog was suffering from a disease of the nervous system. A piece of stick wedging transversely across the mouth between the molar teeth may produce such intense nervous symptoms that the owner, not knowing of the presence of the piece of wood, concludes that the dog has gone mad. Penetration of the skin of the paw by a number of harvest mites, the larvæ of the mites of the family Trombidiidæ, often causes so much local discomfort that the dog, gnawing and biting at the paw, becomes nearly frantic. The mites can only be seen by careful inspection of the part ; this is only possible if the dog is effectively restrained during the examination.

In some instances of hysteria occurring in a group of dogs it appears that the spread of the condition is due to imitation.

REGIONAL ANATOMY

BRAIN AND BRAIN STEM.—The following structures are situated on the ventral aspect of the brain ; their position in relation to the base of the brain is of considerable clinical importance. The spinal cord merges imperceptibly into the brain stem, which consists of three parts. The posterior part of the brain stem is the medulla oblongata ; at the anterior end of the medulla is a transverse band known as the corpus trapezoideum. The central portion is the pons, a transversely elongated mass. The third portion is formed by the cerebral peduncles (crus cerebri) ; these run forward from the pons and separate to pass into the ventral part of the cerebral hemispheres. The space between the two peduncles is known as the interpeduncular fossa ; it is nearly covered by the pituitary body which is connected by the infundibulum to the base of the cerebrum at the tuber cinereum behind which lies the mammillary body. The anterior end of the cerebral peduncle on each side is crossed obliquely by the optic tract, the two tracts joining to form the optic chiasma, from which the two optic nerves originate. At the anterior extremity of each hemisphere is the olfactory bulb connected with the brain by the olfactory tract.

The roots of the twelve pairs of cranial nerves are located as follows. The fibres of the first, or olfactory nerve, enter the curved surface of the olfactory bulb. The second, or optic nerves, meet in the optic chiasma. The third, or oculomotor nerve, arises from the medial part of the cerebral peduncle ; owing to the position of the point of origin the oculomotor nerve is very liable to be involved in lesions occurring in the neighbourhood of the brain stem. The fourth, or trochlear nerve, emerges between the pons and the cerebral hemisphere. The fifth, or trigeminal nerve, arises from the lateral aspect of the pons ; there is a larger sensory root, ventral to which is the smaller motor root. The sixth, or abducent nerve, arises immediately behind the pons from the lateral face of the pyramid of the medulla. The seventh, or facial nerve, and the eighth, or acoustic nerve, arise close together on the lateral extremity of the corpus trapezoideum immediately behind the pons. The ninth, or glossopharyngeal nerve, the tenth, or vagus, and the medullary part of the eleventh, or spinal accessory nerve, are found on the lateral aspect of the medulla in this order, the ninth being the most anterior. Each nerve arises from a series of roots springing from the ventrolateral aspect of the medulla ; these roots join together to form the respective nerves. In the case of the eleventh nerve the medullary root is joined by the spinal root coming forward along the edge of the medulla. The twelfth, or hypoglossal nerve, arises from the posterior part of the medulla at the lateral edge of the pyramid.

The cerebellum lying behind the cerebrum hides the greater part of the medulla and consists of a central lobe and two lateral hemispheres. The cerebral hemispheres are separated one from the other by the longitudinal fissure, which in the cranium is occupied by the falx cerebri. The olfactory bulbs are situated at the anterior poles of the hemispheres. The convolutions on the surface of the cerebral hemispheres are separated from each other by fissures and sulci. The cruciate fissure or sulcus is probably the most important of these. The cruciate sulcus runs laterally on each side from the longitudinal fissure forming a cross with the latter, the point of intersection of the two arms of the cross being approximately at the junction of the anterior and middle thirds of the cerebrum. The cruciate sulcus is not very well marked in the horse, but in the dog is deep and well defined. The cruciate sulcus is important, as it is in this region that the motor areas of the cerebrum are located. The motor areas in the dog and sheep have been defined to some extent, but their accurate localisation in the horse has not been accomplished. It has been suggested that the size of the motor area bears a relationship to the degree of complexity of the limb movements, and so in the horse the motor area is relatively small compared to that in the cat and dog.

If the longitudinal fissure is parted so that the cerebral hemispheres are separated it will be seen that they are connected ventrally by the corpus callosum. This body forms the roof of the lateral ventricles of the brain, and in the median plane is connected with the septum pellucidum, the partition that separates the two ventricles ; laterally the corpus callosum merges with the substance of the cerebral hemispheres. The lateral ventricle is an irregularly shaped cavity in the substance of each of the cerebral hemispheres. The lateral ventricles communicate with the third ventricle through the interventricular foramen (foramen of Monro). The third ventricle is a relatively narrow space lying between the two optic thalami. Posteriorly the third ventricle communicates with the aqueduct of Sylvius, a narrow passage in the mid brain that connects the third and fourth ventricles. The fourth ventricle is the cavity of hind brain (*i.e.* the medulla oblongata, pons and cerebellum). The floor of the fourth ventricle is formed by the medulla oblongata and pons ; the roof is formed by the cerebellum and the lateral wall by the cerebellum and restiform body. The fourth ventricle communicates posteriorly with the central canal of the spinal cord, and by openings in the lateral recess of the ventricle with the cistern that lies between the medulla and cerebellum, a cavity of considerable size within the subarachnoid space.

The thalamus is a large ovoid mass of grey matter resting on the dorsal part of each cerebral peduncle. Anterior to the thalamus and cerebral peduncle lies the corpus striatum, the basal ganglia of the cerebral hemisphere. The principal ganglia are the caudate nucleus and the lentiform nucleus. The caudate nucleus is the larger of the two masses and its ventricular surface forms a portion of the floor of the central part of the lateral ventricle ; the deeper surface is in contact with the internal capsule, a band of white matter that separates the caudate nucleus and the thalamus on the medial side from the lentiform nucleus on the lateral side. In horizontal sections of this portion of the brain the internal capsule is bent at the junction of the caudate nucleus and the thalamus, and this bend is known as the genu or knee of the internal capsule. The internal capsule is a structure of much clinical importance, since the motor fibres from the cerebral cortex pass through it to reach the cerebral peduncle.

It is now convenient to consider the course of the cerebrospinal (pyramidal) tracts. The motor fibres take their origin from pyramidal cells in the region of the cruciate sulcus ; in the corona radiata these fibres converge to pass through the internal capsule. In the internal capsule the motor fibres lie in the anterior two-thirds of the posterior limb and in the posterior part of the anterior limb. It has been shown in the dog and cat that in the posterior limb the order of the fibres from the anterior is eyes, head, mouth, tongue, shoulder, elbow, carpus, digits of the fore-limb, trunk, hip, stifle and digits of the hind-limb. This aggregation of motor fibres in the internal capsule makes the pyramidal tract particularly susceptible to the effects of any lesion causing pressure on the tract. From the internal capsule the motor fibres pass down to the cerebral peduncle, being located in the middle third of its ventral aspect, the fibres for the head being nearest the middle line, then the fibres for the fore-limb and on the outside the fibres for the hind-limb. Before entering the pons the fibres are scattered throughout the pyramidal tract so that a lesion involving the pyramidal tract at this point will not cause isolated paralysis of one limb but a general paralysis affecting the whole of one side of the body. In the posterior part of the medulla the bulk of the fibres cross over to the opposite side, this being known as the decussation of the pyramids. Those fibres which do not decussate continue along the direct pyramidal tract and are probably involved in the production of bilateral or symmetrical voluntary movements.

The pyramidal fibres originating from the cells in the cerebral cortex terminate in the ventral horns of the spinal cord. The term upper neurone has been used to describe the nerve cell in the cerebral cortex, its processes and the fibre that passes down the pyramidal tract to reach the ventral horn of the spinal cord. The lower neurone consists of the spinal cell, its processes and the nerve fibre that proceeds to innervate the individual muscle. Afferent fibres form synapses with the spinal cells, producing a spinal reflex arc. Destruction of the upper neurone removes the inhibitory impulses and the tone of the muscle is raised, and as a result the limb becomes rigid. Destruction of the lower neurone results in flaccidity of the muscles, and with the removal of the trophic impulses the muscles atrophy. Immediately after lower neurone damage a pronounced vasodilatation is observed; this is followed by vascular stasis and imperfect nutrition of the tissues. In the domestic animals there appears to be a considerable development of the reflex arcs involving the brain stem and the spinal cord; in addition the extrapyramidal tracts are functionally more important than in man. In consequence, damage to the pyramidal tracts does not necessarily produce complete paralysis, though there is considerable interference with gait, progression and specialised movements.

Details of the paths taken by sensory nerves have not been so accurately worked out as those for the motor tracts. All afferent impulses reach the spinal cord through the spinal ganglia and dorsal nerve roots. A considerable proportion of the afferent impulses do not reach the higher centres but are concerned with the involuntary spinal reflex functions.

The activity of some of these reflex functions forms a useful indication of the site and extent of a lesion involving the spinal cord ; thus if the micturition reflex is abolished the bladder becomes distended with urine. In the domestic animals the postural spinal reflexes are highly developed, and even in cases of well-established intracranial disease an animal may still be able to maintain an erect standing posture ; thus a horse with dropsy of the lateral ventricles, though dull and stupid and incapable of performing specialised movements, can still stand and walk slowly. In addition to sensory impressions of pain, heat and cold that are appreciated in the higher centres, afferent stimuli play an essential part in the appreciation of posture, position and movement. These afferent stimuli not only arise from superficial tissues, such as the skin, but also from more deeply seated tissues, such as muscles, tendons and joints.

A knowledge of the distribution of the peripheral nerves is important in distinguishing between localised disease of the peripheral nerves and central disease involving the brain and spinal cord. In order to achieve this the reader should be familiar with the course and distribution of the nerves of the trunk and limbs. Details of the distribution of the nerves of the trunk and limbs can be found in standard text-books on Anatomy.

The points of origin of the twelve pairs of cranial nerves from the brain have been mentioned in the description of the brain and cord. The cranial nerves may be divided according to their function into three groups : (I) the afferent nerves ; (II) the efferent nerves ; and (III) the mixed nerves. This distinction will be found useful during the clinical examination of the functional activity of the cranial nerves. The nerves falling into each group are as follows :

I. *Afferent Nerves.*
   First (olfactory) ; Second (optic) ; Eighth (auditory).
II. *Efferent Nerves.*
   Seventh (facial) ; Eleventh (spinal accessory) ; Twelfth (hypoglossal).
III. *Mixed Nerves.*
   Third (oculomotor) ⎫
   Fourth (trochlear) ⎬ Motor and sensory to the muscles of the eye.
   Sixth (abducens) ⎭
   Fifth (trigeminal) ; Ninth (glossopharyngeal) ; Tenth (vagus).

DEFINITIONS

A number of terms are used to describe defects of the nervous system. A clear definition of these terms is of obvious value.

Paresis (relaxation) is used to describe the state of a muscle when its power of contraction is weaker than normal. Paresis may be local, involving a muscle or group of associated muscles. It may, however, be general, when it may be indicative of a general weakness such as that following a debilitating illness, or it may be indicative of a degree of coma manifested, in addition to the other signs of coma, by a general weakness of muscle action.

Paralysis is a term used to describe loss of motor power or sensation. Paralysis may be local, *e.g.* paralysis of the ciliary muscles so that the power of accommodation of the eye is lost, and paralysis of the recurrent laryngeal nerve causing roaring in horses. Paralysis may involve the spinal cord or vital centres in the brain and medulla.

Paraplegia is the term used to describe paralysis of the posterior part of the body and the hind-legs. Hemiplegia implies paralysis of one side of the body. Paraplegia, hemiplegia and paralysis cannot be diagnosed in comatose animals with any degree of accuracy. It may seem that one limb is more limp than the corresponding one, but it is unwise to form a diagnosis of any of these conditions in a comatose patient unless there is a marked difference between the two sides of the body.

CLINICAL EXAMINATION

It will readily be realised that symptoms and clinical signs may arise from the brain, the cord, the meninges, the cranial nerves, the peripheral nerves and the autonomic nervous system ; an examination of the nervous system must therefore include a consideration of these divisions of the nervous system.

GENERAL EXAMINATION

Before commencing a detailed examination of the nervous system it is of vital importance that a thorough general examination of the patient should have been performed, for it is by this method alone that the clinician can appreciate the presence of any of the disease conditions that cause nervous symptoms. It may be that the preliminary general examination has suggested the likelihood of a disease of the nervous system. This undoubtedly justifies a detailed examination of the nervous system, but it is no justification for the clinician failing to complete a thorough general examination of the patient.

BEHAVIOUR.—The behaviour of the animal should be studied without, if possible, disturbing the animal. If as a necessary preliminary to examining the animal it has been disturbed, it should be left at peace for a sufficient time to allow any alterations in its behaviour, due to such disturbances, to settle down. For instance, a partially comatose animal may have been aroused and temporarily appears normal, but if left alone will relapse into its original comatose state. The animal may be dull, depressed and show little sign of appreciating the approach of the clinician, but becomes more alert when handled. If the animal is in a state of deep coma it cannot be aroused. Dullness, depression and coma may be clinical evidence of disease of the nervous system, but these symptoms may equally well be evidence of a general condition, such as milk fever in the cow, or toxæmia. It is sometimes found that an animal that was quite quiet when recumbent becomes acutely excited when compelled to rise ; cows suffering from a mild degree of hypomagnesiæmia display this combination of symptoms. If the animal is excited and hypersensitive it will be seen that it is restless and uneasy ; when approached and handled it displays signs of fear, crouches, tries to get away or may become aggressive. Abnormal muscular movements can be observed ; if approached and handled the animal may momentarily control these movements, or it may be they are accentuated as is the case in tetanus, hypomagnesiæmia and strychnine poisoning. If the animal is recumbent an attempt should be made to cause it to rise ; there may be no response to this attempt or the animal may respond, but it becomes obvious that some local condition is preventing it rising, for instance paraplegia. It must be realised that recumbency may be due to a fracture or dislocation in a limb, and an examination should be conducted with a view to eliminating such a possibility.

The appearance of the animal may present evidence of disturbance of consciousness. The facial expression and the appearance of the eyes ' in a rabid dog are peculiar and strikingly pronounced. Frenzy will not fail to attract attention, but the interpretation of its cause is obviously essential ; a horse fighting for breath because of an obstruction in the upper air passages may well be frantic, as also is the horse suffering from acute gastric distension.

POSTURE.—The posture adopted by the animal is sometimes a useful guide to the nature of nervous disease. A sheep with an intracranial parasitic cyst holds its head twisted to one side. A sheep in the early stages of scrapie holds its head with the nose in an abnormally elevated position. A horse suffering from chronic hydrocephalus stands in a stupid condition, and if the legs are placed in an abnormal position no attempt may be made to restore them to the normal position ; thus if one foreleg is drawn across the other the animal will remain standing with its legs crossed. In tuberculosis of the brain or its coverings cattle may stand with the head pushed into a corner. In coma the posture is often one of complete lateral recumbency. Cattle and sheep, if lying flat on their side, rapidly become tympanitic.

GAIT.—The gait of an animal very often provides useful diagnostic information in relation to involvement of the nervous system. Indeed the gait of the animal provides the only useful means of investigating the degree of muscular co-ordination in the domestic animals. If, therefore, the animal can walk it should be made to do so in order that abnormalities of the gait may be seen. Alterations of the gait may, of course, arise from conditions not due to disease of the nervous system ; for instance, the gait of a horse suffering from laminitis, or a case of equine paralytic myohæmoglobinuria. That the alteration of the gait is due to a local condition should have been realised when the general examination was completed. In less acute cases of tetanus the gait is stiff and stilted, and can be most conveniently seen if the horse is walked away from the observer. In more acute cases of tetanus the greater stiffness and more marked inco-ordination of the muscular movements makes progression difficult, and it may not be possible for the animal to move backwards. Louping-ill of sheep is manifested by trembling due to tremors of muscles and groups of muscles, and progression is made by a series of jumps. In scrapie of sheep the gait has a hackney-like stilted action. In transit tetany the gait resembles that of tetanus.

In the horse a special examination is necessary to determine the presence of stringhalt and shivering. In stringhalt when the horse is turned sharply the affected leg is lifted abnormally high and the foot is brought down to the ground with a sharp stamping action. The animal should be turned in both directions as stringhalt may only affect one leg, and its presence is only shown when the horse is turned in one direction and not when turned in the opposite direction. Shivering consists of an irregular spasmodic contraction of groups of muscles that interfere with the horse's normal movements. If after a period of rest in the stable the horse is suddenly made to move over in the stall, the spasmodic movements of muscles may make the horse move over awkwardly. Another way of testing a horse for shivering is to make it move backwards for a distance, when the tail may be elevated in a series of spasmodic jerks, and the further the horse is made to move backwards the more difficult it becomes for it to do so ; in advanced cases the horse is not able to move backwards for more than a few paces.

Any inco-ordination of the gait should be carefully studied with a view to ascertaining its origin. Ataxia or inco-ordination of gait must be distinguished from the swaying movements of an animal that is suffering from muscular weakness. It will be necessary to find out if the ataxia involves all the limbs ; this can be done by making the animal move in different directions. If one limb is affected that limb must be examined to see if there is any local lesion interfering with the normal use of the limb. This examination must include the whole of the affected limb, and a comparison with the normal limb should be made.

When the consideration of these preliminary points has been completed, the detailed examination of the nervous system should be carried out. This may conveniently commence with an examination of the functional activity of the cranial nerves.

CRANIAL NERVES

FIRST CRANIAL NERVE OR OLFACTORY NERVE.—The majority of tests of the olfactory nerve depend on the co-operation of the patient for their successful performance ; obviously such tests cannot be applied to the domestic animals. It is sometimes noticed that an animal does not show any appreciation of the presence of food until it actually sees the food, indicating that it probably has lost the sense of smell. Any test in connection with the use of food may be rendered useless by the animal recognising sounds connected with the provision of food, such as the rattle of a bucket or any noise made by placing the food in a dish. Before concluding that there is any interference with the sense of smell temporary local conditions, such as nasal catarrh, should be excluded. Gross tissue damage, resulting from a tumour involving the bones of the face and nose, will interfere with the sense of smell. The presence of a lesion of this character will be revealed by inspection and palpation of the face and nose.

SECOND CRANIAL NERVE OR OPTIC NERVE.—The decussation of the fibres of the optic nerve at the optic chiasma results in the optic tract on the right side containing fibres from the inner half of the retina of the left eye and the outer half of the retina of the right eye, the optic tract on the left side containing fibres from the inner half of the retina of the right eye and the outer half of the retina of the left eye. These tracts terminate in the optic centres, and from them a system of nerve fibres, known as the optic radiation, originates and conducts impulses to the cortex. It follows that impulses from the left half of the field of vision are received on the cortex of the right side of the brain, and that of the right half of the field of vision on the left side of the cerebral cortex. If conduction by the optic nerve is prevented by a unilateral lesion anterior to the optic chiasma the eye on that side alone will be deprived of vision. Lesions posterior to the chiasma necessarily lead to impairment of the vision of both eyes. In the domestic animals tests of the functional activity of the optic nerve are confined principally to an examination of the visual acuity. Any test that depends on the reaction of the pupils to light includes a test of the functional activity of the third cranial nerve or oculomotor nerve as well as the optic nerve, and is therefore discussed at a later stage in the description of the examination of the third pair of cranial nerves.

Tests of the visual activity in the domestic animals depend on a demonstration of the animal's appreciation of the presence of objects the existence of which can only be recognised by the animal seeing them. If the observer stands in front of the animal and slightly to one side he may be able to appreciate whether the animal has seen him, and when the observer moves the animal should follow his movements by moving the eyes and head. The test should then be repeated with the observer standing in a comparable position in relation to the opposite side of the head. The accuracy of this test is reduced by the fact that the animal frequently realises the approximate position of the observer by the senses of smell and hearing. In the dog it is often possible, from a position in front of the animal, to determine either that the animal is following the examiner's movements with its eyes or that it is following the movements by the aid of its sense of smell. If it is by means of the sense of smell, the dog elevates his nose and sniffs while the eyes have a vacant look. If one hand, with the forefinger held erect and the other fingers and thumb clenched, is slowly brought up towards each eye in turn, the observer can demonstrate by the animal's reactions the approximate position at which the animal perceives the finger. Rapid movement of the hand must be avoided since this will create a current of air that, impinging on the animal's face, causes it to flinch and so creates a false impression that the animal has seen the finger. If the animal is otherwise normal its ability to perceive and avoid objects in its path should be tested by causing it to walk past a series of obstructions that have been placed in its way. In the dog it is useful to test the animal's ability to ascend and descend a stair with which the dog is not familiar. An observant owner may be able to relate incidents that indicate imperfect vision on the part of the animal ; the accuracy of these observations can be checked by comparing them with the findings of the examination conducted by the clinician himself.

Blindness, whether partial or complete, may be due to lesions of the eye itself. If these lesions are of a gross type they will be seen immediately the eyes are inspected. An examination of each eye must be conducted in the manner described under examination of the eye to eliminate any lesion of the eye that would account for blindness before it is concluded that a lesion of the optic nerve or optic tract is present.

GROUP CONSISTING OF THIRD, FOURTH AND SIXTH CRANIAL NERVES.— Though independent nuclei are described for the third, fourth and sixth nerves, the three centres really constitute a column of grey matter that is responsible for the control of the movement of the eyes. The oculomotor nerve supplies the sphincter pupillæ muscle, the ciliary muscle, the levator of the upper eyelid and all the external muscles of the eyeball except the external rectus which is supplied by the sixth cranial nerve and the superior oblique, which is supplied by the fourth cranial nerve. A large proportion of the fibres of the third, fourth and sixth nerves are afferent, and the combined action of their sensory and motor functions is to control the position of the eyeballs. If defects in this function develop the movement of the eyes will become abnormal. The third nerve also supplies tissues within the eye. It is, therefore, convenient to consider the action of the fourth and sixth nerves immediately after those of the third nerve.

THIRD CRANIAL NERVE OR OCULOMOTOR NERVE.—As the third cranial nerve supplies through its divisions three main groups of muscles, peripheral paralysis may be confined to those muscles supplied by one division only, whereas central paralysis will probably result in a loss of function in all tissues supplied by the nerve.

I. Isolated local paralysis most often affects the fibres supplying the muscle levator palpebræ superioris with resulting ptosis—inability to raise the upper eyelid.

II. It is uncommon that the fibres supplying the extrinsic muscle of the eye are alone deprived of their function, but if this did occur the movements of the eyeball would be very restricted ; practically the only movement possible in these circumstances would be for the eye to move in a downwards and outwards direction.

III. (i) *Accommodation.*—Paralysis of the branch supplying the ciliary muscle and the sphincter pupillæ muscle deprives the animal of the power of accommodation and of contraction of the pupil. It is impracticable to test alterations in the power of accommodation in the domestic animals since all available tests depend for their success on the subjective co-operation of the patient. (ii) *Pupils.*—The examination of the pupils constitutes a most important part of the clinical investigation of any case of nervous disease. As the investigation does not require active voluntary co-operation on the part of the patient, it is one that can be satisfactorily performed in all the domestic animals. The size of the pupil is dependent on a balance between the sphincter pupillæ muscle and the dilator pupillæ muscle, the former being supplied by the parasympathetic fibres in the oculomotor nerve and the latter by sympathetic fibres originating in the superior cervical ganglion ; these reach the eye along the short ciliary nerves after passing through the ciliary ganglion in which the sympathetics do not have a cell station. Abnormalities of the sympathetic supply to the pupil are exceedingly rare.

In an examination of the pupil attention should be paid to the size and the reaction to light. The size of the two pupils should be compared ; slight inequalities in size are sometimes seen in normal animals, but any marked difference in size is abnormal. If the pupils are different in size a decision must be taken as to which is the normal. The brightness of the light in which the animal is being examined will give some indication of the size to be expected, and thus will serve as a guide as to which eye is probably normal. If a decision cannot be based on this observation, the pupil which shows the greater mobility during the subsequent examination should be regarded as the normal. Bilateral dilatation of the pupil is present in extreme exhaustion, but the pupil still retains some mobility. Irregularities in the shape of the pupil are caused by adhesions between the iris and the lens resulting from previous inflammatory conditions of the eye. Distortion of the iris may result from an old-standing iritis.

N

The reaction of the pupils to light depends on impulses conveyed by the afferent fibres in the optic nerve from the eye passing through an intermediate cell station in the corpora quadrigemina and returning to the eye by the efferent fibres in the oculomotor nerve. Failure of the pupil to react to light may be due to a lesion on any part of this reflex arc. In the normal animal the effect of light on one eye and the pupil of that eye is reflected in the other eye, bright light shining on one eye causing some contraction of the pupil of the other eye ; if light is cut off both pupils show dilatation. This bilateral reaction of the pupils appears to be due to the decussation of the fibres of the optic nerve and has been referred to as the consensual reaction of the pupils ; it may be absent in the case of lesions of the optic nerves, the oculomotor nerves or their centres.

The reaction of the pupil to light should be tested by covering one eye with the hand so that all light is excluded, the eye being kept covered for at least half a minute. As soon as the eye is uncovered the reaction of the pupil should be observed. On exposure to light the pupil should almost immediately contract ; it appears to contract rather more than is necessary and then dilates a little, and after a phase of decreasing contraction and dilatation the pupil settles down to the position necessary to control correctly the brightness of the lights reaching the retina. The source of light for the examination requires to be reasonably bright ; the light may be used directly on the eye, or if it is found more suitable may be reflected into the eye by means of a mirror. The test is applied to both eyes. The speed with which the pupil responds to light should be noted and also the amplitude of the response. The pupil is often found to respond very slowly to alterations in the intensity of the light reaching it. In other cases, though the light is strong, the pupil remains dilated.

THE FOURTH CRANIAL NERVE OR TROCHLEAR NERVE.—This nerve supplies the superior oblique muscle of the eye. Paralysis of the fourth cranial nerve interferes with downward movement of the eye so that the eye is turned inwards instead of downwards.

THE SIXTH CRANIAL NERVE OR ABDUCENT.—This nerve supplies the external rectus muscle of the eye and the retractor muscle of the eyeball. The principal evidence shown by paralysis of this nerve will be inability to move the eye outwards.

THE FIFTH CRANIAL NERVE OR TRIGEMINAL.—This nerve consists of sensory, motor and secretory fibres and, as the name trigeminal implies, is divisible into three main branches. The first two branches, the ophthalmic branch and the maxillary branch, are purely sensory nerves ; the third, the mandibular branch, contains a mixture of sensory, motor and secretory fibres.

The details of the three branches that are of importance in clinical diagnosis are as follows :

I. *Ophthalmic Branch.*—This consists of the lachrymal nerve, the frontal nerve and the naso-ciliary nerve. These nerves supply sensation to the eye, the lachrymal glands, the upper eyelid and the skin of the temporal region and forehead.

II. *Maxillary Branch* consists of the zygomatic nerve, the spheno-palatine nerve and the infraorbital nerve. These nerves supply sensation to the lower eyelid, the mucous membrane of the nose, the hard and soft palate, the teeth of the upper jaw and the mucous membrane of the nasopharynx.

III. *Mandibular Branch* consists of the masseteric nerve, the deep temporal nerve, the buccinator nerve, the pterygoid nerve, the superficial temporal nerve, the mandibular alveolar nerve and the lingual nerve. Sensation is supplied by the mandibular branch to the lower part of the face, the side of the head, the lower lip, the ear, the tongue and the lower teeth. Motor fibres from the mandibular branch go to the muscles of mastication, the tensor palati and the tensor tympani.

Paralysis of all three branches of the fifth nerve would cause a loss of sensation in the tissues detailed above ; there would also be inter-ference with mastication. Owing to the loss of sensation in the con-junctiva and cornea trophic change in the eye may develop. The application of tests to the fifth nerve in the domestic animals is limited compared with what may be achieved in human patients. The sensory functions of the cornea, conjunctiva, eyelids, nose and mouth, the teeth and the skin of the area concerned can be tested.

The conjunctival reflex is tested by lightly touching the conjunctiva, when the eyelids should immediately close. The corneal reflex is tested by gently touching the surface of the cornea with some soft object that will not damage its surface ; a rapid and forceful closure of the eyelids should ensue when the cornea is touched. The conjunctival and corneal reflexes may conveniently be tested simultaneously. Tests of the sense of taste are difficult to apply with accuracy in the domestic animal. It may appear that the animal prefers certain foodstuffs or refuses food containing unpleasant tasting adulterants, but such tests would be devoid of significance if the substances used for the test possessed odours that were either pleasing or displeasing to the animal. The sensibility of the skin of the area supplied as well as the mucous membrane of the gums and lips may be tested with digital pressure ; if the response is very poor the point of a fine needle may be used.

The motor functions being principally concerned with the muscles of mastication, the movements of the lower jaw should be examined. A bilateral paralysis of the fifth cranial nerve leads to paralysis of the jaw and the animal is unable to close its mouth. A one-sided paralysis of the fifth nerve causes an unequal closure of the lower jaw ; the muscles on the paralysed side are less prominent than on the healthy side, and when the mouth is opened the lower jaw tends to deviate towards the side on which the nerve is paralysed.   The loss of secretory function due to paralysis of the fifth nerve will cause some dryness in the mouth, but owing to secretions reaching the mouth from tissues in receipt of another nerve supply the reduction of secretion may not be very appreciable.

THE SEVENTH CRANIAL NERVE OR FACIAL NERVE.—This nerve is entirely motor in function at its origin, but in its course it receives a small number of sensory fibres.   Its principal function is to provide the motor supply of the muscles of the face, lips, cheek, nostril and external ear. Because of the tone maintained in these muscles by this nerve it has been spoken of as the nerve of expression.

Paralysis of the seventh nerve produces a typical facial expression. On the affected side the ear droops but the eye remains open, the upper lip is drawn towards the healthy side, the lower lip hangs down on the affected side and saliva dribbles from the mouth.   The face on the affected side has a stupid appearance and the animal looks vacant.   In the horse the facial nerve has an important function in connection with respiration in that it supplies the muscles controlling dilatation of the nostrils.   A horse suffering from bilateral paralysis of the facial nerve develops severe dyspnœa on strenuous exertion owing to the failure of the nostrils to dilate.   It will be appreciated that in facial paralysis there will be difficulty in prehension ; and food and saliva will drop from the mouth when the animal is chewing.

THE EIGHTH CRANIAL NERVE OR AUDITORY NERVE.—The eighth cranial nerve may almost be regarded as consisting of two nerves, these being the auditory nerve that is concerned with the function of hearing and the vestibular nerve that is concerned with the maintenance of equilibrium.   The auditory nerves convey impulses from the cochlea and terminate in the ventral cochlear nucleus and in the tuberculum acousticum ; from there secondary auditory tracts arise and after a partial decussation pass to the cortical centres of hearing.   The vestibular nerve arises from the vestibular ganglion and terminates in the vestibular nucleus on the floor of the fourth ventricle.   There appear to be connections of the vestibular nerve with centres in the cerebellum and the motor tracts of the spinal cord.   Dysfunction of the eighth cranial nerve may, therefore, lead to interference with hearing and disturbances of equilibrium.   Before making any examination of the power of hearing, it is necessary to exclude the possibility of deafness being due to some abnormality of the external ear.

It is difficult satisfactorily to apply delicate tests of the power of hearing in the majority of the domestic animals.   Highly trained dogs may show to a remarkable degree their power of distinguishing accurately between different sounds.   In the first place the response of the animal to a word of command spoken fairly loudly may be observed. If the animal's hearing is normal it will usually raise its head and turn towards the direction from which the sound came. If the animal's response to such a comparatively loud sound is satisfactory the volume of the sound can be gradually reduced, and it is often possible to determine how small a sound will attract the animal's attention. In horses, cattle, sheep and pigs the movement of the external ear should be watched, since the animal rapidly moves the ears to catch any sound. In dogs with erect ears similar movements of the ears may be detected ; a dog usually turns towards the direction from which the sound comes, even though the sound may be very faint. In the case of trained animals their ability to distinguish between different words of command may be tested. It will usually be better that the commands should be given by someone whom the animal knows, since it may not respond to the commands of a stranger and so a wrong impression will be created as to its powers of hearing.

Tests of equilibrium have already been carried out when considering the animal's behaviour, posture and gait. Destruction of the labyrinth or damage to the vestibular nerve on one side causes the animal to hold its head turned so that the affected side is lower and the animal tends to fall towards the damaged side.

THE NINTH CRANIAL NERVE OR GLOSSOPHARYNGEAL NERVE.—This is a mixed motor and sensory nerve, the latter part constituting the bulk of the nerve. The nerve has three main branches. The first supplies sensory fibres to the mucous membrane of the tympanum and the Eustachian tube. The second is motor to the muscles of the pharynx and sensory to the mucous membrane of the pharynx. The third branch is sensory for the posterior third of the tongue, the soft palate and tonsillar region. Paralysis of the ninth cranial nerve alone very rarely occurs.

It is difficult to test the functional activity of the glossopharyngeal nerve in the domestic animals, as localisation of the part of the tongue in which taste is being experienced is not possible. In only some animals is it practicable to test the sensory reactions of the posterior part of the tongue, the soft palate and the pillars of the fauces. In the dog the mouth can be opened widely and the posterior wall of the pharynx stimulated, when there should occur reflex contraction of the pharyngeal wall.

THE TENTH CRANIAL NERVE OR VAGUS NERVE.—The connections formed by the vagus with neighbouring nerves and with the sympathetic are very extensive, and their importance is reflected in the functional balance of many tissues in the body. From a diagnostic point of view the more important ramifications of the vagus are : (1) The Pharyngeal Branch—This supplies the muscles of the pharynx and the soft palate with the exception of the tensor palati. (2) The Anterior Laryngeal Nerve—This provides sensory nerves for the floor of the pharynx, the entrance to the œsophagus and the anterior part of the larynx; the anterior laryngeal nerve anastomoses with the recurrent laryngeal nerve. The anterior laryngeal nerve provides motor fibres for the cricothyroid muscle of the larynx. (3) The Recurrent Laryngeal Nerve, as its name implies, passes down the neck with the vagus trunk and then turns back to retrace its path up the neck. The recurrent nerve is both motor and sensory. It supplies motor fibres to all the muscles of the larynx except the cricothyroid. It also provides the sensory nerve supply to the trachea and œsophagus and, as already stated, anastomoses with the anterior laryngeal nerve in providing a sensory supply to the mucous membrane of the larynx. (4) Cardiac Branches. (5) Tracheal and Œsophageal Branches—These run with the branches of the recurrent nerve and sympathetic fibres to innervate the trachea, œsophagus and large vessels. (6) Bronchial Branches—These unite with sympathetic fibres and provide a plexus supplying the bronchi and blood vessels of the lungs. And (7) The Dorsal and Ventral Œsophageal Trunks—These pass through the mediastinum and enter the abdomen. In the abdomen the vagus provides the motor nerve supply for most of the abdominal viscera through the various plexuses and ganglia.

The effects of vagus dysfunction will depend on whether the lesion is central or peripheral. The following are the abnormalities attributable to dysfunction of the various divisions of the vagus :

(1) *Pharyngeal Branch.*—The animal may not be able to swallow properly ; this may lead to the animal refusing food, or attempts at swallowing result in the animal rejecting the food, which is regurgitated through the mouth and nostrils.

(2) *Anterior Laryngeal Nerve.*—Unilateral paralysis of this nerve does not usually produce any symptoms. Bilateral paralysis causes relaxation of both vocal cords and the voice becomes hoarse and deep ; but even bilateral paralysis of this nerve can seldom be recognised in the domestic animals.

(3) *Recurrent Laryngeal Nerve.*—A unilateral paralysis of the recurrent nerve is the most common cause of " roaring " in the horse. Recurrent laryngeal paralysis is very rarely encountered in the other domestic animals ; it causes alterations in the position of the vocal cords that can only be recognised if the larynx is inspected.

(4) *Cardiac Branches.*—Since the vagus supplies the inhibitory fibres of the extrinsic nerve mechanism of the heart, the removal of the vagus control will result in acceleration of the heart.

(5) and (6) *Tracheal, Œsophageal and Bronchial Branches.*—The only symptom that could be recognised in the domestic animals as being associated with these branches of the vagus is difficulty in swallowing, and this, as has already been mentioned, would be at least in part due to dysfunction of the pharyngeal branch.

(7) *Dorsal and Ventral Œsophageal Trunks.*—As this portion of the vagus is principally concerned with the supply of motor power to the stomach and intestine, the effects of vagal dysfunction in these trunks produces symptoms that are associated with the digestive system.

THE ELEVENTH CRANIAL NERVE OR SPINAL ACCESSORY NERVE.—The spinal accessory nerve is purely motor. It consists of two parts that are distinct in both origin and function. The accessory part arises from the medulla and supplies motor fibres to the vagus for the pharynx and larynx ; the function of this part has therefore been discussed with that of the vagus. The spinal part arises from the cervical part of the spinal cord ; passing forward and receiving filaments on its track it enters the foramen magnum and leaves the cranium in company with the vagus. The spinal part provides the motor nerve supply to the trapezius and sternocephalic muscles. Paralysis of the spinal part of the eleventh nerve will cause some dropping of the scapula on the affected side, and the head will be slightly turned towards the opposite side.

THE TWELFTH CRANIAL NERVE OR HYPOGLOSSAL NERVE.—The hypoglossal nerve is motor to the tongue. In unilateral hypoglossal paralysis the tongue lies limply over to the affected side ; if paralysis is bilateral the tongue hangs limply from the mouth.

AUTONOMIC NERVOUS SYSTEM

Consisting as it does of the sympathetic and parasympathetic systems, the function of the autonomic nervous system is very diverse. It is important to bear in mind the functional balance that exists between the parasympathetic and sympathetic nerve mechanisms ; this balance is exemplified in regard to the control of the size of the pupil and the control through the extrinsic nerve mechanism of the heart rate. The functional efficiency of the autonomic nervous system is reflected by the activity of the tissues whose essential nerve supply is autonomic in character. Reference has already been made, when discussing the cranial nerves, to the majority of the tissues supplied by the cranial portion of the parasympathetic. A systematic examination of the cranial nerves on the lines already indicated will readily reveal the presence of any dysfunction. Apart from the sympathetic supply to the eye, which will now be considered, the main sympathetic functions that merit attention in diagnosis are concerned with the accelerator mechanism of the heart and vasoconstriction. The sympathetic supply to the eye is important, as it is only through the eye that a satisfactory means exists of testing the functional activity of the cervical sympathetic. Arising from the caudal cervical and cranial thoracic region of the spinal cord, the sympathetic fibres pass to the sympathetic chain and so to the inferior and superior cervical ganglia ; from the superior cervical ganglia the sympathetic fibres pass to the dilator muscle of the pupil. Paralysis of the sympathetic supply to the eye results in constriction of the pupil due to the unopposed action of the sphincter muscle innervated by the oculomotor nerve (para-sympathetic). The pupil does not dilate when the eye is covered to occlude light, nor does the instillation of cocaine cause dilatation of the pupil.

PERIPHERAL NERVES

Since the peripheral nerves fall into the two categories of motor and sensory, the examination of the functional state of the peripheral nerves can conveniently be discussed in two parts, one dealing with motor function and the other with sensory function. This division is necessarily an arbitrary one, and the co-ordination of sensory and motor function must also be considered. Such a co-ordination is obviously necessary to maintain posture and to control equilibrium ; that aspect of the state of the nervous system has already received attention. There remains, however, the examination of certain reflexes which indicate the state of conductivity and reflex activity prevailing in the particular part of the nervous system involved. The examination of these reflexes is described after that of the motor and sensory nerves.

MOTOR NERVE ACTIVITY.—The examination of the animal will already have revealed any unusual features in its posture and gait, and the presence of abnormal actions should also have been noticed. If the animal's posture and gait are normal it may be concluded that there is satisfactory control over motor function. If, however, there is a local lack of control, the nature of this should be investigated. It may be that a limb is not being moved normally, because of a local painful condition. Paraplegia characterised by knuckling of the fetlocks and a spastic condition of the lumbar, sublumbar and gluteal muscles occurs in paralytic equine myohæmoglobinuria. This equine disease admirably illustrates the point that an essential preliminary to any examination of the nervous system is a general examination of the patient, since that general examination should enable the clinician to recognise the cause of the paraplegia.

Local paralysis may be due to a lesion involving only a particular peripheral nerve. A clear example of this is found in radial paralysis, a condition that is not at all uncommon in horses and dogs, though it may occur in any animal. Paralysis of the radial nerve removes the motor nerve supply to the extensors of the fore-limb ; in consequence the elbow drops and the limb cannot be carried forward. As the paralysis involves the lower neurone the muscles are limp and flaccid and rapidly atrophy, the presence of this atrophy being readily demonstrated if a comparison is made with the corresponding muscles of the opposite limb. The presence of muscular atrophy may be seen by inspection, but it is desirable that the muscles should be palpated. In animals with a long coat, especially in small dogs, the presence of muscular atrophy will only be realised if the muscles are palpated and compared with the corresponding muscles on the opposite side of the body. Palpation has the added advantage that it will indicate the tone of the muscle. Muscles deprived of their nerve supply by a lower neurone paralysis are flaccid and provide no opposition to the passive movement of the parts concerned, whereas in upper neurone paralysis the muscle is spastic and any forced movement tends to be permitted by a series of jerky relaxations. The clinician must be on his guard against mistaking the spastic state of muscles presen tin highly strung nervous patients for any type of spastic paralysis. The general reaction of the patient will indicate a highly strung nervous subject.

If abnormal muscular movements have been noticed these should now be thoroughly investigated. It will have already been noticed whether these abnormal movements involve the whole of the body or are localised to a particular part of it. In the majority of cases the abnormality consists of spasms of a muscle or group of muscles. The spasm is described as tonic when it is characterised by continuous muscular tension, though the tension may vary in severity ; tonic spasms are characteristic of tetanus. The spasm is described as clonic when periods of contraction are followed by periods of relaxation ; clonic spasms are encountered in strychnine poisoning, the spasms originating in afferent stimuli to which there is an abnormal response owing to the increased rate of conductivity and the increase in reflex excitability caused by the action of strychnine on the peripheral nerves, the spinal cord and its centres.

Generalised muscular spasms, if powerful, may cause distortion of the whole body. This distortion is seen in tetanus, strychnine poisoning and in dogs in poisoning with hydrocyanic acid. If as a result of the spasm the head is bent backwards, the tail elevated, the four legs extended and the spine from the head to tail forms as nearly as possible a concave arc, the condition is termed opisthotonos. If the body is bent downwards so that the feet are bunched together, the back arched and the head and tail also bent downwards, the condition is termed emprosthotonos. A lateral bending of the body is termed pleurothotonos.

The use of the term *tetany* is restricted to the description of a general disease characterised by a syndrome of tonic symmetrical muscular contractions, usually accompanied by increased excitability, hyperpnœa and sweating. A considerable variation occurs in the ætiology of tetany. Grass tetany of cattle and sheep is associated with a reduction in blood magnesium (hypomagnesiæmia) and is apparently dietetic in origin. Transit tetany in ponies, also associated with a disturbance of the blood mineral balance, appears to develop as a result of prolonged exposure to conditions that provoke intense fear ; it has been suggested that the fear causes hyperpnœa and a measure of alkalosis. Tetany must be distinguished from tremor, an involuntary quivering of muscle. Muscular tremors are frequently observed in the later stages of acute disease when a state of collapse is supervening ; these tremors are coarse in character and are well exemplified by the generalised tremors seen shortly before death in a horse suffering from intestinal torsion. Fine muscular tremors are observed in disease that causes dehydration and chloride starvation of the tissues ; such tremors are seen in grass sickness of horses and in persistent vomiting in the dog, especially those cases caused by acute intestinal obstruction. Hysterical tremors occur in all forms of canine hysteria ; terror may cause tremors in highly strung nervous animals.

Chorea is a nervous disease characterised by involuntary jerking movements of individual muscles or groups of muscles. If the muscular contractions are gross in character they can readily be seen. In some cases the movements are only seen when the animal is resting and the postural tone of the musculature is relaxed so that the contraction is not prevented by the opposing group of muscles ; thus a dog's leg may be seen jerking if it is lying at rest, but the jerking is not visible if the animal is standing. In other cases the choreic movements are visible irrespective of the animal's posture. In severe cases of chorea the whole body may be jerking and there is considerable interference with the gait. If the onset of chorea has been sudden it is often attended with great irritability. The muscular contractions of chorea may be so fine in character that they are more easily felt than seen. The muscles of mastication are very frequently involved in early chorea and, if the hands are gently applied to the head, the fine contractions can be appreciated by palpation when they are practically imperceptible to the eye. Chorea in dogs is very frequently, if not always, a clinical manifestation of central nervous disease caused by the virus of canine distemper. Choreic movements are seen in sheep in louping-ill, scrapie and pregnancy toxæmia.

Convulsions consist of a series of violent involuntary contractions of the skeletal musculature, during which the animal may be unable to retain its balance and consciousness may be lost. Convulsions are often described as " fits." Any history of fits given by an owner should be the subject of careful enquiry, as in many cases the fit has passed before the clinician has had an opportunity of examining the animal. The person who actually saw the fit should be allowed to give his own description of it before any questions are put, since the character of these questions is very apt to colour the description. If the convulsions are still present when the clinician examines the animal he will be able to note for himself the nature of the seizure. The character and extent of the muscular movements should be noted, and it will be seen whether they are largely confined to the head or involve the whole body. It should also be ascertained whether equilibrium is lost and if the convulsions become more severe following recumbency. An endeavour should be made to ascertain if the animal remains conscious during the seizure ; if consciousness is lost fæces and urine may be voided involuntarily. It may be that prior to the onset of the convulsion premonitory signs were observed.

Convulsions may arise from a diversity of causes. It may be found that the general examination of the animal has revealed the presence of a disease that may cause convulsions. It is probably true that among the domestic animals convulsions are most common in the dog. The following are some of the more common conditions associated with convulsions in the domestic animals. In adult cattle convulsions very frequently occur in cases of lead poisoning and acute disturbance of mineral metabolism. So-called grass staggers, associated with a marked reduction of the blood magnesium, is in very many cases manifested by a convulsive seizure or fit with apparent loss of consciousness. Frequently more than one animal is affected and there is a history of the animals being recently put out to grass or changed into a new pasture. In calves convulsions may be associated with lead poisoning, a low blood magnesium or vitamin E deficiency or may be due to a foreign body impacted in the pylorus. In young pigs and puppies convulsions frequently result from a heavy helminth infestation of the intestine, the parasite often being the ascarid specific for the particular animal. In foals intussusception of the intestine may be manifested by convulsions ; such cases nearly always have a rapidly fatal termination. In louping-ill in sheep the loss of equilibrium and struggling that follows attempts to walk or run in the later stages of the disease may be regarded as a form of convulsion. Cases of tetanus that become recumbent usually struggle vigorously, and generalised convulsions develop. Strychnine poisoning, if a sufficient quantity has been ingested, causes, in response to afferent stimuli, a violent simultaneous contraction of both extensors and flexors. This in effect is a convulsion, and during the convulsion the animal remains acutely conscious. Canine hysteria in its many forms is very frequently manifested by fits or convulsions. These vary in severity and frequency. Convulsions are very often a symptom of the nervous form of canine distemper, among other symptoms being chorea and paraplegia. In any animal, but particularly the dog, uræmia in its nervous form is shown by convulsions. In all animals convulsions may be clinical evidence of encephalitis and meningo-encephalitis.

SENSORY NERVE ACTIVITY.—The functional activity of the sensory nerves should now be investigated. In the domestic animals the range of this investigation is necessarily limited, and as far as the sensory function of the skin is concerned is practically restricted to the demonstration of sensibility to pain.

Sensibility to pain should first be tested by palpation. Palpation should be carried out methodically with a view to demonstrating the site of any painful area. It may well be that the examination of the patient has already indicated the probable locus of pain ; for instance, in dogs, paraplegia or ataxia will indicate that an examination of the spinal region should be made, and palpation may reveal indefinite discomfort in the lumbar region. Palpation should first be light and superficial, and then may be succeeded by more firm deeper palpation. In some cases of hypersensitivity light superficial palpation is resented, but firm deep palpation fails to reveal any point of maximum intensity of pain. Palpation will also show whether the skin of the region is of the same temperature as the rest of the body. If pain is revealed by palpation, every endeavour should be made to determine the tissues involved. This may be possible by further palpation ; for instance, it may be found that the pain commences in the lumbar region and follows the tract of the sciatic nerves. In other instances the pain may be found to be localised to a particular area ; in the case of dogs a radiological examination of the region may reveal the causal lesion.

If palpation, both superficial and deep, fails to elicit any response in the tissues under examination, a more stringent test of the sensibility to pain must be applied. For this purpose a pin or hypodermic needle should be employed. At first a superficial prick should be made, and if that elicits no response a deeper prick can be made. It will be found most satisfactory if the pricks are first made at the most remote part of the body being examined, and successive pricks are made nearer the spine and head until a point is reached where sensation appears normal. For example, in examining the hind-quarters, the first prick might be made in the metatarsal region and successive tests made up the limb and along the lumbar region until a point is reached where the prick of the pin is resented, both limbs and both sides of the body being tested similarly. In this way a line may be drawn indicating the point at which sensation ceases. In lesions of the spinal column causing damage to the cord or its afferent roots, the line marking the limit of sensation is usually found to be behind the actual site of the lesion owing to the fact that the nerves leaving the spinal cord do not run at right angles but at a relatively acute angle to the long axis of the body. Pain directly due to a spinal lesion may be located fairly accurately in relation to the site of the lesion, but tends to radiate backwards from the lesion. Pain caused by irritation of nerve roots is referred back along the track of the afferent nerves, and may, therefore, radiate some distance behind the point at which the irritation is occurring. Pressure on the cord or nerve roots gives rise first to pain and finally to a complete absence of sensation in the regions peripheral to the site of the lesion.

It will readily be appreciated that in the domestic animals the demonstration of sensation is dependent on the activity of both sensory and motor fibres, and the nature of the response to the stimulus may provide a useful indication of the site of the lesion, which may be of assistance in prognosis. Thus in a paraplegic animal a deep prick with a needle may provoke no response at all, indicating a complete lack of sensation in the part concerned. The prick may provoke a central response, indicated by the animal emitting some audible indication of pain with possibly a movement of the head and neck showing that the animal resented the painful stimulus ; but, if there is no motor response in the region where the pain was inflicted, the indication is that though the sensory tracts to the region are still functioning, the motor tracts and spinal centres are functionless. It may be found that the painful stimulus provokes not only a central response but also a local motor response indicating that both the sensory and motor functions are still effective, though it may appear from the comparatively small response that there is some impairment of function. The likelihood of a local motor response without a central response to the infliction of pain is limited to the case of an animal suffering from coma or some cerebral disease that does not immediately cause death, *e.g.* dropsy of the lateral ventricles or cranial tumour.

Lesions of the spinal column cause damage to nervous tissue in a number of ways. A fracture-dislocation of the spinal column will inevitably exert pressure on the spinal cord. This, if it amounts only to pinching of the cord, would not necessarily cause irretrievable damage provided the displacement could be promptly reduced. If the over-riding of the displaced parts of the spinal column has been considerable the cord will have been subjected to such pressure that it has been so damaged that there is no possibility of repair occurring. In severe cases the cord is practically severed as by a scissors action between the two bony parts. Disease of the bones of the spinal column (*e.g.* tuberculosis) may exist for a very long time without causing any symptoms, and it is only when subjected to some sudden stress that the bones collapse under the strain and pressure is exerted on the cord with the immediate appearance of symptoms.

Lesions developing within the spinal column, once they attain sufficient dimensions, exert pressure on the spinal cord. In the posterior region of the body the cord does not occupy the whole of the spinal canal, and a lesion must be relatively large before it is of a sufficient size to exert pressure on the cord, though for some time it may have been causing displacement of the cord. The effects of pressure tend to appear quite suddenly and are those of interference with sensory and motor function. Lesions involving the spinal column may cause damage to the cord without effecting direct pressure on it ; this damage may result from pressure of the lesion on the veins within the spinal column, thus causing a vascular stasis and consequent anoxæmia of the part of the spinal cord posterior to the lesion. Owing to the walls of the vein being thin, comparatively little pressure is required to cause occlusion of the lumen, so it follows that a comparatively small lesion within the spinal column may cause the sudden appearance of serious symptoms indicative of a cessation of function of the affected part of the spinal cord.

REFLEXES.—Some of the tests of motor and sensory function already described necessarily involve spinal reflexes—e.g. local motor response to the infliction of pain. There are, however, throughout the body a number of established reflexes that should be tested in the course of an examination of the central nervous system. These reflexes are divisible into three classes :

  I. Superficial reflexes concerned principally with the protection of the surfaces of the body.

 II. Deeper reflexes involving tendons, muscles and joints and concerned principally with equilibrium and locomotion.

III. Organic reflexes concerned with the basal bodily functions of ingestion and excretion.

SUPERFICIAL REFLEXES

Conjunctival Reflex.—The method of testing the conjunctival reflex has already been described. The nerves concerned are the sensory fibres in the ophthalmic and maxillary branches of the fifth cranial nerve and the motor fibres of the seventh cranial nerve.

Corneal Reflex.—The method of testing the corneal reflex has already been described. The nerves concerned are the sensory fibres in the ophthalmic branch of the fifth nerve and the motor fibres in the seventh cranial nerve.

Pupil Reflex.—The testing of the pupil reflex has already been described. The nerves involved are the second (optic) nerve (sensory) and the third (oculomotor) nerve (motor).

Perineal Reflex.—In the recumbent animal the perineal reflex provides a convenient means of testing the functional integrity of the local spinal reflexes. One of the folds of the skin radiating from the anus is pinched between the forefinger and thumb ; this should result in a reflex contraction of the perineal musculature, causing the skin in the region to become tense. The test will be found particularly useful in cattle and horses. In these animals, in cases of recumbency, failure to elicit a response by the perineal reflex must be regarded as a sign of serious import.

Pedal Reflex.—The testing of this reflex in the domestic animals is not necessary unless the animal is recumbent and either cannot rise or cannot stand when assisted to its feet. In the dog and cat if one of the folds of skin between the pads is nipped between the ball of the forefinger and the thumb nail, retraction of the leg should take place. In the normal dog the response is quick and active ; in paraplegic dogs, in which the spinal reflexes are still intact, the movement may be rather sluggish and limited in extent. The absence of any response to the pad reflex indicates a breakdown of the reflex arc.

In cattle and horses the pedal reflex cannot be utilised owing to the protection afforded to the sensitive tissues by the horn of the hoof, but a comparable reflex may be tested by stimulating the skin of the bulb of the heel with a pin or hypodermic needle.

Scratch Reflex.—Much attention has been focussed by experimental physiologists on the scratch reflex in dogs, but the testing of this reflex as part of a clinicial examination of the nervous system is of very little value.

Deeper Reflexes

The number of the deeper or muscle-tendon reflexes that can be tested satisfactorily in the domestic animals is limited. Testing of the muscle-tendon reflexes can only be carried out if the animal is recumbent ; if the animal is standing on its four limbs it will be found impossible to distinguish between voluntary and involuntary response to the stimulus applied. In any case the need of testing these reflexes is principally confined to cases of recumbent animals in which it is desired to investigate the state of the neuro-muscular mechanism. The principal value of testing these reflexes lies in the investigation of cases in which damage to the spinal cord is suspected. If destruction of the cord has occurred the tendon reflexes will be abolished behind the level of the point of damage.

Patellar Reflex.—The hind-limb should be placed in a position with the stifle (knee proper) slightly flexed. The lower part of the limb must be free to move, but if necessary may be supported on a flat surface. When the limb is adjusted in this way the patient must be reassured and made to lie in as comfortable a position as possible ; it is helpful if an assistant handles its head and so attracts its attention. The tendon of the patella must now be sharply struck ; to do this the clinician may use the edge of his hand, or the edge of a ruler, or any firm object that will render a sharp stimulus to the tendon without damaging the skin. In small dogs a flick with the nail of the forefinger very frequently provides a satisfactory method of stimulating the tendon. The effect of stimulating the tendon is to initiate a spinal reflex that results in an immediate contraction of the quadriceps muscle with a consequent extension of the knee and forward extension of the rest of the leg. While this test is satisfactory in the majority of canine patients, it is not nearly so satisfactory in the larger animals owing to the bulk and weight of the limb making it difficult to obtain a satisfactory position.

Tarsal Reflex.—This again is a test that can only conveniently be carried out in a recumbent animal. In order to carry out the test of this reflex the hock (tarsus) must be slightly flexed. If attempts to flex the hock are countered by the animal vigorously extending the limb, it may reasonably be assumed that it is not necessary to perform the test. When the hock has been flexed so that the achilles tendon (tendo calcaneus) is slightly tensed the tendon must be struck a quick sharp blow. A prompt vigorous contraction of the gastrocnemius muscle should result. This also is a test more conveniently performed on smaller animals.

ORGANIC REFLEXES

Some of these reflexes have already received attention during the description of the examination of other systems of the body.

Respiration.—Respiration is a complex muscular movement originating in the respiratory centre in the medulla. Disturbance of respiration may be caused by disease of the respiratory system or may simply be a response to greater demands of the body. Alterations in the respiratory rate and character will result from stimulation or depression of the nervous mechanism controlling the respiratory movements. Depression of the respiratory centre along with other medullary centres occurs in disease resulting in toxæmia and also in disease causing coma. That such a depression of the respiratory centre has occurred will be made manifest by the general examination of the patient. Stimulation of the respiratory centre may be reflex, *e.g.* the stimulation of the centre that occurs in colic as a result of visceral pain ; stimulation of the centre also occurs when the carbon dioxide content of the blood increases. Serious damage to the cervical and anterior thoracic portion of the spinal cord, if interfering with conduction, must result in death from asphyxia.

Circulation.—The extrinsic nerve mechanism of the heart is discussed in the chapter dealing with the circulation.

Deglutition.—Difficulty in swallowing may be caused by an obstruction in the pharynx or œsophagus or a local inflammatory reaction such as acute pharyngitis. The examination of the pharynx and œsophagus carried out when dealing with the digestive system will exclude the presence of an obstruction or local inflammatory process. Difficulty in swallowing is present when there is an inco-ordinate action of the neuro-muscular mechanism ; this occurs in tetanus, strychnine poisoning and tetany. Paralytic conditions may interfere with swallowing, *e.g.* a rabid animal in the later stages of the disease is unable to swallow.

Defæcation.—It is necessary to distinguish between interference with the defæcation reflex and failure to defæcate owing to inability of the animal to assume the normal posture for the act of defæcation. Recumbent animals usually retain the fæces even though the defæcation reflex is normal. Complete destruction of the cord results in a flaccid state of the anal sphincter and fæces are voided passively, producing a state of incontinence of fæces. Irritation of the cord—by early pressure or other causes—may produce a spasm of the anal sphincter that prevents the passage of fæces.

The state of the anal sphincter reflex may be tested by making a rectal examination and observing the tonus of the anal sphincter, bearing in mind that the normal anal tonus differs in the various domestic animals. If the anal sphincter is unusually flaccid, it may be tested further by stimulating the junction of skin and mucous membrane with a pin or needle ; a prompt contraction of the anal sphincter should at once follow such stimulation.

Micturition.—Enquiry will have been made as to whether micturition is being performed normally or not. It is necessary to ascertain if difficulties in micturition are due to inability to adopt the normal posture for this act. It is often found that an ataxic dog that cannot lift one leg without losing its balance will empty the bladder when supported in the normal posture if the process of urination is initiated by expressing some urine from the bladder with manual pressure on the latter through the abdominal wall. Damage to the micturition reflex may result in a relaxation of the sphincter of the bladder so that urine is constantly dribbling through the urethra, without however a complete emptying of the bladder, as the vesical muscle is lacking in tone. If incontinence of urine is present the bladder must be examined in order to ascertain if the incontinence is due to the pressure of urine in a distended bladder overcoming the action of the sphincter.

Trophic Reflexes.—Trophic impulses play an important part in the nutrition of tissues. The absence of trophic impulses is most easily seen in the state of the skin. The removal of these trophic impulses by damage to nerve tissue at first results in a local vasodilatation that produces a temporary increase in the temperature of the parts ; this is succeeded by stasis and the skin becomes colder than that of other parts of the body. With the withdrawal of trophic impulses the skin is particularly susceptible to trauma and the entrance of infection. Animals recumbent on account of posterior paralysis are very liable to develop bed-sores on the skin of the regions from which the trophic impulses have been removed as a result of the paralysis. The rapid development of bed-sores in any part of the body is therefore of significance in regard to the nerve supply of the part.

RADIOLOGICAL EXAMINATION OF THE NERVOUS SYSTEM

Radiological examination of the nervous system is only practicable in the sheep, dog and cat. In sheep the localisation of an intracranial cyst may be facilitated if radiographs are taken in either the dorsoventral or lateral positions. Unfortunately the density of the cyst and its contents

O

is not very much greater than that of the surrounding tissues, and in some breeds, especially Blackfaces, the air sinuses of the skull produce a pattern on the radiograph that seriously interferes with accurate interpretation.   In the dog tumours involving the bones of the cranium may be shown radiologically.   Intracranial tumours do not usually show up at all well on a radiograph, but by pressure they may alter the shape of the lateral ventricles, and a careful comparison of the shadows caused by the ventricles will show that there is a difference between the two sides.   Air introduced into the cerebrospinal spaces by means of a

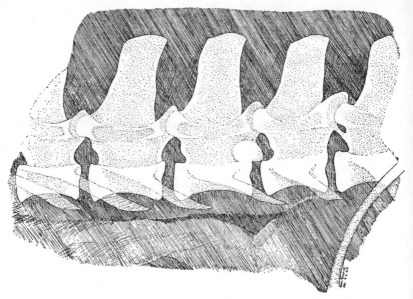

FIG. 17.—Intraspinal Tumour, Lumbar Region Dog.
Drawn from radiograph.   Two-thirds actual size.

needle passed through the atlanto-occipital space into the cisterna magna (cerebello-medullary cistern) will enter the lateral ventricles and enable these to be demonstrated radiologically.   A radiological examination of the spine is seldom carried out except in the dog and cat.   It is useful for the demonstration of fractures, dislocations and disease of the vertebræ causing either rarefaction of bone or the deposition of new bone. By means of radiographs the lesions of ossifying spondylitis can be demonstrated, as also can changes in the substance of the inter-vertebral discs associated with calcification.   In the case of protrusion of the disc substance it may be possible by comparing the width of the inter-vertebral spaces on a radiograph to determine a reduction in width in the affected inter-vertebral joint. It must be remembered that only lesions causing an alteration in the density of the tissues to X-rays will be shown by a direct radiological examination. The intrathecal injection of an opaque substance, such as iodised poppy-seed oil, into the cerebrospinal fluid may make it possible for a lesion causing pressure on the cord to be demonstrated radiologically, the opaque material passing along the spinal cord only as far as the point of pressure. In this way it is possible to demonstrate intraspinal tumours and protrusion of the intervertebral disc substance. In these conditions pressure on nerve tissue causes pain, muscular spasm and subsequently paralysis develops.

Interpretation of Symptoms and Signs arising from the Nervous System

The diagnosis and differential diagnosis of diseases of the nervous system present in not a few cases a problem of considerable difficulty.

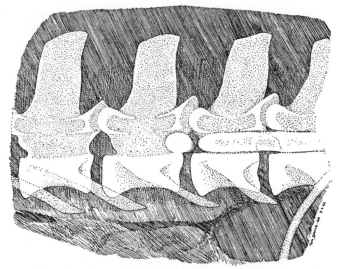

Fig. 18.—Intraspinal Tumour, Lumbar Region Dog.

Drawn from radiograph taken after intrathecal injection of iodised poppy-seed oil. Two-thirds actual size.

An early diagnosis is often desirable since needless suffering may be obviated if the animal is known to be affected with an incurable condition and can be destroyed.

The clinician will find it convenient to divide nervous disease into the categories local and central. Local disease of the nervous system is found to be restricted to those parts of the body supplied by the affected nerves. Trauma to bone, joint, muscle or tendon must be excluded by an examination of the affected parts. The clinician can then proceed to map out the regions that have been deprived of the normal motor and sensory nerve supply. If the site of the damage is located in the spinal cord, the symptoms and clinical signs will be found to relate to the parts of the body posterior to the site of the lesion. The methods of determining the site of the lesion, and to some extent its character, have been discussed under the various headings of motor nerves, sensory nerves and reflexes. If a local nerve lesion exists in the region of the head its locus can be ascertained by a systematic examination of the functional activity of the cranial nerves.

Central disease of the nervous system falls into a number of subdivisions, namely : *Specific diseases, e.g.* tetanus, rabies, louping-ill, nervous complications of distemper, tuberculosis. *Non-specific diseases, e.g.* encephalitis, meningo-encephalitis, meningo-myelitis. *Poisoning, e.g.* strychnine, lead, ergot. *Hæmorrhage, e.g.* cerebral hæmorrhage. *Neoplasm,* intracranial tumours, extracranial tumours causing pressure on the brain by extension through the cranial walls. *Helminthiasis, e.g.* tapeworm cysts within the cranium ; for example, *Cœnurus cerebralis. Degenerative processes, e.g.* degeneration of the optic nerve causing blindness, degeneration of the oculomotor centre interfering with pupil reflex, " sway-back " in lambs associated with a myelin defect of the cerebral white matter.

Before considering the possibility of one of these central diseases being present, the clinician must eliminate the presence of any of the diseases that cause symptoms and clinical signs arising from the central nervous system ; for example, bovine hypocalcæmia and the comparable conditions occurring in the other species of domestic animals, hypomagnesiæmia in cattle and other species, helminth infestations, especially in young pigs and puppies.

SPECIFIC DISEASES

TETANUS.—A disease caused by the inoculation through a wound of *Cl. tetani,* more liable to follow deep punctured or contused wounds. In a number of cases the existence of a wound has escaped notice. The incubation period varies from forty-eight hours or less to as much as three weeks. Generally the shorter the incubation period the more rapid the onset of symptoms and the more intense their character. The disease is characterised by tonic spasms of the skeletal musculature. In a mild case the disease causes generalised stiffness, some degree of trismus (lockjaw) and protrusion of the membranæ nictitantes. In severe cases the muscular spasms are so acute that progression is almost impossible ; the animal sweats profusely and is manifestly distressed ; trismus may be complete ; the eyes are retracted in their sockets and the membranæ nictitantes are in a constant state of rigid protrusion. The muscular spasms may be so severe that the animal loses its balance and when recumbent lies struggling ; generalised convulsions rapidly ensue.

RABIES.—An inoculable disease caused by the bite of a rabid animal. The incubation period is very long ; the average period in dogs is in the neighbourhood of two months, but an incubation period of as much as six months is not unknown. The disease is characterised by disturbance of consciousness and subsequent paralysis. Many animals after a phase of indefinite nervous disturbance suddenly become aggressive (furious rabies) ; during this stage the animal may travel great distances and may attack other animals and human beings, transmitting infection to them by the bites inflicted during the attack. This phase is succeeded by paralysis affecting first the swallowing reflex and later the muscles of locomotion. Even when recumbent the animal may still be able to bite if approached or handled. An animal suspected of rabies must be securely confined ; rabies is usually fatal within ten days of the onset of symptoms. Diagnosis is confirmed by the microscopic demonstration of Negri bodies in the cells of the hippocampus or by animal inoculation.

LOUPING-ILL.—Though a disease most commonly attacking sheep, its incidence in cattle in some areas is quite considerable. Cases have also been confirmed in horses and pigs. The existence of the disease in dogs has not been established. The disease is caused by a virus transmitted by ticks, the most important tick in the British Isles being *Ixodes ricinus*. The introduction of the virus results first in a febrile reaction ; this very frequently has passed before the animal shows the characteristic symptoms of the disease, which are those of meningo-encephalomyelitis. In sheep the symptoms are those of hypersensitivity and fibrillar contractions of the skeletal muscles that causes trembling. The muscular contractions become more intense until there is serious interference with the gait, the animal progressing by a succession of leaps, hence the name louping-ill. Paraplegia develops, the animal dying from inanition and exhaustion. In cattle the nervous symptoms develop suddenly ; the animal may be found standing trembling and hardly able to walk. Generalised paralysis rapidly develops and death follows in a few hours. Cattle showing the nervous symptoms of louping-ill are usually found to have a subnormal temperature. In horses the symptoms are less pronounced, trembling and interference with gait being observed. It appears that at least a proportion of cases in horses recover. Louping-ill is a disease with a very definite geographical incidence, being associated with the activities of ticks infected with the virus of the disease. The incidence of the disease is at its highest following the periods of maximum tick activity, *e.g.* early summer and autumn.

DISTEMPER COMPLEX.—The nervous complications of the distemper complex are chorea, convulsions and paraplegia. Chorea in the dog is very rarely due to any other cause than the invasion of the central nervous system by one of these viruses. Convulsions in dogs, if the nervous complications of this disease, can only be identified as such when it is possible to establish the existence or recent existence of an attack of the disease. Similarly the decision that paraplegia is due to this disease must rest on the recognition of the clinical signs of the disease.

TUBERCULOSIS.—Symptoms arising from tuberculosis of the nervous system are most commonly encountered in cattle and especially in young animals. The symptoms vary somewhat according to the site and extent of the lesions. Epileptiform convulsions may occur in some cases, while in others the animal is in a state of dull stupor ; blindness and disturbance of motor control are also seen. Other clinical signs of tuberculosis may be present that indicate generalisation of the infection.

A positive tuberculin test may be a guide in as far as it indicates the presence of a tuberculous focus in the body. In young calves a clinical examination of the mother may reveal the source of the infection.

In a number of cases diagnosis in life can only be a tentative one that may be confirmed by a post-mortem examination.

NON-SPECIFIC DISEASE

ENCEPHALITIS, MENINGO-ENCEPHALITIS.—There may be a history of disease, septicæmic in type, that by extension could lead to involvement of the brain and its coverings. Acute meningo-encephalitis is accompanied by a high temperature with all the concomitants of fever and intense injection of the conjunctiva. In the earlier stages there is a pronounced excitability and in some cases convulsions. The stage of excitement is succeeded by a stage of depression that may result in coma and death. Frequently there are disturbances of the function of the cranial nerves ; not uncommonly this involves the optic and oculomotor nerves interfering with the pupil reflex, the animal having wide staring pupils that are not responsive to light. Defective vision also occurs. Paralysis may commence in the hind-quarters and become progressively worse until the animal is completely recumbent. The extent of damage caused by the inflammatory process may be defined by a systematic examination of the cranial nerves and the peripheral nervous system.

MENINGOMYELITIS.—Inflammation of the spinal cord and its coverings may cause damage to spinal centres, peripheral nerve roots and the tracts of the spinal cord. The symptoms and clinical signs vary according to the site and extent of the inflammatory process. Initial irritation of the nervous tissue by a local lesion is often succeeded by paralysis. In many cases meningomyelitis is part of an inflammatory process involving the brain, the cord and their coverings.

POISONING

STRYCHNINE.—Strychnine poisoning gives rise to convulsive symptoms in response to afferent stimuli on account of the increased rate of conductivity and the increase in reflex excitability of the spinal cord and its centres. The symptoms may amount to no more than some excitement and quivering of muscles, or on the other hand there may rapidly develop a series of very powerful convulsive spasms that cause the animal to fall and by fixation of the muscles of respiration cause death by asphyxia. Strychnine poisoning is characterised by a rapid onset and rapid development of symptoms. Death may take place within five minutes.

LEAD.—The clinical manifestations of lead poisoning in cattle are very variable. The following have been observed in proven cases of lead poisoning : peculiar behaviour suggesting mental aberration, nervous excitement amounting to mania, violent muscular activity shown by plunging violently in all directions and attempts to climb the walls of buildings, blindness and terminal convulsions. In one outbreak of lead poisoning causing the death of all seven of a group of young bulls, the leading sign in the early stages was diarrhœa.

Rarer manifestations that have been reported are extensor paralysis and in the horse paralysis of the recurrent laryngeal nerve causing roaring.

BRACKEN.—In horses bracken poisoning is due to a thermo-labile anti-thiamine factor causing an acute thiamine deficiency. The clinical manifestations are those of progressive inco-ordination, muscular tremors, inability to maintain a standing posture and finally generalised muscle spasms.

EQUISETUM.—In both horses and cattle equisetum poisoning causes diarrhœa, signs of nervous excitement and a peculiar stringhalt-like gait.

ERGOT.—In addition to the vasoconstrictor and ecbolic effects of ergot, this substance may cause serious central nerve damage. This is made manifest by excitement and muscular trembling ; later paralysis may develop.

CEREBRAL HÆMORRHAGE

In the domestic animals, with the exception of cases due to trauma, cerebral hæmorrhage is rare. In both traumatic and non-traumatic cases there may be loss of consciousness, and on recovery of consciousness it is seen that paralysis has occurred. The site of the hæmorrhage can be deduced by tracing out the tracts in which interference with conduction has occurred. Local paralysis may occur without loss of consciousness. It is necessary to emphasise that in the domestic animals hæmorrhage in the region of the pyramidal tracts does not cause as much interference with locomotion as might be expected. No reliable statistics are available of the incidence of cerebral hæmorrhage as a cause of sudden death in the domestic animals. The clinical picture of these cases is one of more or less sudden loss of consciousness followed by involvement of the vital centres and death.

Neoplasm

Intracranial tumours may be present for a very considerable time before they cause any symptoms. It is a remarkable fact that in very many cases symptoms due to an intracranial tumour appear suddenly and the animal dies within a few hours of the onset of symptoms. The symptoms attributable to an intracranial tumour vary according to its site. Very often the first symptoms observed are those of a disturbance of posture and gait. The animal stands with its head turned to the affected side ; if made to move it staggers round in a circle ; it may lose its balance and will have great difficulty in regaining its feet. Interference with vision is very common. The extent to which the cranial nerves are involved can be traced by a systematic examination. Similarly other symptoms and clinical signs can be co-related with damage to the motor areas and tracts.

In small animals a radiological examination may prove helpful.

Helminthiasis

In cattle and sheep sturdy or gid is caused by the presence within the cranial cavity of the cystic stage of *T. multiceps*, known as *Cœnurus cerebralis*. The cyst causes locomotor disturbances by pressure. The animal holds its head towards the affected side and turns in a circle. The gait is staggering and the animal frequently loses its balance. Blindness is common and the animal stumbles over any obstruction in its path. Sheep may fall into a ditch and be unable to climb out of it. Cattle are often found pressing the head against some fixed object. Affected animals are unable to feed properly and soon become exhausted, dying from starvation. Softening of the bones of the cranial vault by pressure from a cyst lying superficially in the cranium is sometimes observed.

Location of the cyst is sometimes assisted by a radiological examination. Failure to demonstrate the cyst by X-rays does not exclude its presence.

Degenerative Processes

The toxic effects of various drugs appear to have a selective action on certain nerve tissues. Oil of Chenopodium in toxic doses frequently causes deafness in dogs. Certain arsenic compounds may cause blindness due to degeneration of the optic nerve. In many cases there is no known cause of the degeneration. The symptoms are entirely dependent on the structures involved; very frequently it is one of the pairs of cranial nerves that is involved, and perhaps most commonly the optic, oculomotor or auditory nerve.

Sway-back is a disease of new-born lambs of unknown ætiology. It is characterised by a demyelination of the cerebral white matter. The symptoms may be noticed at birth, but in some cases do not become manifest until the lambs are from two to six weeks of age. The predominant symptom is ataxia; this varies from a slight weakness of the hind legs to complete paraplegia. In severe cases the cerebral white matter may be completely liquefied; in milder cases histological examination of the brain may be necessary to establish a diagnosis.

CHAPTER VIII

SKIN

General Discussion. Clinical Examination :—Macule—Papule—Vesicle —Pustule— Ulcer — Scab — Desquamation — Scar — Hyperkeratin- isation — Keratosis — Pigmentation
Mode of Extension—Secondary Changes
Parasitic Skin Diseases :—Larger Animal Skin Parasites—Smaller Animal Skin Parasites—Ringworm—Favus
Non-parasitic Skin Diseases

THE incidence of skin disease in the domestic animals is high. Many of the skin diseases are contagious, therefore prompt and accurate diag- nosis is of vital importance in their control and eradication. Sheep scab and equine parasitic mange (sarcoptic and psoroptic) are diseases scheduled under the Diseases of Animals Acts, the procedure for dealing with the disease being detailed in the Sheep Scab Order and Parasitic Mange (Horses) Order.

Skin diseases fall into two main categories, parasitic and non-parasitic. Parasitic skin disease may be caused by either animal or vegetable parasites. The animal parasites include the larger ectoparasites, such as lice, fleas, keds and ticks, and the small animal parasites include the mange mites, the principal genera being Sarcoptes, Psoroptes, Chorioptes (Symbiot), Demodex, Otodectes and Notoedres. In sheep the action of larvæ (maggots) of the blow-flies may also be considered as an example of the effect of animal parasites. The vegetable parasites of the skin cause ringworm and favus. The severity of parasitic skin disease is often found to be related to the nutrition the animal is receiving. If the nutritional level is low, or if there is a lack of an essential element in the diet, parasitic disease may rapidly become generalised with the develop- ment of extreme debility.

Parasitic skin diseases of the domestic animals are of importance in public health, as a number of these diseases are transmissible to man. The larger ectoparasites are chiefly of importance from an æsthetic point of view, since their multiplication on the human skin does not occur. Sarcoptic mange in any animal is transmissible to man and may prove to be a very troublesome condition. Ringworm and favus are also transmissible to man. The clinician must remember this infectivity for mankind when examining cases of skin disease in the domestic animals, since he may himself become affected unless he takes reasonable pre- cautions ; it is, of course, necessary to extend these precautions to include those responsible for the control and handling of animals affected with skin diseases that are capable of affecting man.

Non-parasitic disease of the skin includes those diseases caused by the invasion of the skin by micro-organisms, e.g. acne and impetigo. In this category there must also be placed the skin manifestations of systemic disease, e.g. the skin lesions of swine erysipelas, and the reaction of the skin in anaphylaxis, e.g. urticaria and also disturbances of the nutrition of the skin causing alopœcia (baldness). In the disease of sheep known as " Scrapie " there develops an intense progressive pruritus without a macroscopic lesion of the skin ; self-inflicted lesions result from the sheep rubbing itself against fixed objects. Non-parasitic disease may be directly related to a nutritional deficiency, so in the examination of cases of skin disease a full clinical examination should be made and an accurate history of the diet obtained. Skin diseases are frequently attributed to hormone deficiency, but it is often difficult if not impossible to establish a definite relationship to any specific hormonal defect. In diabetes mellitus in dogs skin lesions are sometimes encountered that are apparently related to defective nutrition of the skin. There are a number of non-parasitic skin diseases of unknown ætiology, e.g. acanthosis nigricans (keratosis nigricans).

CLINICAL EXAMINATION

The majority of skin diseases can be regarded as an inflammatory reaction to irritation of the skin by a pathogen, the character of the inflammatory reaction depending principally on the causal agent ; but it also depends to some extent on the species of animal affected, for the skin response varies, an outstanding example of this being the difference between the lesion of ringworm in cattle and the lesion of the same disease in dogs.

The early minute lesions of skin disease may escape visual detection owing to their being hidden by the coat or fleece, but in many cases attention is quickly attracted by the animal showing evidence of skin irritation. The clinician must, therefore, make careful enquiry concerning any evidence of skin irritation ; this may not be constantly in evidence but the information may be elicited that when the animal is resting it is disturbed by skin irritation ; such irritation is more intense if the skin is warm. The animal will show evidence of irritation by rubbing, scratching and biting the part ; this leads to further damage to the skin, and inspection of the area concerned will show not only the lesion of the disease but evidence of the self-inflicted damage. Skin irritation may be localised, e.g. a patch of acute moist eczema in a dog or chorioptic mange in a horse's hind-leg ; or it may be generalised, e.g. sarcoptic mange affecting the greater part of the body. Inspection of the skin may suggest that the skin disease is confined to the area to which attention was attracted by evidence of irritation, but palpation of the skin may reveal very small lesions in neighbouring or remote parts of the body. It is, therefore, necessary in cases of skin disease to examine both by inspection and palpation not only the immediate site on which attention has been focussed but also the rest of the skin, in order to determine the extent of the disease.

An early sign of skin disease in some cases is the erection of a tuft of hair ; inspection and palpation of the part will reveal the presence of a small lesion that is disturbing the lie of the hair. An inflammatory reaction in the skin may interfere with the nutrition of the hair or wool ; the fibres become brittle and the hair breaks, leaving an area in which truncated hairs are seen protruding through the products of the inflammatory reaction. The skin inflammation may result in such damage to the hair follicles that the skin becomes entirely denuded of its normal covering. Congestion causes reddening that is visible in non-pigmented skin ; though most readily appreciated in those parts of the body not covered by the coat or fleece, erythema can be seen if the hairs of the coat are divided so that the skin can be inspected, or if the hair has been lost as a result of skin disease.

Many skin diseases are accompanied by an unpleasant smell ; though there are marked differences in these smells it is very doubtful if the character of the smell alone should be considered as of diagnostic value. The squamous form of demodectic mange in the dog has a rather well-defined musty odour, but a diagnosis of demodectic mange can only be established by the microscopic demonstration of the parasites. Favus also has a quite distinct mouldy or musty odour, but diagnosis is based on the characteristics of the favus cup and, if need be, confirmed by the demonstration of the parasitic fungus.

When the area of skin involved has been defined, it should be examined with a view to identifying the primary lesion. Very often the appearance of the primary lesion has been altered by secondary changes ; these may be due to invasion of the devitalised skin by the organisms normally present in the skin, or the secondary lesions may have been caused by trauma inflicted by the animal licking, biting or scratching the parts. Sometimes the secondary lesions are mainly due to the action of skin dressings that have either been unsuitable or have been excessively irritant in their action.

In order that the lesion may be identified it is necessary to consider the variations in form that may represent successive stages in the inflammatory reaction of the skin. For instance, the stages characteristic of the lesion of variola vaccinia (cow-pox) are papule, vesicle, pustule, scab and scar, but if the lesion is subjected to trauma its appearance may be changed—e.g. in a cow-pox lesion on a cow's teat damage inflicted during the process of milking causes early rupture of the vesicle and the development of an ulcer that in its turn may be invaded by secondary infection.

The lesions that may be encountered and points that require notice are as follows :

MACULE.—A discoloured stain or spot on the skin that is not raised above the surface of the surrounding skin. Many skin diseases commence as a small red spot. The initial lesion of variola occurs as a rose-red spot and has been termed roseola. A macule or spot due to congestion of the skin as in variola can be obliterated by pressure, but if due to hæmorrhage, as in the bite of a large ectoparasite, such as a tick or louse, the spot cannot be obliterated by pressure. Though maculæ may appear at first as isolated discrete spots, if numerous they may by extension become confluent to form a large erythematous area. The increase in size of maculæ is often very rapid, and the individual spots may lose their identity in a larger area very soon after the commencement of the inflammatory process in the skin.

PAPULE. A circumscribed solid elevation of the skin formed by the proliferation of the epithelial cells of the skin. Papules are small lesions not larger than a pea. Larger lesions of the skin are described as nodules. The presence of a papule in skin covered with hair disturbs the lie of the coat and the site of the papule may be marked by an erect tuft of hair. Papules can be felt if the skin is palpated, and the impression gained is that of small areas raised above the surface and firmer than the surrounding skin. The form of the papule may be of assistance in diagnosis ; in acne the papule has a pointed peak, whereas in parasitic disease of the skin the papule tends to be flattened ; the papule in eczema is rounded. The papule may be comparatively superficial, painless and surrounded by a small area of infiltration as in the lesion of impetigo ; or if the lesion be of a more deeply seated inflammatory reaction in the skin there will be a correspondingly greater infiltration and the lesion will be painful as in the severe form of contagious acne of horses.

VESICLE.—A vesicle is formed by the elevation of the horny layer of the skin epithelium with serum. The vesicle represents a further stage in the inflammatory process. Vesicles may be simple in character or they may be septate, containing numerous fine strands that divide up the cavity. Simple vesicles develop by extravasation of serum as a result of the irritation of the skin by mange mites. A septate vesicle is encountered in the variolæ ; in cow-pox retraction of the septa in the centre of the vesicle produces a depressed area, and a vesicle of this form is sometimes spoken of as an umbilicated vesicle. The base of the vesicle may be surrounded by a zone of hyperæmia, indicating that underlying the vesicle is a marked inflammatory reaction, which may be of considerable diagnostic value. In true cow-pox (vaccinia) the vesicles are not numerous on the udder and teats, but are surrounded by a marked area of hyperæmia ; in false cow-pox the vesicles are numerous, very superficial, non-septate and surrounded by very little inflammatory reaction.

Large blister-like lesions are encountered in some skin diseases; these are called *bullæ* or *blebs* and vary in size from that of a hazel-nut to that of a walnut. Bullæ develop on the course of the lymphatics in farcy of equines (the cutaneous form of glanders) and in equine epizootic lymphangitis. In urticaria (nettle-rash) the lesion is formed by the extravasation of serum into the malpighian layer (stratum mucosum); a true vesicle is not formed, the serum being dispersed between the cells, producing a firm, slightly elevated patch.

PUSTULE.—A small elevation of the skin containing pus. The pustule may be superficial with comparatively little infiltration of the surrounding skin. The walls of the superficial pustule are largely formed by the elevated horny epithelium; they are comparatively thin, so that there is little tension in the pustule and the surrounding area. The lesion of impetigo is an example of a superficial pustule. The pustule may be deep-seated with a correspondingly greater zone of infiltration. The wall of a deep-seated pustule is formed by the inflamed surrounding skin; there is considerable tension and the part is painful. Deep-seated pustules are encountered in acne, pustular dermatitis, sarcoptic and demodectic mange, and in pyobacillosis in sheep due to *Actinobacillus lignièresi* (*B. purifaciens*).

ULCER.—Ulceration results from the breakdown of a vesicle or pustule. This may occur as part of the inflammatory reaction or it may result from trauma to the lesion. The characters of the ulcer are often of assistance in determining the nature of the disease causing it, and the following details should be observed: the depth, the character of the floor, the form of the edge of the ulcer, the nature of discharge from the ulcer, and the reaction in neighbouring tissues, including lymphatic glands.

The depth of the ulcer will indicate whether the skin lesion from which it arose was superficial or whether it was deep-seated in the skin proper, or whether a subcutaneous lesion breaking through the skin has led to ulceration.

The character of the floor is distinctive in some skin diseases. The floor of the ulcer of equine ulcerative cellulitis rapidly fills with granulation tissue. The ulcer in farcy is more indolent and the floor does not show the same evidence of profuse granulation.

The edge of the ulcer may be clear-cut, almost as though a piece of skin has been punched out. This form of ulcer may be seen in the bulbs of the heel in foot and mouth disease. The edges of the ulcer may be ragged; the ulceration round the angles of the mouth in contagious pustular dermatitis of sheep (orf) has a ragged appearance. The edge of the ulcer may be inverted as occurs in the lesion of equine epizootic lymphangitis.

The discharge from an ulcer will vary in character to some extent according to the state reached in the inflammatory process when the ulcer is examined. In a superficial ulcer the discharge is seldom other than clear and serous. In acute moist eczema the discharge is serous. In more deeply-seated ulcers the discharge tends to be purulent and to some extent the type of pus may give an indication of the cause of the ulceration. In farcy the discharge has a grey, gleety appearance ; in epizootic lymphangitis the discharge to begin with is thick and yellow, later it becomes clear and serous. Any discharge from an ulcer may have admixed with it traces of blood shed from the floor of the ulcer. In many skin diseases the discharge from an ulcer has a distinct odour ; very frequently this is unpleasant in character. Thus mange, in any form with ulceration, has a very pronounced and not too pleasant smell.

The reaction in the neighbouring tissue and lymphatic gland will indicate whether the ulcer is merely a minor local incident or whether it is part of a more general disease of skin and underlying tissue. Thus in farcy the ulcer is found on the course of a lymphatic vessel which is distended ; the lymphatic gland to which the lymph vessel passes will be enlarged and usually there is a good deal of subcutaneous œdema in the area drained by the lymphatic vessel.

Finally the ulcer should be examined for the presence of any gross parasites. In sheep the ulceration may be caused by the activities of the larvæ of the blow flies. In any animal running out-of-doors in warm weather skin sores may attract flies that lay their eggs on or near the sore, the maggots emerging from the eggs proceeding to feed on the exposed tissue.

SCAB.—The discharge from a vesicle, pustule or ulcer dries to form a scab consisting of, in addition to the dried discharge, epithelial cells, fibres of the coat and extraneous debris. The scab in some skin diseases is so characteristic in appearance that diagnosis can often be based on the appearance of the scab. Probably the classical examples of scabs having definite and characteristic forms are those of ringworm in cattle and favus in dogs, cats and rabbits. In bovine ringworm the scab is distinctly elevated above the surrounding skin with a clearly defined margin. The scab is greyish white in colour, tough in consistence, firmly attached to the underlying tissues and tending to shed off fine flakes—indeed very much the colour and appearance of asbestos. Closer examination of the scab will show truncated hairs sticking up through the scab. In favus the scab takes the form of a cup or shield. This has a sharply raised margin and de-pressed centre. The edges of the scab are silver grey and the centre lemon yellow ; in the centre of the cup are stumps of hairs that appear dusty, due to the threads of the favus fungus enwrapping the hair. If the crust is broken it has a strong musty odour. The scab of impetigo is very lightly attached to the underlying tissue and rapidly separates, leaving a smooth shining surface formed by a very thin covering of newly formed epithelial cells covering the site of the original lesion. In many skin diseases the scab is firmly attached and cannot be separated until healing has been completed under the scab ; if forcibly removed tissue damage is inflicted and bleeding occurs.

DESQUAMATION.—When in a skin lesion healing has progressed and the scab has been shed, proliferation of epithelial cells takes place at an abnormally rapid rate for some time, the surface of the lesion being covered with scales until the skin has regained its normal condition. If the skin disease has not proceeded beyond the stages of macule and papule no scab is formed, but the surface layers of epithelial cells are shed and the skin is covered with loose scales. Desquamation may be localised to an area where a skin lesion has been situated or it may be widespread over the body in generalised conditions. In animals that have been in poor condition and have then begun to thrive, a diffuse scaly condition of the skin often develops and may last for some time. Demodectic mange of the squamous type in the dog causes marked desquamation of the skin epithelium without the development of any gross lesion other than the almost complete loss of hair from the affected part.

SCAR.—Scar formation will not result from superficial lesions of the skin. The deeper layer of the skin (*i.e.* the true skin) must be involved in the inflammatory process with damage resulting in ulceration, before a scar is formed. Small scars, though devoid of hair, are hidden under the animal's coat and are not discernible unless the fibres of the coat are separated and a search made for the scar ; small scars are, however, noticeable in the domestic animals when they occur on hairless portions of the skin. The scar marking the site of a cow-pox lesion remains distinct for many months after the original lesion has healed. A deep-seated lesion of the skin that has resulted in a slough will heal with a scar of sufficient dimensions to be visible even on the portions of the body covered with hair.

HYPERKERATINISATION.—Thickening of the keratinised layers of the skin is a local feature of certain generalised diseases. Thus, in so-called paradistemper, the skin of the pads and nose may become thickened and hard, hence the colloquial name " hard-pad disease." Examination of the skin covering the pad shows that it is many times thicker than normal and that the thickening consists of keratinised tissue. Sometimes this layer of hyperkeratinised tissue is shed off leaving a smooth soft surface layer of new cells, this being gradually replaced by normal keratinised cells. In other cases, the central zone of the pad subjected to pressure and friction is worn away by walking and there persists a rim of hard horny material surrounding the edge of the pad. These skin lesions of paradistemper are not important of themselves but the lesions are useful in assisting differential diagnosis.

In cattle, hyperkeratosis of the skin has been observed in many parts of the world as a disease manifested by digestive and reproductive disturbances. This is commonly found to be associated with the ingestion of chlorinated hydrocarbon compounds which interfere with the health of epithelial surfaces, possibly by interfering with vitamin A metabolism. The substances incriminated include wood preservatives, additions to lubricating oil, seed dressings and fumes formed by the combustion of chlorinated hydrocarbons. The skin becomes thickened and hard and affected areas may peel off in strips. Other signs include lachrymation, diarrhœa, abortion and infertility.

KERATOSIS.—A condition of the skin characterised by thickening of the horny layer with loss of hair is known as keratosis. The surface of the affected skin may be irregular. Frequently, the affected skin is dark coloured and the condition is then known as keratosis nigricans; an alternative name is acanthosis nigricans.

PIGMENTATION.—The pigment deposited in the skin is nearly always red, purple or black ; when red or purple it is due to hæmatin compounds, and when black it is usually due to deposits of melanin in the skin. Pigmentation must be distinguished from reddening of the skin caused by congestion during an inflammatory process ; deposition of pigment is more permanent in character than the reddening of congestion and invariably indicates a long-standing disease of the skin. The normal colour of the skin may obscure pigmentation and the pigmented area may be covered by the animal's coat ; frequently, however, the area is devoid of hair.

MODE OF EXTENSION.—The manner in which the skin disease extends is important. In ringworm the periphery of an active lesion is marked by a wheal that is reddened and slightly moist and raised above the surrounding skin. This wheal often surrounds the lesion in the form of a more or less complete ring ; within the centre of the ring the skin is denuded of hair and has a covering of scales that may be aggregated into a scab formed by dried serous discharge. Owing to the dense scab formed in bovine ringworm, it is nearly always impossible to see the active peripheral ring, but the ring can usually be seen in the dog, cat and pig. In sheep scab (psoroptic scab) the active edge of an extending lesion is swollen, hot and red ; from the surface there exudes a thick yellow sticky discharge that mats the wool together ; in the older part of the lesion the discharge has dried to form a tough scab. The spread of otodectic mange from the ear in a dog is made obvious by loss of hair on the skin of the head below and in front of the ear ; the skin is dry and scaly ; it may be excoriated by scratching.

In some forms of skin disease the original lesions remain discrete and extension of the disease results from the development of a further crop of lesions. The lesions of cow-pox, acne and impetigo are examples

P

of skin disease in which the lesions remain discrete. Occasionally discrete lesions may become confluent, giving rise to a large area that is involved in the inflammatory reaction. Thus in the malignant form of acne encountered in horses, an area formed from a number of confluent lesions may be the site of gangrene of the skin.

It should be realised that many cutaneous infections can be transferred to other parts of the body by the animal licking or scratching the affected part and then transferring its attention to other portions of the skin.

SECONDARY CHANGES.—A variety of gross changes may develop in the skin as a result of disease. The skin may become thickened and hypertrophied, great folds of skin being formed; sarcoptic mange in horses, cattle and dogs, if long-standing and active, produces massive folds of skin in the region of the neck. The skin may become toughened and leathery, losing its elasticity; this occurs in various forms of chronic skin disease, but it may also result from the irrational application of strong sulphur preparations. Large crust-like scabs may develop over the site of chronic skin disease. Symbiotic mange affecting the lower parts of the legs—especially the hind-legs—of heavy horses causes profuse epithelial proliferation with the formation of dense crusts firmly attached to the underlying skin. Grease (chronic seborrhœa), also a disease affecting the lower part of the legs of heavy horses, causes a great thickening of the skin, with a thick greasy discharge exuding from the sebaceous glands in the skin.

SUBCUTANEOUS TISSUE.—Inflammatory and other changes involving the subcutaneous tissue must be distinguished from those involving the skin. Subcutaneous œdema is common in the domestic animals, and there are many conditions causing it; for instance, œdema of the dewlap in traumatic pericarditis in cattle, œdema of the intermaxillary space in liver-fluke infestation of sheep, œdema of the limb in equine sporadic lymphangitis, œdema of the lower parts of the chest and abdomen in cardiac failure in the dog. It is possible to recognise œdema of the skin by palpation if a fold of skin is grasped and raised from the underlying parts. Though subcutaneous œdema may ultimately involve the skin, the existence of subcutaneous œdema will indicate that probably the disease is not merely a local skin disease.

Emphysema of the skin does not occur, but subcutaneous emphysema is not uncommon. When the skin is handled crackling is felt under the fingers. Penetrant wounds of the axilla often lead to subcutaneous emphysema as the movements of the foreleg produce a bellows action that draws air in through the wound and forces it under the skin. Rupture of the interstitial tissue in acute pulmonary interstitial emphysema following acute bovine pulmonary œdema may permit air to enter and pass through the mediastinum to reach the subcutaneous tissue of the neck whence it may spread under the skin of the trunk. Perforation of the œsophagus in cattle following choking leads to subcutaneous emphysema. The gas under pressure in the rumen is forced up the œsophagus and by way of the perforation in the œsophagus finds its way along the connective tissue planes into the loose tissue of the neck, from there spreading under the skin of the neck, chest and back. Subcutaneous emphysema may be a clinical sign of infection of the tissues with one of the gas-forming organisms; black quarter of cattle is manifested by the development of a crepitant swelling, the skin covering the swelling, at first hot and painful, becoming cold, leathery and painless when necrosis has taken place.

EXAMINATION FOR PARASITES

As so many of the skin diseases of the domestic animals are parasitic in origin, the clinician will frequently find it necessary to eliminate the possibility of a parasitic disease before he can proceed to make a definite diagnosis. There are some non-parasitic diseases in which the lesion is sufficiently characteristic to enable a diagnosis to be reached by inspection of the lesion, for instance acute moist eczema ; but in others the lesion sufficiently resembles that of a parasitic disease to necessitate a search being made for parasites before assuming that the disease is non-parasitic in origin.

The examination for parasites can be considered under three headings : examination for the larger animal parasites by the naked eye, microscopic examination of material for the presence of the smaller animal parasites, and the special diagnostic procedures required for the demonstration of ringworm fungus and favus fungus.

THE LARGER ANIMAL SKIN PARASITES

LICE.—There are a number of biting and sucking lice that infest the domestic animals. The lice specific to one host are normally found only on that host, multiplication only taking place on the specific host. The morphology of lice is shown in the figures. The eggs are laid and attached to the base of the hair, and as the hair grows the eggs are carried farther away from the skin. The distance of the egg from the skin and the number of eggs on a hair gives some indication as to whether the infestation is long-standing or recent.

Both biting and sucking lice cause irritation of the skin that makes the animal rub, scratch and bite the affected parts, when considerable damage may be inflicted. The continued irritation causes an excessive epithelial proliferation and the skin becomes scurfy ; in some cases epithelial scales become aggregated with serum or blood to form scabs. Even when the lice have been destroyed or removed the pruritus may persist for a quite considerable time.

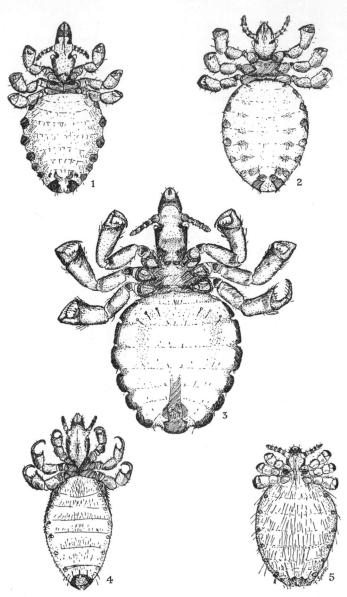

FIG. 19.—Lice.

1. *Hæmatopinus asini* (Horse).   2. *Hæmatopinus eurysternus* (Cattle).
3. *Hæmatopinus suis* (Pig).
4. *Linognathus vituli* (Cattle).   5. *Linognathus piliferus* (Dog). × 20.

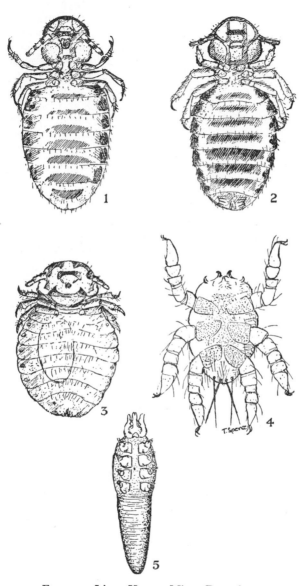

FIG. 20.—Lice. Harvest Mite. Demodex.

1. *Bovicola equi* (Louse, Horse). × 20.   2. *Bovicola bovis* (Louse, Cattle). × 20.
3. *Trichodectes canis* (Louse, Dog). × 20.   4. *Trombidium holosericeum* (Harvest Mite). × 75.
                    5. *Demodex folliculorum.* × 100.

Infestations with lice are seen especially in winter and on animals with long heavy coats. Heavy infestations with lice cause the animals to be restless and to interfere with feeding so that the animals lose bodily condition, and in dairy cows the milk yield is reduced. Lice on calves cause them to lick the skin and swallow loose hairs, thereby predisposing to the formation of hairballs in the abomasum. Diagnosis is dependent on finding the lice, which, if the infestation is heavy, will be found on practically any part of the body covered with long hair. In less heavy infestations the lice are found principally on fine portions of skin, especially where some protection is afforded, such as on the skin behind the elbows. Warmth increases the activity of lice and makes them more easy to detect. If a horse infested with lice is brought out into sunlight, the warmth and strong light facilitates their detection.

FLEAS.—Fleas are principally encountered as parasites of the dog and cat, but the flea is not specific in respect to its host, and fleas frequently suck blood from species other than the usual host. Fleas are flattened laterally and have a tough dark brown chitinous covering ; they have great powers of motility and can jump considerable distances. Fleas do not usually lay their eggs on the host, but deposit them in dirt or dust ; any eggs laid on the host drop off the host as the eggs do not adhere to the hair. The bite of the flea is very irritating ; dogs and cats may be made very restless, and some loss of condition may result. The skin may be further damaged by biting and scratching. The active habits of the flea make it quite easily seen, but it is sometimes difficult to catch a specimen for definite identification.

TICKS.—In the British Isles ticks are usually found on animals grazing on rough hill pastures. They are thus most commonly parasitic on sheep, but infestation of cattle on hill grazings is not uncommon. Horses and dogs having had access to tick-infested land are often found to be carrying a number of ticks. Ticks may attack any part of the body, but in cattle in light infestations they are often found on the finer portions of skin in the armpit and groin.

While the ingestion of blood by a large number of ticks may cause a considerable loss of blood from the host, the principal importance of the tick is as an insect vector transmitting the causal parasite of disease. The virus of louping-ill, a disease of sheep that may occur in cattle, pigs and rarely horses, and the rickettsia of tick-borne fever of sheep are transmitted by ticks. *Babesia bovis*, the parasite of British bovine hæmoglobinuria, is transmitted by ticks. Tick pyæmia of lambs, in which there may be extensive involvement of joints, results from the inoculation of staphylococci at the sites of the tick bites. The deep penetration of the skin by the tick so damages the skin that cutaneous infection often leads to suppuration at the site of the tick bite. Ticks, being large, characteristic parasites, are easily identified.

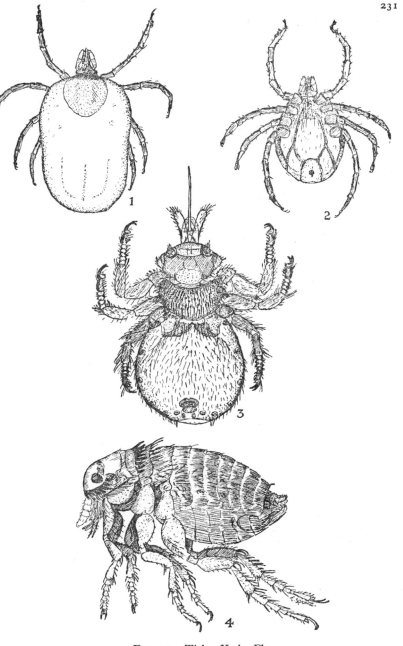

FIG. 21.—Tick. Ked. Flea.

1. *Ixodes ricinus*, female, dorsal view (Castor-bean Tick). × 5.
2. *Ixodes ricinus*, male, ventral view.   "   "   × 20.
3. *Melophagus ovinus* (Sheep Ked). × 8.
4. *Ctenocephalides felis* (Cat Flea). × 15.

KEDS.—The sheep ked (*Melophagus ovinus*) is an obligate parasite of the sheep. It is an aberrant fly, being wingless ; it has a hairy, leathery body. The parasites live in the sheep's fleece ; they suck blood, and in doing so cause intense irritation of the skin. Keds are usually easily found in the wool.

MYIASIS IN SHEEP.—The " blow flies," *e.g. Lucilia sericata*, deposit their eggs on carcases, wounds or dirty wet wool, apparently being attracted to the spot by the smell of the moist material on which the eggs are placed. The larvæ hatch from the eggs in from eight hours to three days and at once commence to feed. The larvæ grow rapidly and attain maturity as full-grown maggots in two days or more.

The affected sheep may bite at the part, but very often attracts attention to a lesion on the buttocks by wriggling its hind-quarters and wagging its tail. Closer inspection will reveal a moist area from which evil-smelling purulent material is exuding. The larvæ are found burrowing into the tissues, and when the area is exposed it is found to be acutely inflamed and bounded by a ragged edge. Extensive myiasis may cause death of a sheep. Diagnosis is based on the discovery of the maggots.

THE SMALLER ANIMAL SKIN PARASITES

MICROSCOPIC DEMONSTRATION OF PARASITES.—The diagnosis of mange is based on the microscopic demonstration of the parasite. For this purpose a skin scraping must be made. The scraping is made with a sharp knife and should penetrate the skin until blood is just oozing from the site of the scraping. Parasites will be found more readily if the scraping is made from an active lesion, that is to say one that is acutely inflamed and has a surface moist with recently extruded exudate. Parasites are more difficult to find in hard dry scab-covered lesions. The scraping may be made without any preparation of the skin, but the collection of the scraping is facilitated if the surface of the skin is moistened with a 10 per cent. solution of caustic potash. The material obtained by scraping the skin may be examined by one or other of three methods.

(*a*) *Direct Smear*.—This is the method most often employed, and in the majority of cases the parasites can be demonstrated by it. The material is placed on a glass slide and moistened with 10 per cent. liquor potassæ and then triturated with the blade of a knife until a homogeneous suspension is formed. A cover-slip is then lowered on to the material and with gentle pressure the suspension is evenly dispersed between the slide and cover-slip. Alternatively another glass slide may be used instead of a cover-slip. The preparation is then examined microscopically, using a two-thirds objective and a 10 diameter eyepiece.

(*b*) *Sedimentation*.—The material obtained by scraping is transferred to a test-tube and digested in 10 per cent. liquor potassæ in a water bath until a homogeneous syrupy liquid is formed. This is spun in a centrifuge until a deposit is formed in the bottom of the tube. The supernatant fluid is drawn off with a pipette and smears are made from the deposit. The smear is covered with a cover-slip and the preparation examined in the same way as a direct smear. Alternatively the material obtained by scraping may be boiled in 10 per cent. liquor potassæ until homogeneous. Care must be taken when boiling the material to avoid loss by spurting ; excessive boiling must be avoided as it leads to unnecessary disintegration of the parasites.

(c) *Sugar Flotation.*—The material is prepared by the same method as described under sedimentation, but when the supernatant fluid has been removed, the centrifuge tube is half-filled with water and then completely filled with a saturated solution of cane sugar. The tube is again spun in the centrifuge ; the parasites are then brought to the surface of the tube. A slide or cover-slip is brought in contact with the top of the fluid in the tube and the fluid lifted on the cover-slip is examined microscopically.

SARCOPTIC MANGE.—Sarcoptic mange may affect any of the domestic mammals and the disease can be transmitted to man. As the mites *Sarcoptes scabiei* can be transmitted from one species of host to another it is considered that evolution has produced a variety adapted to the individual animal species, *e.g. Sarcoptes scabiei var. equi.* The female parasite burrows in the skin, forming a tunnel in which she lays her eggs. The larvæ hatch in from about three to seven days. The activity of the parasites cause an intense inflammation of the skin which is reddened and covered with exudate that dries to form scabs and crusts. The affected parts are violently itchy, and the animal by attacking the parts increases the damage to the skin. Widespread lesions of sarcoptic mange rapidly reduce the animal's bodily condition ; emaciation and death from exhaustion may occur in neglected cases.

In horses the disease appears to have a predilection for the head and neck, but if the disease is neglected it rapidly extends to involve the whole of the body except the lower parts of the limbs, which are not involved. In the dog early lesions are often found on the bridge of the nose, the sides of the face, base of ears, inner aspect of the forelegs and in the region of the hocks. Sarcoptic mange extends rapidly and the whole of the surface of a dog's body may be affected. In cattle sarcoptic mange sometimes affects the hind-quarters, and if transmitted to dairy workers produces in them a condition known in some districts as " dairyman's itch." In well-nourished cattle sarcoptic mange tends to be a relatively benign local condition, but if an animal's resistance is lowered by malnutrition the disease rapidly becomes generalised with the development of extreme debility. The lesions of sarcoptic mange may remain hidden under the long hairs of the winter coat for a considerable time. In pigs sarcoptic mange is seen chiefly on the limbs and on the ears especially on the inner aspect of the external ear but the greater part of the body may be involved in bad cases.

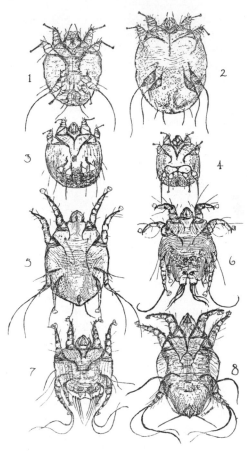

FIG. 22.—Mange Mites.

1. *Sarcoptes scabiei*, male.	2. *Sarcoptes scabiei*, female.
3. *Notoedres*, female.	4. *Notoedres*, male.
5. *Chorioptes*, female.	6. *Chorioptes*, male.
7. *Otodectes*, male.	8. *Otodectes*, female.

× 50 (approx.).

The lesion of sarcoptic mange appears as a red papule on an intensely inflamed base. The papule rapidly develops into a vesicle ; this ruptures, discharging a thick yellow oily exudate which dries to form scabs. The skin becomes wrinkled and by hypertrophy heavy folds of skin are formed. The hair is lost from affected parts.

The characteristics by which *Sarcoptes scabiei* is identified are : The parasite is roughly circular in outline. The posterior legs (pairs 3 and 4) are short and do not project beyond the margin of the body. The stalks of the suckers on the legs are not segmented. The anus is terminal. In the male the first two pairs of legs terminate in suckers, the third pair terminates in bristles and the fourth pair in suckers, *i.e.* the formula of the legs is S.S.B.S. In the female the first two pairs of legs also terminate in suckers and the third and fourth pairs terminate in bristles, *i.e.* the formula of the legs is S.S.B.B.

PSOROPTIC MANGE.—Psoroptic mange is principally of importance in horses and sheep ; in the latter animal the parasite *Psoroptes communis ovis* is the cause of the more important form of sheep scab. The parasites of the genus *Psoroptes* are specific for the host on which they are found ; thus *Psoroptes communis ovis* causes scab in sheep but not in other animals. The psoroptic mites pierce the skin to feed on lymph but do not themselves burrow in the skin like sarcoptes. The injury to the skin caused by the mites feeding stimulates an inflammatory reaction that appears as a swollen area of the skin from which serum exudes ; this dries to form a scab.

Equine Psoroptic Mange.—The lesions of psoroptic mange in the horse very much resemble those of sarcoptic mange. Pruritus is perhaps not so intense and the extension of the disease over the surface of the body is less rapid. The disease usually commences in the region of the neck, withers or the base of the tail, these being regions protected respectively by the mane, saddlery and the folding of the skin at the base of the tail. Once established, psoroptic mange may spread to other parts of the body. Psoroptic mange does not produce such marked thickening of the skin as sarcoptic mange ; in consequence the development of dependent folds of skin is not seen. Diagnosis and differential diagnosis is entirely dependent on demonstration of the mites.

Sheep Scab.—The lesions of sheep scab occur on any part of the body covered by the fleece. The early lesions are usually found in the region of the withers, along the back and at the base of the tail. The inflammatory reaction due to the punctures made by the mites causes the affected part of the skin to be swollen and reddened, and serum oozes from it ; in older lesions the serum has dried to form a tough scab embracing the wool, which parts easily from the skin. The lesion is usually at least five days old before scab formation has occurred. The lesion is itchy and the sheep bites and rubs at the affected parts. When the fleece is broken and scab formation has occurred detection of an affected sheep is not difficult. But if the disease has been partially checked by dipping or dressing, or if the disease is still in its early stages without gross damage to the fleece, detection of the affected sheep may be singularly difficult. Detection of the sheep with dormant lesions is obviously fraught with difficulty.   If sheep have been gathered from the pasture and are then confined in a fold so that they are kept close together the warmth thus engendered stimulates the activity of the mites and attention will be attracted to any sheep that is showing evidence of itchiness.   If such a

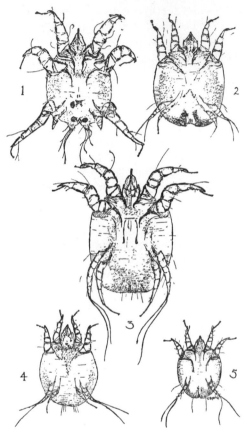

Fig. 23.—*Psoroptes communis ovis* (Sheep-scab Mite).

1. Male.	2. Pubescent female.
4. Nymph. 3. Ovigerous female.	5. Larva.
× 50 (approx.).	

sheep is caught and the skin carefully examined, lesions may be found by inspection if the fleece is methodically parted.   Early lesions may sometimes be detected if the skin is palpated, the fingers being gently drawn over the skin exposed by parting the fleece.

Diagnosis and differential diagnosis depend on the microscopic

demonstration of the parasites. Preparations made from the dry scab
are often found to be rich in mites, but if the sheep has been repeatedly
dipped or dressed mites may not be numerous in the scab. If mites
cannot be found in the scab or if the lesion is an early one a scraping
should be taken, preferably from a lesion having the form of a papule
undergoing softening and just exuding serum, as such lesions should
contain mites if the disease is sheep scab.

Psoroptic Mange in Other Animals.—Psoroptic mange may occur in
goats, when it is found to affect the ears and the contiguous skin. Scab-
like lesions at the base of the tail and on the udder of cattle may be found
to be due to *P. communis bovis.*

The characteristics by which the Psoroptes are identified are : The
parasites are oval in outline. The posterior legs (pairs 3 and 4) are long
and project beyond the margin of the body. The stalks of the suckers
on the legs are segmented. In the male the first three pairs of legs
terminate in suckers on jointed pedicles, and the fourth (posterior) pair
of legs terminate in bristles, *i.e.* the formula of the legs is S.S.S.B. In
the female the first two pairs of legs terminate in suckers on jointed
pedicles, the third pair of legs terminate in bristles and the fourth
(posterior) pair of legs terminate in suckers on jointed pedicles, *i.e.* the
formula of the legs is S.S.B.S.

SYMBIOTIC MANGE.—Symbiotic or chorioptic mange is only of
importance in the horse. The parasite *Chorioptes equi* is a scale-eating
mite. Symbiotic mange affects the lower parts of the legs of horses and
is found chiefly on the hind-legs. The condition is common in heavy
draught horses with coarse hairy legs but is rare in fine-skinned light
horses. The activities of the parasites cause intense itching ; the horse
rubs and scratches the affected parts and stamps and kicks. The pruritus
appears to be worse if the horse is warm in the stable, and the horse's
rest may be interfered with, leading to some loss in bodily condition.
Damage to the shoes and hoofs also occurs. The skin of the legs
become thickened and covered with crusty scabs, the lesions usually
being dry. *Chorioptes bovis* occasionally causes lesions in cattle on the
legs and base of the tail.

Diagnosis depends on the demonstration of the parasites in the
scabs ; they usually are quite numerous. The strict localisation of the
lesions assists diagnosis.

The characteristics by which the parasites may be identified are :
In form they resemble Psoroptes, but the stalks of the suckers on the
legs are not segmented. In the male all four pairs of legs terminate in
suckers, *i.e.* the formula of the legs is S.S.S.S. In the female the first
two pairs of legs terminate in suckers, the third pair terminate in bristles
and the fourth pair in suckers, *i.e.* the formula for the legs is S.S.B.S.
(see Fig. 22).

OTODECTIC MANGE.—*Otodectes cynotis* is a parasite causing parasitic ear canker in the dog, cat and fox ; it closely resembles Chorioptes, but one can be distinguished from the other by the source of the material (see Fig. 22). Otodectes live in the external ear, and by irritation of the lining membrane cause an inflammatory reaction that is characterised by considerable exudation. In the dog the inflammation of the external ear rapidly becomes purulent, but in the cat the exudate tends to remain dry and waxy except in very severe cases. The presence of the disease causes the animal to shake its head and scratch at the ear. Violent scratching may damage the blood vessels of the external ear leading to the development of a conchal hæmatoma. Sometimes the animal holds its head turned to the more seriously affected side, and may turn in a circle. Reflex nervous symptoms are sometimes seen in dogs ; these may take the form of epileptiform convulsions. The parasites may extend their activities to the skin in front of and below the ear. Diagnosis depends on the demonstration of the mites. In the dog old dry crusts and scabs should be gently removed and some fresh exudate obtained from the surface of the lining membrane of the ear. In the cat some of the waxy discharge should be gently removed from the surface of the lining membrane.

NOTOEDRIC MANGE.—*Notoedres cati* is a very small mite that causes mange on the face and ears of the cat. A similar parasite causing mange on the head of rabbits is probably a different variety. In the cat hard brittle scabs rapidly develop on the surface of the lesions ; these become cracked and secondary infection leads to suppuration. Infection of the feet may occur by scratching. The cat rapidly becomes debilitated and emaciated. The parasites closely resemble Sarcoptes, but distinction between the two genera can be made partly on the source of the material and on the position of the anal opening which is dorsal in Notoedres and not terminal as in Sarcoptes (see Fig. 22).

DEMODECTIC MANGE.—The genus *Demodex* contains a number of species named after the host on which they are pathogenic. Though morphologically there is very little difference except in size, each species appears to be specific for its own particular host. Though demodectic mange does occur in cattle, sheep, goat and pig, it is rarely that the disease is encountered in this country.

Demodectic mange in the dog is a condition of considerable clinical importance. Two forms of the disease occur : the dry, scaly or squamous form, and the pustular form. The mites penetrate into the hair follicles and sebaceous glands, both of which may be completely packed with parasites. The presence of the parasites causes a chronic inflammation of the skin, which becomes thickened ; there is great epithelial proliferation and practically complete loss of hair on the affected parts. If secondary bacterial infection occurs, pustules form. In demodectic mange in the dog a peculiar odour develops. The disease usually commences on the face, especially the bridge of the nose and round the lips, on the legs and on the feet. It extends slowly, but in neglected cases a very considerable area of the body may become affected. Factors such as distemper or debility due to helminthiasis may contribute to the spread of the disease.

In the squamous form deep scrapings are required if the parasites are to be demonstrated microscopically. In the pustular form, if the contents of a " ripe " pustule are squeezed directly on to a slide, the parasites may be found easily, as they are usually present in large numbers in the contents of the pustule. The parasites are elongated and cigar-shaped. A small head is succeeded by a thorax which carries four pairs of short legs. The abdomen is elongated and tapers to a blunt posterior end ; striations transverse the abdomen (see Fig. 20). The eggs are spindle-shaped.

FORAGE ACARI.—The forage acari that grow readily on vegetable foodstuffs must be distinguished from the pathogenic mange mites. Forage acari are both much larger and have much longer legs than the mange mites ; they are reddish in colour and the body is richly furnished with hairs. Forage acari are not infrequently found in scrapings taken from skin disease of a scaly type, especially in horses during the late summer. It is debatable if they are pathogenic. They may merely be saprophytes feeding on the epithelial debris of a pre-existing skin disease ; on the other hand it is possible that the irritation caused by their activities is a contributory factor in the development of the skin disease. The scaly skin disease of the horse associated with their presence has been colloquially termed " summer itch."

HARVEST BUGS OR HARVEST MITES.—The family *Trombidiidæ* contains the harvest mites ; these are brilliantly coloured scarlet, red, orange or yellow. The nymphs and adults are free-living forms feeding on invertebrate or vegetable material. The larval forms are parasitic on man or the domestic animals. The larvæ are picked up by animals moving through infested herbage in the late summer and autumn, when they attach themselves to the skin of the host and suck blood, causing very marked irritation at the site of their attachment. In a few days they drop off the vertebrate host in order to moult. In horses, the parasites may be found in the region of the head and neck, and also in the bulb of the heels, the coronets and fetlocks. In the dog the lower parts of the limbs and feet are the parts in which the parasites are usually found. The parasites may be recognised by their bright colour, the presence of three pairs of long legs, the tarsi of the legs having three claws, the middle one being the longest (see Fig. 20). *Trombicula autumnalis* and other species of this genus include the more common mites of this family.

RINGWORM

Ringworm is a contagious disease of the skin caused by a fungus. It appears to be generally accepted that two distinct genera of fungus are involved in the production of ringworm, though some maintain that the two forms, distinct though they may be, are merely varieties of a single genus. Favus, though also caused by a fungus, is a disease clinically distinct from ringworm and is therefore dealt with separately. Ringworm not only affects the domestic animals, but man can become affected from animal lesions.

The two genera of fungi causing ringworm are :

1. Trichophyton, and 2. Microsporum.

The classification of these is based chiefly on the macroconidia which are developed in cultures on suitable media. Certain other secondary characters in culture are also of use in determining the genera and species of the particular fungus isolated.

1. *Trichophyton.*—The macroconidia, 10-50μ long and containing 2-6 segments, are cylindrical, thin-walled and smooth. Some species only rarely produce macroconidia so that generally other features are used in practical mycology. Several species cause disease in animals. The size of the arthrospores differs in the various species and they tend to be arranged in chains along the hairs.

2. *Microsporum.*—The macroconidia, 40-150μ long and containing 5-15 segments, are fusiform, thick-walled and develop superficial tubercles. Two species are important in animals. The arthrospores are small and arranged somewhat irregularly.

The fungi confine their activities to the outer layers of the skin, particularly to the hair follicles. Some species invade the length of the hairs in the follicles and are referred to as " endothrix," while others form masses of spores on the surface of the hair, filling the hair follicle with spores giving the hair a sheathed effect. These are " ectothrix " types. The spores may be small or large depending on the species of fungus involved. Death of the hairs occurs in each case. The fungus also develops in the upper layers of the skin, spreading just below the keratinised epithelium. On parts of the skin poorly provided with hair the lesion of ringworm appears as a superficial inflammation with but scanty exudation, though epithelial proliferation is marked. On parts of the skin covered with the coat the lesion at first appears as a little erect tuft of hairs ; these hairs soon become brittle and break over, leaving an area that looks as though it had been closely cropped. Epithelial proliferation in the area with but scanty exudation produces a scaly condition of the skin ; the scales may be aggregated together to form a scab or crust.

Cattle.—The common ringworm of cattle in Britain is caused by *T. discoides*—a large spore, ectothrix species.

The predilection sites for ringworm in cattle are the head, neck and root of the tail in that order of frequency ; less commonly lesions are found on the chest, abdomen or croup. The limbs are not affected, even in cases in which a considerable area of the body is affected. The lesion in cattle develops into the typical asbestos-like crustaceous scab firmly adherent to the underlying skin. Starting as a small spot over which the hair is ruffled and the skin covered with greyish white scales, the lesion increases in size until in ten to fourteen days it may attain the size of a sixpenny piece, and in six to twelve weeks may be as large as a small tea-plate. Diagnosis is usually based on the naked eye inspection of the lesions. It is rarely that microscopic examination of material from the lesion is necessary. If confirmation of diagnosis is required, hairs must be plucked from an active part of the lesion. A large quantity of the asbestos-like material is quite useless for diagnosis. It is worth while spending a little time selecting suitable material. Affected hairs have a whitish sheath at the lower end when plucked from the follicles.

Horse.—In horses both Trichophyton and Microsporon are encountered as the causal agents of ringworm. Only one species of Microsporon has been described, but four species of Trichophyton have been named. The disease usually attacks the shoulders, the side of the chest and flanks ; parts of skin covered by harness are particularly liable to become affected. A round patch appears as though the hair had been clipped ; the truncated hairs sticking up through a crust of scales appear dirty, due to their being enveloped in a network of mycelial threads. Ringworm in the horse is rarely accompanied by marked irritation unless the hair follicles have become infected and pus formation has ensued, although marked prurition has been noted in cases affected with *T. equinum.* Diagnosis cannot be satisfactorily based on the appearance of the lesion and should be confirmed by the microscopic demonstration of the fungus.

Sheep.—Ringworm in sheep is a rare disease. It is said to be due to Trichophyton, and crustaceous scab lesions have been described.

Pig.—Ringworm in pigs is uncommon.

Dog.—In the dog ringworm may be caused by either Microsporon or Trichophyton. Microsporon infections appear to be the more common. The disease commences on the head, neck and limbs, but may spread to other parts of the body. Children are liable to contract ringworm when handling affected dogs. Different forms of lesion appear in the dog ; (1) A sharply defined scaly patch, up to about two inches in diameter, from which the hair is lost ; (2) on comparatively hairless parts of the skin, *i.e.* the skin of the abdomen and inside the thighs, the lesion may appear as a red circular area but little raised above the surrounding skin ; or

Q

(3) also on hairless portions of skin the centre may be scaly and the growing periphery of the lesion is marked by a reddish wheal on which there are very small vesicles. Except in the third type of lesion, in which the ring-like wheal of the growing periphery of the lesion is characteristic, diagnosis must be confirmed microscopically.

Cat.—There is some evidence that cats may act as carriers of ringworm without showing visible lesions. The circular lesion seen in dogs and other animals may not be very noticeable in cats. Sometimes the lesions are small and scaly ; they look very much as though a little cigarette ash had been dropped amongst the hairs of the coat. The lesions are usually found in the head, neck and chest.

DEMONSTRATION OF RINGWORM FUNGUS.—Material may be taken directly from a suspected area and prepared for microscopic examination ; but careful selection of material is required if the fungus is to be demonstrated. An affected hair removed by epilation forceps may prove the best material for microscopic examination. In order to detect the affected hairs the suspected part of the skin should be moistened with chloroform applied by means of a swab. When the chloroform evaporates the affected hair appears white as though covered with hoar frost. This method is effective for both Trichophyton and Microsporon. Hairs affected with Microsporon can be detected by means of ultra-violet rays passed through Wood's glass. Wood's glass is specially prepared glass of a dense purple colour ; it contains nickel oxide. The piece of Wood's glass should completely cover the opening in the hood of the ultra-violet ray lamp so that the only illumination is that supplied by ultra-violet rays that have passed through the glass. The examination is conducted in a dark room, and may be made directly on the patient's coat or on material previously removed. Hairs affected with Microsporon show a peculiar greenish-yellow fluorescence ; any hairs so detected are then removed for microscopic examination. The fluorescence must occur on the hair and not on the skin, as normal epithelial scales from the skin may show a fluorescence that has a rather bluish-white tint. Hairs covered with a film of vaseline give a somewhat similar fluorescence, but it is yellower in tint. It should be realised that this is only a method for detecting hairs that may be affected with the ringworm fungus, and these must then be examined microscopically.

If an affected hair or hairs is the material selected for microscopic examination, these are placed on a slide with a small quantity of 10 per cent. liquor potassæ ; a cover-slip is lowered on to the surface of the preparation which is gently warmed over a bunsen. The material on the slide is inspected with $\frac{2}{3}$ inch objective and a 10 diameter eye-piece to locate likely hairs. Then a $\frac{1}{6}$ inch objective is used to examine the material. The light should be reduced to an optimum by either closing the iris diaphragm of the microscope substage or by simply lowering the substage condenser. The characteristics that enable the presence of ringworm fungus to be established are that the broken hair has a frayed end, not a clean transverse break; the spores are greenish in colour and refractile. Mycelial threads will not readily be seen by this method, as they are not sufficiently opaque to show up without being stained. Suspected hairs may be stained before examination, using a modified gram method as described by Lewis or by the Hotchkiss McManus stain. Generally speaking, staining is unnecessary for ordinary clinical diagnosis.

REFERENCES

LEWIS, E. F. (1950). *Vet. Record*, vol. lxii, p. 94.
HOTCHKISS and McMANUS (1951). *Amer. J. of Clinical Pathology*, p. 86.

FAVUS

Favus is a skin disease caused by a fungus that occurs in the dog, cat, rabbit, rats and mice. Human beings, especially children, may acquire favus infection from cats, these animals in their turn having been infected by rats or mice. Two species of favus fungus are encountered in the domestic animals; they may be simply varieties of the same species. *Trichophyton schönleinii* is the favus fungus of man, *Trichophyton quinckeanum* is the favus fungus of the mouse.

The fungus grows into the hair follicles as well as over the exterior part of the hair; it also penetrates between the layers of the epidermis. The response of the skin to the invasion by the fungus is the development of the very characteristic favus cups or shields. These are most often found on the face, ears, head and paws. The lesion appears as a small round yellowish-grey spot slightly raised above the surrounding skin; this gradually increases in size, the margins become raised and the centre is rough and concentrically cracked. The fully developed favus cup has a raised margin that is silver grey in colour; the centre of the cup is depressed, sulphur yellow in colour and crusty. Standing up in the centre of the crust are stumps of dusty hairs. The centre of the cup is very brittle, and if broken a characteristic musty odour is emitted.

Diagnosis based on the characteristic appearance of the favus cup is probably justified, but if thought desirable material may be examined microscopically in order to demonstrate the parasitic fungus. A small piece of scab removed from the centre of the lesion should be placed on a slide and triturated with liquor potassæ until a clear uniform emulsion is obtained. The preparation is covered with a glass slip and examined with a $\frac{1}{6}$ inch objective. The mycelial threads can be seen embracing and penetrating the substance of the hair. The mycelia are branched. The spores are large and may be found in groups or in chains.

NON-PARASITIC SKIN DISEASES

The following brief details may be of assistance in the differential diagnosis of non-parasitic skin diseases.

PRURITUS.—In very many cases pruritus (itching) is a symptom of skin disease. Occasionally pruritus occurs as an apparent anomaly of skin function. Before a diagnosis of pruritus can be accepted all probable causes must be excluded. As parasitic infestations are manifested by pruritus, the skin should be examined for the presence of parasites and early minute lesions of mange ; if any lesion, however small, is found, a scraping should be taken and examined microscopically for the presence of mites.

ERYTHEMA.—Erythema, or reddening of the skin due to congestion, is in many cases the first stage of an inflammation of the skin. In some cases the inflammatory process does not proceed beyond the stage of congestion, and it is these cases that may be termed erythema. Secondary erythema occurs in the course of some specific fevers, e.g. the reddening of the skin in swine fever and swine erysipelas. Before making a diagnosis of erythema it is necessary to eliminate the possibility of the reddening of the skin being the initial stage of some other skin disease.

ECZEMA.—The skin disease termed eczema takes the form of a well-defined type of inflammatory reaction in the skin that may be compared with catarrhal inflammation of a mucous membrane. Eczema is characterised by a sudden onset and a course that tends to be chronic. All animals suffer from eczema, but the disease is most common in dogs. In moist eczema the affected part is intensely inflamed, being red and swollen, and is covered with a viscid yellow discharge. The discharge may have dried to form a tough scab, matting the hairs over the part. There is marked irritation in the lesion and the area is often exquisitely sensitive. The margins of the lesion are poorly defined. The progressive stages in the development of the lesion may be visible ; they are an initial erythema, a papule, a vesicle or pustule, exudation of viscid yellow discharge and the formation of scab or crust. Trauma inflicted on an area of acute eczema by the animal attacking the part may introduce infection into the deeper layers of the skin, causing an acute cellulitis in the part.

In so-called dry eczema the reaction of the skin is less violent and there is much less exudation. In one type the surface of the skin lesion is covered with scales aggregated by exudate to form thin scabs ; in the other type the scales are aggregated by excess secretion from the sebaceous glands to form a layer that has a greasy feeling. These two forms of so-called dry eczema are probably better designated squamous dermatitis and seborrhœic dermatitis. Removal of the scab or greasy layer of scales reveals an area that is devoid of hair and covered with a fine epithelial pellicle.

Diagnosis of moist eczema is based on the characteristic features of the lesion; it will be necessary to effect a distinction between eczema and cellulitis. Many cases of so-called dry eczema resemble one or other of the parasitic skin diseases, and it is a wise precaution to take a skin scraping and eliminate the possibility of parasitism.

ACNE.—The term acne is applied to an inflammatory disease of hair follicles and associated sebaceous glands, in which the inflamed glands form either small red nodules or pustules. The lesions vary in size from a pin-point to the size of a bean. Lesions may occur on practically any part of the skin; they are painful and involve the deeper layers of the skin. The surrounding skin is infiltrated and thickened. Contagious acne of horses is caused by a variety of *Corynebacterium ovis* (*B. Preisz-Nocard*). Staphylococcal infections are not uncommon in dogs, they may follow an infestation of the hair follicles with *Demodex folliculorum*.

As acne is due to a number of different infections, bacteriological examination of material will only be of assistance if it is desired to confirm the presence of a particular organism.

IMPETIGO.—An inflammatory disease of the skin characterised by the development of discrete isolated pustules. The pustules are superficially situated on the skin; they have very thin walls and rupture readily; a thin scab covers the lesion. Recurrent crops of pustules give the disease its chronic nature. While more common in the comparatively hairless parts of the skin, impetigo may occur on the parts of the body covered with hair; matting of the hair in the scab causes irritation, otherwise impetigo does not as a rule cause much irritation.

PITYRIASIS.—A name applied to a skin disease characterised by the production of bran-like scales. This condition of the skin may only be a symptom; for instance, in chronic iodine poisoning the skin is literally covered with masses of bran-like scales. The condition is also termed dandruff, and may be evidence of a disturbance of the skin metabolism. Not a few cases of dandruff are associated with, or the sequel to, parasitic infestation of the skin, *e.g.* lousiness. Dirt is also a contributory factor.

URTICARIA.—Urticaria or nettle-rash is a skin disease characterised by the sudden appearance of roundish, smooth, slightly elevated patches in the skin in consequence of infiltration of the malpighian layer with serum. Urticaria occurs most often in horses, cattle and pigs, and only rarely in sheep, dogs and cats. The lesions may be confined to a small local area of the skin, but very often in horses and cattle large areas of the body are affected. The lesions maintain their characteristic appearance, except in dependent parts of the body such as the lips, where they may become confluent, producing a diffuse œdematous swelling that may persist for some days. The lesions of urticaria frequently disappear as quickly as they appeared.

ALOPECIA.—Alopecia or baldness must be distinguished from loss of hair occurring as a symptom of skin disease, such as mange. Alopecia implies the loss of hair without visible disease of the skin to account for it. If the baldness is confined to more or less circumscribed patches, it is known as alopecia areata. The general condition of the animal and its recent history must be taken into account before a diagnosis of alopecia is formulated ; a skin scraping should be examined for parasites, especially in dogs, as the squamous form of demodectic mange may be mistaken for alopecia. In aged male dogs considerable loss of hair is frequently found to be associated with atrophy of the testicles ; in bitches baldness may be associated with disturbance of the œstrus cycle. Temporary loss of hair is often seen in lactating mares and bitches.

ACANTHOSIS NIGRICANS.—Acanthosis nigricans, or as it is sometimes termed, keratosis nigricans is a skin disease seen principally in dogs. Any part of the body may be affected but lesions are most common in the neighbourhood of the axilla or groin. The lesion consists of marked thickening of the keratinised layers of the skin, the affected area of the skin being so heavily pigmented as to appear black. Starting as a small area the lesion may progress to attain quite large dimensions. Acanthosis nigricans must be distinguished from a melanotic tumour of the skin. In the latter the skin involved in the lesion is greatly thickened in consequence there is a definite ridge at the edge of the lesion where it encroaches on normal skin. As a rule the surface of a melanotic tumour of the skin is nodular whereas the surface of the acanthosis lesion is smooth.

CHAPTER IX

THE LYMPHATIC SYSTEM

Regional Anatomy :—Horse—Cattle—Sheep—Pig—Dog
Clinical Examination—Local Conditions involving the Lymphatic
System

THE lymphatic system constitutes an important part of the body's defences against invasion by infective agents. This system consists of the lymphatic vessels and the lymphatic glands located along the course of the lymphatic vessels. The lymphatic glands form a barrier to the progress of infection along the path of the lymph stream ; an inflammatory reaction in a lymph gland indicates the presence of a defensive reaction. The presence of this reaction may be of valuable assistance in ascertaining the nature and distribution of a disease process. In addition to inflammatory reactions arising from bacterial infections, changes due to tumour formation occur in lymph glands.

REGIONAL ANATOMY

It is only necessary here to refer to those parts of the lymphatic system that can be examined clinically. Many of the lymphatic glands can only be palpated if they are enlarged. There is unfortunately some confusion in regard to the nomenclature of the lymph glands, especially in the region of the head and neck.

HORSE.—The submaxillary lymph glands form two elongated groups in the posterior part of the mandibular space ; anteriorly the two groups converge. The submaxillary lymph glands are covered only by skin and fascia and can be palpated in the living animal. These glands receive lymph from the greater part of the nasal cavity, the lips, cheeks, the anterior part of the tongue, the lower part of the mouth and the jaws.

The pharyngeal lymph glands form two groups. One group, the parapharyngeal, lies immediately dorsal to the posterior extremity of the submaxillary lymph gland ; it is subparotid in position (hence the name subparotid lymph gland). The other group, the supra-pharyngeal, lies dorsal to the pharynx.

The cranial cervical lymph glands are small in size and inconstant in number and position. The middle cervical lymph glands form a small variable group on the dorsal face of the trachea. The caudal cervical lymph glands constitute a large group at the entrance to the chest, lying immediately below the trachea.

The prescapular lymph glands are situated immediately anterior and dorsal to the shoulder joint, lying on the cranial border of the anterior part of the deep pectoral muscle.   The axillary lymph glands form a group lying in the axilla under cover of muscle masses that render accurate palpation impossible.   The cubital lymph glands form a group on the distal part of the medial aspect of the humerus ; they are also largely protected by muscle.

The precrural lymph glands form a group on the anterior border of the muscle tensor fasciæ latæ, the group lying some inches dorsal to the

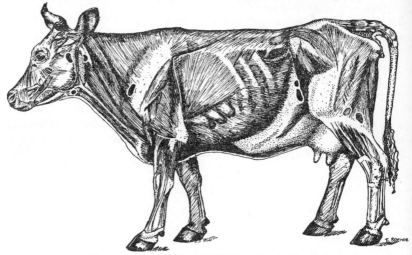

FIG. 24.—Cow.   Superficial Lymphatic Glands.
(Popliteal and Supramammary Glands shown in projection.)

fold of skin extending from the hind-limb to the abdominal wall.   The superficial inguinal lymph glands consist in the male of an elongated group on either side of the penis ; in the female the group is aggregated together and lies dorsal to the mammary gland.   The deep inguinal lymph glands are located in the upper part of the femoral triangle between the pectineus and sartorius muscles.   The deep surfaces of the glands are in contact with the femoral vessels.   Dorsally they are related to the inguinal ligament ; they are covered by skin and fascia.   The popliteal lymph glands are deeply embedded between the biceps femoris and semitendinosus caudal to the origin of the gastrocnemius.

The following lymph glands cannot be examined directly, but clinically they are of some importance.   The bronchial lymph glands form a group lying round the terminal part of the trachea and the commencement of the bronchi.   The posterior mediastinal lymph glands are small and form a diffuse group on the terminal part of the thoracic portion of the œsophagus, being mostly dorsal to that organ. The mesenteric lymph glands are very numerous, forming a chain in the mesentery lying in the majority of places near the root of the mesentery. Other groups in connection with the intestine are the cæcal and the colic lymph glands ; they are disposed along the course of the vessels supplying these organs.

CATTLE.—Though less numerous the individual lymph glands in cattle are on the whole larger than in the horse ; in some places a single gland takes the place in cattle of a group in the horse.

The submaxillary lymph gland on each side lies between the sterno-cephalic muscle and the lower part of the submaxillary salivary gland ; the ventral face of the gland is, if the gland is at all enlarged, in contact with the skin. A second smaller gland may be present ; its position in relation to the larger gland is variable. The parotid lymph gland lies on the posterior part of the upper half of the masseter muscle ; a considerable portion of the lymph gland is covered by the parotid salivary gland.

The retropharyngeal glands lie between the ventral straight muscles of the head and the dorsal wall of the pharynx. These glands receive lymph from the tongue, floor of the mouth, the palate, the pharynx and the posterior part of the nasal cavity. If grossly enlarged they can be both seen and felt through the skin in a thin animal. In some animals a second smaller gland is present on each side. The parapharyngeal glands are small and are found on the surface of the lateral wall of the pharynx. The atlantal lymph gland on each side lies under cover of the wing of the atlas. The cranial and middle cervical lymph glands form small variable groups lying in contact with the trachea. The caudal cervical lymph glands form a group at the entrance to the chest ; the larger mass is situated immediately dorsal to the manubrium of the sternum. The prescapular lymph gland is situated immediately under the skin at the cranial border of the supraspinatus muscle, about four or five inches above the level of the shoulder joint. The axillary lymph glands are quite small and are situated deeply under cover of muscles.

The precrural lymph gland lies four or five inches above the patella, usually in contact with the anterior edge of the muscle tensor fasciæ latæ ; it lies directly dorsal to the fold of the flank. The gland is elongated, its long axis being nearly perpendicular. Sometimes a second smaller gland is present either above or below the larger gland. The precrural lymph glands can be palpated through the skin in the normal animal.

In the bull the superficial inguinal lymph glands lie caudal to the spermatic cord in the pad of fat found at the neck of the scrotum. In the cow the corresponding glands form the supramammary lymph gland, the two glands usually being wholly or partly fused. The fused gland lies dorsal to the udder, but its relation to the posterior border of the

udder is variable.   If the gland is situated near the posterior border it
may be palpated without any difficulty.   But if the gland is situated
further forward and the udder is closely attached to the tissues above,
palpation of the gland may not be possible.   In a cow with a dependent
udder and a manifest " neck " dorsal to the udder, palpation of the
gland is usually possible irrespective of its position in relation to the
posterior border of the udder.   Only the posterior part of the udder is
drained by the supra-mammary lymph gland, which also drains part of the
perineum and the vulva.   The remainder of the udder is drained by the
inguinal lymph glands.   The deep inguinal lymph gland is found at the
point of origin of the circumflex iliac artery from the external iliac ; being
thus situated within the body cavity it cannot be palpated except by rectal
examination and then only if greatly enlarged.

The popliteal lymph gland is found in a mass of fat lying on the
upper part of the gastrocnemius muscle between the biceps femoris
muscle and the semitendinosus muscle, approach to the gland being
made between these two muscles.

The following lymph glands, though they cannot be examined directly,
are of clinical importance ; the anterior mediastinal glands form a group
partly ventral to the trachea and partly dorsal and partly ventral to the
œsophagus.   The posterior mediastinal lymph glands are situated on and
around the œsophagus behind the aortic arch.   The largest gland of the
group may be six to eight inches in length and lies dorsal to the œsophagus.
Enlargement of this gland may occlude the lumen of the œsophagus
causing recurrent or chronic tympany of the rumen.   There are usually
three or four bronchial lymph glands.   The mesenteric lymph glands
consist of a very large number of lymph nodes ; these for the purposes
of anatomical description are conventionally described as occurring in
groups related to the divisions of the intestine.   In addition to these lymph
glands there are many others that are of importance in connection
with post-mortem examination of carcases in meat inspection, but are
of only very minor importance in a clinical examination of the living
animal.

SHEEP.—The disposition of the lymph glands in the sheep is very
similar to that in cattle ; there are few points of difference meriting
attention.   There are usually two submaxillary lymph glands on each
side ; these are placed behind the angle of the mandible.   The parotid
lymph glands lie on the posterior border of the masseter muscle approximately halfway between the angle of the mandible and the mandibular
joint.   The retropharyngeal lymph glands lie on the dorsal wall of the
pharynx.   The mesenteric lymph glands consist of long narrow masses.

PIG.—There are usually two submaxillary lymphatic glands on each
side, one is large and the other quite small.   The parotid lymph glands
form a group on each side consisting of four larger glandular masses

and a number of smaller masses. One of the larger masses on the posterior border of the masseter muscle is partly covered by the parotid salivary gland. Another mass is entirely subparotid in position. The remaining two lymph nodes are related to the external maxillary vein. The retro-pharyngeal lymph glands consist of two fairly large masses on each side and these are situated on the dorsal wall of the pharynx.

A group forming the middle cervical lymph glands is disposed on the course of the external jugular vein. The caudal cervical lymph glands are situated just within the entrance to the chest ventral to the trachea. The prescapular lymph gland is situated at the cranial border of the anterior deep pectoral muscle. Neither axillary lymph glands nor cubital lymph glands are usually present; a few scattered lymph nodes may be present, but even if hypertrophied these cannot be palpated.

The precrural lymph gland lies on the anterior border of the muscle tensor fasciæ latæ on a level approximately midway between the coxal tuber and the patella. The gland is large, about two inches in vertical length and an inch wide. A large number of small lymph glands form the superficial inguinal group disposed in an extensive area around the external inguinal ring. The popliteal lymph glands are very small.

The lymph glands in connection with the stomach and bowel are numerous and are disposed along the course of the mesentery.

Dog.—There are at least two, and often four or five, small sub-maxillary lymph glands on each side, lying in the angle between the masseter muscle and the submaxillary salivary gland. They are immedi-ately below the skin and can be accurately palpated. The parotid lymph gland is usually very small. The retropharyngeal lymph glands are large; they lie dorsal to the pharynx, with the anterior extremity in contact with the occipito-mandibular muscle, and extend backwards for about two inches in a fairly large dog (e.g. Airedale).

The cranial, middle and caudal cervical lymph glands are not present as definite masses of lymphatic tissue. The prescapular lymph glands are found at the anterior border of the supraspinatus muscles. The axillary lymph gland lies in a mass of fat and can usually be palpated if the foreleg is abducted.

The superficial inguinal lymph glands are disposed around the external inguinal ring, being related to the penis in the male and the inguinal mammary glands in the female. The popliteal lymph gland is situated relatively superficially and is therefore more easily palpated than in any other animal. The mesenteric lymph glands consist of a number of small nodes and two elongated masses lying in the root of the mesentery; these large masses, if enlarged, can be palpated through the abdominal wall. The lymph glands of the colon are small; the majority are found in the short meso-colon, the remainder in connection with the transverse and terminal colon.

CLINICAL EXAMINATION

The usual method to employ in the examination of the superficial lymph glands of the body is palpation. Inspection is useful when a lymph gland is so grossly enlarged that the normal contours of the region are altered. Enlarged lymphatic glands may interfere with contiguous tissues, and so give rise to symptoms discernible by the clinician. Enlarged retropharyngeal lymph glands in cattle, by pressure on the pharyngeal wall, distort the shape of the respiratory passages and cause snoring respirations. Enlarged posterior mediastinal glands in cattle, by pressure on the œsophagus, prevent the eructation of gas from the rumen and cause tympany.

By palpation it is hoped to determine if the lymphatic gland is the site of any inflammatory or other change. In acute inflammation of a lymphatic gland the tissues are swollen, hot and painful ; frequently there is a zone of œdema partly or wholly surrounding the affected gland. In chronic inflammation the gland is hard, fibrous, not hot and usually painless. In tumour formation at first there is little or no pain, but later by involvement of neighbouring tissues in the tumour mass pain may be caused. The tumour mass is usually firm and does not yield to pressure.

If the resistance of a lymphatic gland to an acute infection is overwhelmed pus formation occurs, the gland softens, becomes fluctuating and finally ruptures to discharge its purulent contents. In tuberculosis the classical changes of necrosis, caseation and calcification occur in areas usually situated in the depth of the gland ; ultimately the gland hypertrophies.

The spread of disease by the lymphatic system is indicated by the involvement of successive lymphatic glands. The extent to which a disease such as tuberculosis has spread throughout the body can be estimated if the degree of involvement of lymphatic glands is known. If a lymphatic gland is found to be involved at least the neighbouring glands should be examined, but very often it is also desirable to examine glands remote from that first found to be involved. The discovery of a symmetrical, firm, painless enlargement of any pair of lymphatic glands in the body should be followed by a systematic examination of all the superficial and other lymphatic glands of the body that can be palpated. If there is evidence of disease of the upper air passages, the submaxillary and pharyngeal glands should be examined. In disease of the udder examination of the supramammary lymph gland should be carried out. Acute fever and lameness in a horse indicate the necessity of an examination of the lymphatic system of the affected leg.

Examination of the lymphatic vessels is carried out by palpation and inspection. If the coat is long or the skin pigmented it may not be possible to see the lymphatic vessels. Where the skin is only sparsely covered by hair, or where the coat is short and fine, swollen subcutaneous lymphatic vessels may be seen standing out as tense cords. If the skin is thin and non-pigmented an inflamed lymphatic vessel appears as a red streak or cord. Palpation of the affected parts will enable the clinician to detect the presence of swollen painful lymphatic vessels, provided the effect of the local lymphangitis has not been to cause sufficient œdema of the parts to completely " bury " the lymphatic vessels.

If infection is not retained at the site of entrance to the body the regional lymphatics are invaded ; the infection is then conveyed to the first regional lymph gland in which a defensive reaction occurs. If that lymphatic gland is not able to restrain and destroy the infection, it may then progress along the proximal portion of the lymphatic vessels until the next regional lymph gland is reached. If, finally, the last lymphatic gland guarding the part of the body wherein lies the site of infection is overwhelmed, infection gains access to the blood stream.

LOCAL CONDITIONS INVOLVING LYMPHATIC SYSTEM

Involvement of the lymphatic system following traumatic infection should not present any difficulty in differential diagnosis, since the lesion caused by the trauma will indicate both the portal of entry and possibly the probable type of infection.

Infections involving mucous membranes very frequently cause a local inflammatory reaction in both the lymphatic vessels draining the area and the associated lymphatic glands. For example, equine strangles is characterised by catarrh of the upper respiratory passages and an involvement of the submaxillary and pharyngeal lymph glands that in the majority of untreated cases terminates in abscess formation. During the course of the illness acute fever develops ; the febrile symptoms usually abate when the purulent material is evacuated from the abscess. The lesion in the lymphatic gland is typically that of acute inflammation. The gland is hot, swollen and painful, and œdema of the surrounding tissues develops. As liquefaction of the gland occurs, the centre of the swollen area becomes soft and a point of fluctuation indicates the place where the abscess will ultimately rupture. Necrosis of the skin covering the abscess takes place, and when the continuity of the skin is broken the purulent material escapes, the pus being thick and yellow. If the lymphatic defences of the pharyngeal region are overwhelmed, the caudal cervical lymphatic glands are involved. Should the lymphatic system fail to restrain the infection and the blood stream become involved, pyæmia results, when abscesses may form in almost any part of the body. In other types of catarrhal infections involving the upper respiratory passages in the horse, the reaction in the lymphatic gland does not proceed beyond the stage when the gland is hot, swollen and painful. When the attempted invasion of the body has been repelled the reaction in the gland abates.

Equine lymphangitis (sporadic lymphangitis) is characterised by a severe local lymphangitis accompanied by fairly intense symptoms of fever. The febrile symptoms may be present for some little time before the local lymphatic changes are manifest. In an acute case the animal soon becomes very lame (in the majority of cases a hind-limb is involved), and examination shows the deep inguinal gland to be swollen, hot and extremely painful. The lymphatic vessels on the inside of the leg are distended and can be seen and felt as tense painful cords. Œdema of the limb commences in the lower part and extends upwards ; if the case is severe the whole limb may be uniformly swollen till it is two or three times the size of the normal limb.

Epizootic lymphangitis is a contagious form of equine lymphangitis caused by *Cryptococcus farciminosus*. Though the leg is the commonest site, other parts of the body may be affected. The lymph vessels of the infected part are inflamed and stand out as prominent cords. Nodules develop on the course of the inflamed lymphatic vessels ; these nodules soften and burst, discharging thick creamy pus. The ulcer that results has inverted edges and heals slowly. The affected parts may be very œdematous. It is clear that infection of the lymphatic system has occurred, but before diagnosis can be completed the causal organism must be identified, this being done by the microscopic examination of the pus.

Farcy is the cutaneous form of glanders caused by *Pfeifferella mallei*. Farcy may result from a local infection or it may be a local manifestation of generalised glanders. Farcy is essentially a chronic inflammation of lymphatic vessels and glands. The lymphatic vessels are corded, farcy buds develop, these soften, the contents become purulent, forming an abscess that ruptures to discharge oily pus. The ulcer has an angry red depressed centre and the margins are thickened. Great œdema of the limb may develop. Differential diagnosis may be based on the reaction to a mallein test or the causal organism may be demonstrated in the purulent discharge from the lesion.

In glanders affecting the upper respiratory passages the submaxillary gland is commonly affected. The chronic inflammatory process renders the gland hard, fibrous and adherent to the jaw. Very often it is only the gland on one side that is affected. Glanders in the donkey may run a very acute course, when the lesion in the submaxillary lymphatic gland resembles that described as occurring in strangles.

Tuberculosis spreads in the body mainly through the lymph stream ; consequently lesions of lymphatic glands are an important clinical sign of this disease. Infection may enter the body through a mucous membrane without causing any noticeable lesion, the first evidence of the disease being found in the regional lymph gland. From the gland first involved infection may be carried by the lymph stream to the next, and so on until glands remote from the original portal of entry are affected. The blood stream may receive tubercle bacilli if the organisms in the lymph stream eventually reach the thoracic duct, or infection may enter the blood stream when a tuberculous lesion ruptures into a blood vessel. The pathological changes in lymphatic glands due to tuberculosis vary in the different domestic animals. In cattle the lesion in the gland becomes caseous and is ultimately calcified; the gland itself is enlarged in proportion to the severity of the lesion and the length of time infection has survived in the gland. Caseation and calcification occur more rapidly in lymphatic glands in the pig than in cattle. Caseation and calcification do not as a rule occur in the lesions of tuberculosis in the horse, but the gland tissue is replaced by thick white pus that is often very rich in tubercle bacilli. In the dog and cat caseation and calcification of lymphatic glands very rarely occur. In some cases lesions of tuberculosis in lymphatic glands in dogs and cats have a firm tumour-like consistency, the cut surface being pale and the lesion may seem macroscopically to resemble that of a lymphosarcoma. In other cases the centre of the gland breaks down to form pus. Whatever the character of the lesion, tuberculosis in any animal causes enlargement of the affected lymphatic glands. Since the reaction in the gland is chronic, the gland is not hot; there is no surrounding œdema and pain is usually absent, but if present is not severe. If a group of regional lymphatic glands are found to be enlarged the neighbouring regional glands must be examined, and it is usually desirable that all other superficial lymphatic glands should also be examined. Though a chronic non-painful enlargement of the lymphatic glands is very often caused by tuberculosis, further evidence is required before it can be decided that the lesion in the gland is tuberculous. There may be other clinical signs of tuberculosis, *e.g.* a chronic cough, progressive emaciation, etc. A tuberculin test may be applied, or the causal organism may be demonstrated in sputum, milk, fæces or urine. The supramammary lymphatic gland is not found to be constantly involved in cows with tuberculosis of the udder; if enlargement of the supramammary gland is found it is an additional and useful clinical sign, but if no enlargement of the lymphatic gland is found the possibility of tuberculous mastitis is not negatived. The symptoms and clinical signs attributable to tuberculosis of the posterior mediastinal gland in cattle have already been discussed. Tuberculosis of the mesenteric glands in horses and dogs may produce enormous lesions; in the former animal these may be palpated per rectum and in the latter they may be palpated through the abdominal wall. In cattle and pigs palpation of tuberculous lesions in the abdomen is difficult if not impossible.

Lymphatic leukæmia is not uncommon in dogs and is occasionally encountered in cattle. The disease is characterised by a progressive non-painful symmetrical enlargement of all the lymphatic glands in the body. There is a steady loss of bodily condition until the animal becomes extremely emaciated. The superficial lymphatic glands are easily palpated, as the glands are not only hypertrophied but very firm. Frequently the spleen is greatly enlarged. The total white cell count is increased and the lymphocytes may constitute 95 per cent. or more of the white cells.

There appears to be some doubt if the disease of man known as Hodgkin's disease does occur in the domestic animals, though a comparable condition macroscopically similar occurs in dogs. The blood picture is variable, there may be a moderate increase in the number of leucocytes, but there is no lymphocytosis.

Tumours may arise or metastatic growths may occur in lymphatic glands. Lymphosarcomata often arise in the bronchial and mediastinal glands. The mass formed by the tumour in the chest will ultimately cause collapse of the neighbouring lung tissue by pressure. The early symptoms resemble those of chronic bronchitis, the cough having a peculiar brassy note. The great veins may be occluded causing venous congestion and œdema. As the tumour does not always develop symmetrically in the mid-line, the heart may be displaced. Pressure on the œsophagus may interfere with swallowing, preventing the passage of solids which are regurgitated a few moments after they have been ingested. Radiological examination of the chest in the dog is of material assistance in establishing a diagnosis in these cases. Carcinomata produce metastases chiefly by lymphatic spread, therefore involvement of the lymphatic system gives a valuable indication of the degree to which extension has taken place.

Examination of the lymphatic system is an important part of a post-mortem examination. In the acute septicæmic form of swine fever, diagnosis cannot be completed until a post-mortem examination has been made ; among other characteristic lesions are the changes in the mesenteric lymph glands, these being swollen and œdematous with a zone of congestion. In meat inspection, the decision regarding a carcase is very frequently based on the degree of involvement of the lymph glands, e.g. tuberculosis in a bovine carcase and caseous lymphadenitis in the carcase of a sheep. The classification of tuberculosis as advanced or not advanced within the meaning of the Tuberculosis Order is based on the findings of the post-mortem examination and may in certain cases be based on the extent to which the carcase lymph glands have been involved in the disease.

CHAPTER X

SENSE ORGANS

Eye :—Anatomy — Clinical Examination — Conjunctiva — Cornea —
Anterior Chamber—Iris—Lens—Fundus—Ophthalmoscope
Ear :—Anatomy—Clinical Examination

THE EYE

THE superficial examination of the eye has already been discussed, and
the presence of conjunctivitis and conjunctival discharge will have been
noted. The tests of the functional activity of the optic nerve, the oculomotor nerve, the trigeminal nerve and the facial nerve were carried out
when testing the conjunctival, corneal and pupil reflexes. It is now
necessary to describe the further examination of the eye required for
the purpose of general diagnosis.

ANATOMY

The cornea is covered with stratified epithelium ; the greater part of
the thickness of the cornea is made up of fibrous connective tissue. The
inner aspect of the cornea is covered by a homogeneous elastic layer
known as Descemet's membrane. The anterior chamber of the eye is
bounded in front by the cornea and behind by the iris and anterior face
of the lens ; the posterior chamber is a small space formed by the posterior
surface of the iris, the ciliary body and the anterior face of the lens.
The anterior and posterior chambers of the eye contain a clear fluid
(the aqueous humour) formed by filtration from the blood stream.
Pressure in the anterior chamber is regulated by drainage through the
angle of the anterior chamber formed between the iris and the posterior
surface of the cornea at the corneo-scleral junction, fluid escaping by
way of the spaces of Fontana into the canal of Schlemm.

The iris is a musculomembranous curtain intervening between the
anterior chamber of the eye and the lens, the central aperture in the iris
forming the pupil. In the horse, the upper edge of the iris bears small
granular masses known as the granulæ iridis or corpora nigra ; similar
masses, though smaller, may occur on the lower edges of the iris. The
lens is held in position by its suspensory ligament ; the tension on the
ligament is controlled by the ciliary muscle and thereby accommodation
of the eye is adjusted to suit the immediate circumstances.

The globe of the eye is formed by three coats ; from without they
are the sclerotic coat, the choroid and the retina ; the cavity of the

globe is filled with the vitreous humour.   The optic nerve enters the posterior surface of the eye just below the median horizontal plane and slightly lateral to the central vertical horizontal plane ; blood vessels entering the eye do so with the fibres of the optic nerve.

CLINICAL EXAMINATION

CONJUNCTIVA.—The presence of any conjunctival discharge has been noted.   If there is a copious quantity of exudate present the eyes should be cleansed with a swab of gauze or cotton-wool, using clear water or a bland eye lotion.   When the eye has been cleansed it will be possible to determine the severity of any conjunctivitis present.   In conjunctivitis the membrane is injected and the vessels distended, the mucous membrane being dull red in colour and the vessels pursue a twisted, tortuous course.   The injection is greatest on the eyelids and in the cul-de-sac, where the mucous membrane is reflected from the posterior surface of the eyelid on to the globe of the eye ; it diminishes round the edge of the cornea.   Conjunctivitis may be a local clinical sign of a general febrile disease, e.g. equine influenza, swine fever, canine distemper.

CORNEA.—The cornea should be examined for evidence of inflammatory changes (keratitis) ; these are indicated by a bluish-white discoloration of the surface of the cornea and by the development of blood vessels running radially across the surface of the cornea from the conjunctiva.   The presence of ulceration should be looked for with particular care.   An endeavour should be made to determine the depth of any ulcer. If the ulcer has penetrated through the connective tissue layers so that only Descemet's membrane remains intact and can protrude through the cavity in the substance of the cornea, the condition is known as Keratocele.   If rupture of Descemet's membrane has occurred with protrusion of the contents, the condition is termed Staphyloma.

The cornea should be examined for the presence of opacities.   These may occur as white spots or as pigmented areas ; they indicate a previous keratitis.   It is well to try and ascertain if the opacity is superficial or penetrates into the deeper layers.   This can be done by looking at the cornea obliquely from the side of the eye with adequate illumination, which may be conveniently provided by means of a small electric torch.

ANTERIOR CHAMBER.—The anterior chamber is inspected for the presence of opaque fluid ; this is usually found in the lower part of the chamber.   Pus in the anterior chamber is known as Hypopyon.

The tension of the anterior chamber should be estimated.   This is done by inspection for any signs of bulging of the cornea and by applying gentle digital pressure to the surface of the eye through the eyelids.

IRIS.—Examine the iris for evidence of inflammatory changes.   If iritis is present the eye appears diffusely coloured, the shade being pink rather than red.   It is necessary to distinguish between iritis and conjunctivitis ;   in iritis the injected vessels pursue a straight course and do not have the twisted, tortuous course occurring in conjunctivitis.

Old-standing inflammatory changes in the iris cause distortion of the edges of the pupil.   If small distortions are seen and there is doubt of their significance, a few drops of a 1 per cent. solution of homatropine sulphate may be instilled into the eye in order to dilate the pupil ; dilatation of the pupil usually increases the distortion due to these changes.

LENS.—The object of examining the lens is to detect cataract.   The presence of an opacity in the lens necessarily interferes with vision. Cataract may indicate that past or present illnesses have disturbed the nutrition of the lens.   In the horse opacities of the lens may appear after a severe attack of equine influenza ;   in the dog opacities of the lens commonly occur in chronic interstitial nephritis and diabetes mellitus. Opacity of the lens is also a common occurrence in old age.

In very many cases cataract can be detected by a direct inspection of the eye in a reasonably good light, when it will be seen that the lens is wholly or partly white and opaque.   It is necessary to differentiate between a white opacity of the cornea and cataract ;   examination of the eye obliquely from the side will readily show whether the opacity is superficially situated on the cornea or deeply seated in the lens.   Small opacities of the lens will be detected when an examination of the fundus is being made with an ophthalmoscope.

FUNDUS.—In order to examine the fundus of the eye an ophthalmoscope must be employed.   Various patterns exist, and these fall into two main types ;   (1) An ophthalmoscope fitted with a mirror that reflects light into the eye to be examined, and (2) an ophthalmoscope provided with a source of electric light that is projected by a prism into the eye to be examined.   Whichever pattern of ophthalmoscope is used the principle is the same, namely that the observer looking through a small aperture behind the mirror or prism is able to see along the beam of light projected into the fundus of the eye and so inspect it.   The ophthalmoscope is usually provided with a number of lenses that can be interposed between the observer's eye and the aperture in order to correct errors of refraction.

OPHTHALMOSCOPE

The Simple Ophthalmoscope.—The animal should be placed in a dull or dim light with a source of light behind it ;   this may be daylight or artificial light.   The observer then stands in front of the animal, but a little to the side on which is the eye he is going to examine.   The light reflected by the ophthalmoscope mirror is then directed on to the animal's eye. Some practice will be found necessary before the beam of light can be directed on to the eye and any movements made by the animal followed.

The Electric Ophthalmoscope.—It will be found that the electric ophthalmoscope gives the most satisfactory results if it is used in relative darkness. An advantage of the electric ophthalmoscope is that the beam of light can be projected into the animal's eye more easily than with the simple ophthalmoscope, where it is necessary to maintain the relationship between the source of light, the mirror and the animal's eye. Many electric ophthalmoscopes are provided with a means of adjusting the position of the electric light bulb in relation to the prism so that the divergence of the beam of light may be regulated to suit the method for which the ophthalmoscope is being used.

There are two methods of using an ophthalmoscope, the indirect method and the direct method.

THE INDIRECT METHOD.—This method has the advantage of providing at one time a view of a large part of the fundus, and therefore for diagnostic purposes in medical cases it provides a suitable method. But it has the disadvantage that in a restless patient it may be found almost impossible to keep the beam of light centred on the eye for a sufficient length of time to permit examination of the fundus. It will, however, be found a very satisfactory method if the animal keeps still, as the whole of the fundus can be rapidly examined.

For the purpose of examining the fundus by the indirect method the simple form of ophthalmoscope fitted with a mirror one or two inches in diameter should be used. The ophthalmoscope is held by the observer at a distance of not less than two feet from the animal's eye. When the beam of light is projected into the eye the entire pupil should be illuminated ; if there is opacity of the lens this illumination of the pupil will not take place, or if there are small opacities in the lens they will show up as specks or streaks in the substance of the lens.

The colour of the light reflected from the retina varies in the different animals. Very frequently the light impinges on the tapetum, and a brilliant colour, blue or green in tint, is produced. The tapetum (tapetum lucidum) is the iridescent pigment epithelium of the choroid of animals which gives their eyes the property of shining in the dark ; the tapetum forms an extensive semilunar area which in the horse occupies the upper two-thirds of the fundus. In some dogs a reddish reflection from the retina may fill up the whole pupil ; in others the reflected light has a golden colour.

When the fundus has been illuminated a convex lens is placed between the animal's eye and the ophthalmoscope at a point about two or three inches from the animal's eye ; the lens is then moved backwards or forwards until a clear picture of the fundus presents itself. It will be found that considerable practice is necessary before the knack can be acquired of maintaining illumination of the fundus while simultaneously keeping the convex lens in position to maintain a clear focus. If the patient is restless, this may be found almost impossible. If, when the convex lens has been interposed, the magnification is found insufficient a convex lens with a focal length of 20 inches (*i.e.* $+$ 1D) may be placed behind the ophthalmoscope mirror, there usually being a fitting on the ophthalmoscope to receive a lens in this position.

THE DIRECT METHOD.—In using a simple ophthalmoscope by the direct method, the same method of illumination is employed, but a small oblique mirror is fitted to the ophthalmoscope. The observer adjusts his position in relation to the animal so that his eye and the ophthalmoscope are about two inches from the animal's eye. The fundus is illuminated, and then in order to bring the structures into focus the observer must allow his own accommodation to relax. Many people find it impossible to do so, and therefore cannot obtain a clear picture of the fundus. To overcome this difficulty a concave lens may be placed behind the mirror, the power of lens required varying with each individual ; most often a lens $-$2D or $-$3D is found effective ; the lenses provided with the ophthalmoscope usually have a range from $-$1D to $-$4D or $-$5D.

If the electric ophthalmoscope is used the same adjustment for accommodation will be required. Many electric ophthalmoscopes have a range of convex and concave lenses fitted to a revolving disc whereby a suitable power of lens is readily brought into use. The illumination provided by the electric instrument is of limited power, and the examination must be conducted in very dim light or in darkness.

If ophthalmoscopy is performed in circumstances that do not permit a bright light to enter the animal's eye, except from that directed into it by the ophthalmoscope, it is nearly always possible to examine the eye without resort to any means of dilating the pupil. If, however, it is found that the pupil contracts forcibly and so prevents a satisfactory examination, a few drops of a 1 per cent. solution of homatropine sulphate may be instilled into the eye, or a mixture of 1 per cent. homatropine sulphate and 1 per cent. cocaine hydrochloride may be used ; in a few minutes the pupil will be artificially dilated. When the examination has been completed the mydriatic effect of these drugs can be neutralised by instilling a few drops of a 1 per cent. solution of pilocarpine nitrate.

When the fundus has been illuminated and brought into clear focus the structures can be examined. In the horse the tapetum shows a brilliant tint of blue, green or yellow ; in cattle and sheep the tint is blue, and in the dog a golden colour is most common ; in the cat green predominates.

The optic disc or optic papilla is that part of the retina where the optic nerve enters the eye. In the horse this is found as an oval light rose-coloured area just below the lower border of the tapetum ; the optic disc in horses is quite sharply defined. In cattle the optic disc is much smaller and is not so sharply defined. In dogs the optic disc is within the area of the tapetum but at its lower edge, the disc varies in shape from nearly circular to almost triangular. In optic atrophy the disc appears pale. In glaucoma the disc is pale and appears as though it was depressed.

Blood vessels radiate from the optic disc ; the arteries are narrower than the veins and are not so dark in colour. Pulsation of the arteries should not be appreciable in normal animals. Pulsation may be seen in cases of increased intra-ocular pressure. Hæmorrhages appear as blotches if large, or as discrete spots if small ; they may appear to be spreading around a vessel. In cases of increased intracranial pressure the veins are distended and appear to pursue a twisted course ; at places the course of the vein may be hidden by hæmorrhage or exudation.

THE EAR

Tests of hearing have been discussed when the tests of the cranial nerves were described.

ANATOMY

The external ear of horses, cattle, sheep, pigs and cats is erect ; in dogs the shape and form of the external ear varies, being erect in some breeds, e.g. Alsatians, and in others the flap is dependent, e.g. Spaniels.

The external meatus is relatively long in all animals, and therefore direct inspection of the eardrum is not possible. In dogs and cats not only is the external meatus long but there is a right-angled turn at the bottom, the meatus running practically horizontally at the terminal part approaching the tympanum. The external meatus is lined by skin richly supplied with glands ; in any animal a certain amount of waxy secretion is always found in the external ear.

CLINICAL EXAMINATION

It is necessary to examine the ear in any animal that is found to be holding its head to one side, or is observed to be shaking its head, or in which there is a suspicion of deafness. The external ear must first be inspected. Inspection is facilitated if the light from an electric torch is shone into the ear.

In the smaller animals an auroscope is a useful instrument for inspection of the ear. This consists of an electric bulb with a reflecting shade that projects light through a speculum into the external ear, the eye of the observer being placed at an aperture behind the source of light. A convex lens placed in the apparatus assists inspection by magnifying the tissues seen in the field of vision. This instrument is of value in showing inflammation and ulceration of the lining membrane in ear canker. In place of an electric auroscope a speculum may be used with a concave inspection mirror to reflect light through the speculum. The inspection mirror has an opening in the centre through which the observer looks.

Any excess or abnormality of the secretion in the ear must be noted. The state of the lining membrane must also be noted. If an inflammatory reaction is present in the lower part of the external meatus no visual sign may be noticed on inspection, but if the lower part of the meatus is compressed with the fingers a clicking sound may be produced by the exudate, when the ear is allowed to relax. Palpation of the ear will reveal pain if present.

If there is any sign of itching, and especially if the material in the ear contains a lot of epithelial debris bound together with waxy secretion, a microscopic examination must be made for the presence of mange mites.

Rupture of the tympanum, whether due to trauma or the result of suppuration, causes acute pain, and the animal holds the head turned towards the affected side. Diagnosis of rupture of the eardrum must be based on indirect signs unless the tissues are exposed so that the tympanum can be inspected.

CHAPTER XI

GENITALIA AND MAMMÆ

Male :—Scrotum—Testicles—Spermatic Cord—Inguinal Canal—Prepuce and Penis
Female :—Vagina—Uterus—Ovaries—Mammæ

For the purposes of this work the description of the examination of the genital organs is restricted to that necessary to determine the presence of disease that may be affecting the general health of the animal and therefore may be of significance in differential diagnosis. The more detailed examination required in the investigation of infertility or sterility is beyond the scope of this work.

MALE

Scrotum, Testicles and Spermatic Cord.—Acute inflammatory conditions involving these tissues may cause a very marked febrile disturbance. The tissues should be examined for the cardinal signs of inflammation—pain, heat and swelling. Orchitis and epididymitis are very painful conditions and cause considerable reflex acceleration of pulse and respiratory rates.

Inguinal Canal.—Strangulated or incarcerated hernia is frequently the cause of acute colic in horses, especially stallions. The examination of a case of acute colic in a stallion or colt foal should always include an examination for the presence of hernia. The swelling caused by the hernia can be palpated as a hot, painful, turgid mass.

Prepuce and Penis.—Lesions of the prepuce and penis may interfere with the outflow of urine. In any case of retention of urine these organs should be examined.

Suppurative balanitis, if severe, causes some general disturbance of health, and there may be a slight febrile reaction.

FEMALE

Vagina.—Acute vaginitis causes severe discomfort shown by restlessness and possibly straining ; there is reflex acceleration of pulse and respiratory rate, and not infrequently some rise in temperature. Inspection of the vagina will show the inflamed state of the mucous membrane.

Uterus.—The state of the uterus in relation to pregnancy may have an important bearing on differential diagnosis. In addition to obtaining the history of the animal in regard to œstrus and service an examination may be required to determine if conception has occurred. In the larger animals this examination consists of a vaginal and rectal examination. In mares a specimen of urine may be obtained for biological examination with a view to determining if the animal is pregnant. This biological examination is not dependable until ten weeks after conception. In the test devised by Cuboni the presence of œstrogens in the urine of pregnant mares is demonstrated chemically. This test is not dependable until 120 days after conception. The accuracy of the Cuboni test is rather less than that of the biological test. These tests cannot be applied in any of the domestic animals other than mares.

For further details of the clinical and laboratory methods employed in the diagnosis of pregnancy in the larger domestic animals reference should be made to standard works on the subject.

In the smaller domestic animals the existence of pregnancy may be determined by abdominal palpation. A radiological examination may be of value in the later stages of pregnancy ; it is not possible with certainty, consistently to demonstrate the existence of pregnancy before the 49th day in bitches, as up till then the ossification of the fœtal bones is insufficient for them to produce a radiographic shadow. Repeated radiological examination of pregnant bitches should be avoided in view of the lethal effect of X-rays on the fœtus.

Phantom pregnancies may present a problem in differential diagnosis that can only be solved when the normal period of gestation has elapsed and the apparent pregnancy terminates.

The recent occurrence of parturition is often of importance in diagnosis ; if a history cannot be obtained, a vaginal and rectal examination should be made to determine evidence of recent parturition. Acute metritis and pyometra are diseases that cause profound toxæmia. The external genitalia must be examined for evidence of discharge, and a vaginal and rectal examination made to ascertain the state of the uterus. In the smaller animals abdominal palpation may enable the enlarged uterus to be felt. Uterine sepsis may be reflected by a muco-enteritis of a rather severe character in addition to the other signs of general toxæmia.

OVARIES.—Cystic ovaries causing nymphomania may be associated with acute nervous excitement that in some cases simulates hysteria. In maiden bitches that are upwards of five years of age acute nervous symptoms sometimes occur during the œstral period. Tachycardia is sometimes encountered in bitches before, during and for a period after the œstral period.

MAMMÆ

Cow.—In the differential diagnosis of the various forms of bovine mastitis a broad division into two main categories may be made on the presence or absence of signs of septicæmia. It is, therefore, important that a general clinical examination of the animal should accompany the detailed clinical examination of the udder.

Acute infections of the udder are usually associated with loss of appetite, suspension of rumination, elevation of temperature and acceleration of pulse and respiration. In cows, in the absence of other obvious cause, an examination of the udder should always be made in any febrile disease. In acute mastitis the affected quarter is hot, painful, swollen and turgid ; the secretion is markedly altered in character, varying according to the causal organism. An acute tuberculous mastitis may be encountered. This takes the form of a diffuse inflammation leading to general enlargement of the quarter which, on palpation, is found to be very hard. This may develop rapidly, appearing in as short a time as ten or twelve days, though it usually takes longer. There is little or no pain in the quarter. To begin with the milk is unchanged in macroscopic appearance, but later it becomes thin and watery, and finally dirty yellow, a heavy deposit settling out on standing. The secretion usually contains tubercle bacilli in very large numbers.

Chronic mastitis is not usually accompanied by any general systematic reaction. In pronounced cases the milk is obviously altered in character, but quite distinct daily variations in the appearance of the milk are observed. In less pronounced cases the presence of small clots and flakes can only be detected by the use of the strip cup, when these are seen against the black background of the plate of the cup. In old-standing cases of mastitis, fibrosis of the gland may be detected by palpation of the udder after all secretion has been removed by milking. In the early stages of chronic tuberculous mastitis no lesion is demonstrable by palpation, and the milk is unaltered in macroscopic character. It is only in the later stages that the milk becomes thin and watery ; finally the secretion may consist of a small quantity of straw-coloured fluid. Enlargement and induration of the udder develops slowly ; in old-standing cases the enlargement of the quarter is such as to destroy the normal symmetry of the udder. As the demonstration of fibrosis by palpation is not possible in an udder distended with milk, it is desirable that examination of the udder of cows in full milk should be carried out after milking. At the commencement of milking the strip cup should be used, and the secretion examined for macroscopic changes, e.g. the presence of clots, changes in colour, presence of blood and an abnormal smell. If any abnormality is noticed in the strip cup, a specimen of milk should be obtained from the affected quarter or quarters. The teats are cleansed with 70 per cent. alcohol and allowed to dry ; the sample is drawn directly into a wide-mouthed clean sterile bottle. In obtaining such samples for microscopic examination it is usually desirable to discard the first few jets of milk. By this method the fore-milk is obtained for the demonstration of the organisms of non-tuberculous mastitis. As

—except in advanced cases—the lesion of tuberculous mastitis can only be detected in an udder that is empty of milk, it is usually found most convenient to collect the strippings of the udder for the demonstration of cell groups and tubercle bacilli. Further details will be found in Chapter XIV.

In cows approaching parturition, the udder may be so congested as to render palpation unsatisfactory ; in some heifers and cows a considerable measure of subcutaneous œdema may be present ; this renders palpation of the udder tissue impossible. In these cases examination of the secretion is of vital importance.

The udder should be inspected for uniformity of the quarters, the forequarters being compared one with another and the hindquarters similarly. A comparison should not be made between fore and hindquarters. The quarters of the udder are then palpated, each quarter being thoroughly examined. By palpation it will be possible to determine the presence of heat, pain and swelling in an acute inflammation, or of fibrosis in chronic inflammation of the udder. During the examination of each quarter the teat is examined for evidence of recent injuries and for signs of fibrosis resulting from injuries ; the presence of lesions of any specific disease on the teats should also be noted, *e.g.* the vesicle of cow-pox. The orifice and sphincter of the teat must be inspected for any signs of abnormality. The supramammary gland should, if accessible, be palpated.

In addition to the clinical examination of the cow or cows, enquiry should be made regarding the incidence of mastitis in the herd, the methods of milking and the standard of dairy hygiene, this information being particularly useful in assessing the causal factors in cases of chronic mastitis.

Laboratory examination of samples of milk by cultural methods takes a considerable time ; it is usually desirable that specific treatment should be initiated without delay. The clinician can, in a high proportion of cases, make an accurate diagnosis of the type of mastitis if the clinical findings are co-related with the results obtained by the following simple methods of examining a sample of the secretion from the affected quarter. Samples of milk, that do not show any abnormality by the strip cup examination, may be tested for increased alkalinity. A definite increase in alkalinity is regarded as evidence of mastitis, but the absence of this increase in alkalinity unfortunately does not eliminate the presence of mastitis. The indicators used for this purpose are either brom-cresol-purple or brom-thymol-blue. A few drops of the indicator may be added to some of the milk in a test-tube or a few drops of the milk are applied to paper or gauze impregnated with the indicator. The increased alkalinity is in the case of brom-cresol-purple indicated by the appearance of a purple colour, and in the case of brom-thymol-blue a bluish-green or green colour.   Microscopic examination of the sample of milk made on a smear prepared from the deposit obtained by centrifuging non-incubated milk is of little value, except in the case of tuberculosis ; much more satisfactory results are obtained by the microscopic examination of a smear made from incubated milk.   It is not essential for the sample of milk to be kept in an incubator, since adequate multiplication of the organisms will take place if the sample of milk is kept in a warm room for eighteen hours.   In addition to searching the smear for organisms, the cell content of the smear should be carefully examined.   The presence of polymorpho-nuclear leucocytes is indicative of the inflammatory reaction associated with both acute and chronic non-tuberculous mastitis. Details of the method of preparing, staining and examining smears of incubated milk and smears of the deposits obtained by centrifuging milk are given in the chapter on clinical bacteriology, Chapter XVI.

It is possible to decide on examining a smear of incubated milk whether the causal organism is *Streptococcus*, *Staphylococcus* or *Corynebacterium*.   At one time about 80 per cent. of streptococcal infections were due to *Streptococcus agalactiæ* ; infections with this organism will show distinct evidence of infectivity, but with the use of antibiotics this proportion has been markedly reduced.

Cases due to *Streptococcus dysgalactiæ* are usually found to be associated with lowering of the resistance of the udder tissue by injury or other cause.

Acute mastitis due to *Staphylococcus* or *Corynebacterium* infections are usually associated with a considerable degree of septicæmia.

The diagnosis of tuberculous mastitis is considerably facilitated if a search is made for cell groups and the neighbourhood of these examined with the oil-immersion lens for tubercle bacilli.   Definite diagnosis of tuberculous mastitis can only be made if the tubercle bacillus is demonstrated in the secretion from the affected quarter.   If microscopic methods are unsuccessful, a biological examination should be carried out, especially if the clinical findings are suggestive and cell groups have been found. Biological examinations can only be carried out in established laboratories.

A tuberculin test is not a dependable method of differential diagnosis of tuberculous mastitis.

In some cases, in both cows and goats, the milk may be heavily tinged with blood, but neither by means of a smear of incubated milk nor by cultural methods, can any causal organism be demonstrated, but a sample taken some days later may reveal organisms.

SHEEP.—Gangrenous mastitis in the lactating ewe, of staphylococcal origin, is commonly associated with septicæmia.

GOAT.—Staphylococcal and streptococcal mastitis of goats is encountered clinically, the condition being one of chronic mastitis.

MARE.—Mastitis of indeterminate ætiology occurs in mares during lactation. Mastitis may also occur in a mare when the foal has been weaned and the tension of the udder is not relieved at intervals by hand milking.

Sows AND BITCHES.—Mastitis may affect one or more of the mammary glands ; the ætiology is variable.

In bitches mammary tumours are of common occurrence. In many cases the tumours are benign and multiple, occurring in several of the mammary glands. These tumours are well defined and sometimes are cystic. Malignant tumours are frequently found to be ill-defined and on palpation give the impression of an actively spreading neoplasm. The regional lymphatic glands may be involved and metastasis in other parts of the body are common. Such malignant tumours are frequently adeno-carcinomata.

CHAPTER XII

LOCOMOTOR SYSTEM

Muscles—Bones—Joints—Feet

MUSCLES.—The examination of the nervous control and functional activity of muscles is discussed in the description of the tests of nerve function. Inspection and palpation of muscles indicates the general tone of the muscular system, while a comparison between corresponding muscles and groups of muscles is required in order to determine the presence of local lesions. In local paralysis there rapidly develops atrophy of the muscles supplied by the damaged nerve. The interference with function will be reflected in the limitation of movement ; thus in radial paralysis the extensor group of muscles is deprived of its nerve supply, the elbow is dropped and the carpus flexed, and the muscles atrophy. Muscular atrophy also occurs from diseases of bone and joint ; this may occur from some mechanical interference with movement, for instance, anchylosis of the elbow joint or from some painful condition leading to voluntary limitation of movement as occurs in arthritis of the hip.

In animals in good bodily condition the contours of the muscles are smooth and rounded, in wasting diseases the borders of the muscles become more prominent ; this is sometimes particularly evident in the muscles of the head. Spasms of muscles occur in tetanus and strychnine poisoning and these throw the muscles into prominent relief. Tremors of muscle are observed in dehydration and chloride starvation.

Certain diseases cause characteristic lesions in muscle, and the recognition of these lesions is necessary in diagnosis. Thus in paralytic equine myohæmoglobinuria the lumbar and gluteal muscles are involved in a characteristically hard board-like lesion ; the history of the case and the recognition of the discoloration of the urine with myohæmoglobin assist the clinician in diagnosis. In black quarter in cattle the animal is noticed lame and is found to be acutely ill; an examination of the muscles of the affected limb is made to determine the presence of an emphysematous lesion.

Muscular dystrophy of calves is a condition associated with deprivation of vitamin E. The muscles involved do not have the elasticity of normal muscle and on section are found to be pale and translucent. Affected calves are stiff, they get to their feet with difficulty and are unwilling to walk. Badly affected calves may be unable to rise. In some cases, the muscles forming the attachments of the fore-limbs to the chest are those most seriously affected ; in consequence, the chest drops and the cartilages of the scapulæ protrude above the ridge of the spine. Lesions in the heart muscle may be responsible for sudden death.

REFERENCES

BLAXTER, K. L. (1953). " Muscular Dystrophy." *Vet. Record*, vol. lxv, pp. 835-837.
SHARMAN, G. A. M. (1954). " Muscular Dystrophy of Beef Calves in the North of Scotland." *Vet. Record*, vol. lxvi, pp. 275-279.

BONES.—In the examination of bones it is necessary to ascertain whether there is present a generalised condition affecting the bones throughout the skeleton, or whether the disease of bone is a local lesion. Inspection and palpation of bones has as its object the recognition of alterations in contour and form, as well as changes in the texture and consistency of bone.

In abnormalities of bone, secondary to general disease, it is frequently found that the bones first involved are those of the face. The head is, therefore, examined for signs of distortion of its normal contours, and the bones are palpated to determine softening, fragility or other abnormalities. Decalcification of the membranous bones of the head in the dog causes a flexibility that permits the bending of these bones. Lesions involving the periosteum of the long bones of the limbs and sometimes the metacarpals, metatarsals and digits are seen in the condition known as pulmonary osteoarthropathy. These lesions have been encountered in both dogs and horses in association with either tuberculosis or tumour of the lung. The periosteal lesions cause swelling and pain ; X-ray examination shows periosteal new bone formation.

Local disease of the jaw in cattle is frequently due to *Actinomyces bovis* : the lesion causes a large deformity with rarefaction of the bone and the development of pockets of pus that ultimately rupture into the mouth or to the outside through the skin.

Examination of the long bones of the body in young animals is frequently directed to determine the presence of abnormalities of bone formation. In advanced cases of rickets the deformity and bending of the long bones is readily appreciated on inspection. Inspection and palpation of the epiphyseal region reveals a broadening of the bones in this region. As the costo-chondral junctions are enlarged in rickets, these are examined for signs of this abnormality. It not infrequently happens in cases of rickets that the animal shows lameness and pain in a particular joint ; in such cases the recognition of the general involvement of the bones is a necessary factor in diagnosis. Precise diagnosis of rickets may not be possible without a radiological examination of the affected bones. In rickets the blood calcium is lower than normal, and

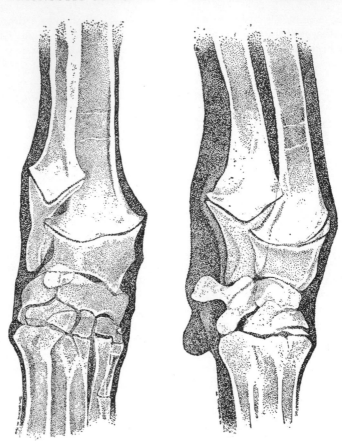

FIG. 25.—Dog. Drawing from radiograph of radius and ulna (anterior
view)—Rickets.

FIG. 26.—Dog. Drawing from radiograph of radius and ulna (lateral
view)—Rickets.

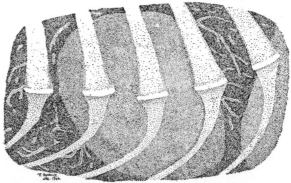

FIG. 27.—Dog. Drawing from radiograph of costo-chondral functions—Rickets.

if the reduction is marked, muscular tetany may occur. Tetany of this type is most frequently seen in calves, piglets and puppies.

When the absorption and utilisation of calcium in a young animal has been defective the deciduous teeth may be found to be translucent and to have a peculiar blue colour ; the formation of the permanent teeth is in these cases also defective.

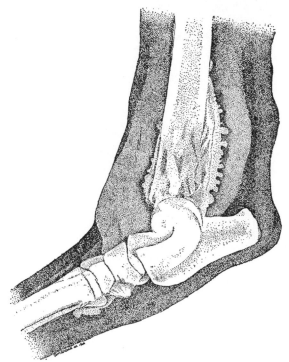

Fig. 28.—Dog. Drawing from radiograph showing telangiectic osteogenic sarcoma.

Fragility of bone is encountered in young growing animals and may be due to dietetic deficiencies, but cases occur, especially in dogs, in which, though the diet is adequate, there is an imperfect development of bone, the cortex of the long bones being excessively thin. A radiological examination of the bones may assist diagnosis. Fragility of bones develops in certain types of chronic poisoning, for example, chronic fluorine poisoning.

The distinction between traumatic damage to bone and tumours of bone, *e.g.* osteosarcoma, is important, in view of the pronounced malignancy of the majority of the tumours of bone occurring in the domestic

S

animals. This distinction is frequently only possible by means of a radiological examination of the lesion. Osteosarcomata usually affect the ends of long bones ; two forms occur. In one the tumour develops within the cavity of the bone, destroying the surrounding cortical bone, beyond which the tumour mass extends, this form being known as a telangiectic osteogenic sarcoma. Tumours of this type develop very

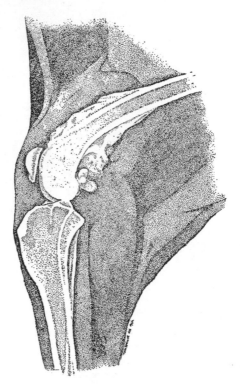

FIG. 29.—Dog. Drawing from radiograph showing sclerosing osteogenic sarcoma.

rapidly. The fragility of the bone permits fracture as a result of relatively slight trauma. The radiographic appearance is that of an osteogenic tumour exploding outwards. In the other type, though malignant, the tumour develops more slowly. The tumour may be described as a sclerosing osteogenic sarcoma. There is sclerosis of the affected bone and the development round it of dense new bone with irregular spicular margins. Fibromata may develop in association with the periosteum and lead to erosion of bone.

Among the domestic animals tuberculosis of bone occurs most frequently in the horse and cat. In the horse the most common site is the cervical vertebræ, where a rarefying ostitis causes stiffness of the neck ; there may be no other clinical signs of tuberculosis, but diagnosis may be facilitated by a positive reaction to a tuberculin test. In the cat the lesion may occur in the vertebræ or in the bones of a limb, the rarefying ostitis in some cases leading to a complete breakdown of the bone. A radiological examination of the bone will show the nature of the lesion. Sometimes a sinus communicates with the lesion, and bacteriological examination of the discharge from this sinus demonstrates tubercle bacilli. Tuberculosis of the spine leading to ataxia and paraplegia is seen in pigs. The exact nature of the condition can only be determined by post-mortem examination.

In dogs ataxia and paraplegia may be caused by anchylosing spondylitis—inflammation of the vertebræ leading to spinal anchylosis—or by ossification of the intervertebral discs. These conditions can only be diagnosed with certainty by means of a radiological examination. In anchylosing spondylitis the radiograph shows deposits of new bone which appear as outgrowths causing fusion of the vertebræ. These are more commonly found in the posterior part of the spine, especially the lumbar vertebræ. Ossification of the intervertebral discs is shown radiologically by opacity of the intervertebral spaces, commonly this is only visible in one or two of the intervertebral spaces but post-mortem examination reveals degenerative changes in many, if not all, of the intervertebral discs. Prolapse of the intervertebral disc substance by pressure causes intense pain. In part the pressure is due to the inflammatory reaction provoked by the prolapse. If the inflammatory reaction subsides recovery may take place. If, however, pressure is maintained the phase of pain and spasm is followed by flaccid paralysis. Diagnosis may be assisted by a radiographic examination as described on page 210.

JOINTS.—Inflammatory conditions of joints may arise as a result of local trauma. An infected joint may be the primary focus responsible for septicæmia or pyæmia. Inflammatory involvement of joints occur in toxæmia, septicæmia and pyæmia. Arthritis in an acute form is encountered in navel-ill in foals, calves and lambs, which is due to a variety of organisms. A severe, painful form of arthritis, involving particularly the tarsus, is frequently seen in septic metritis and acute mastitis in cows. In pigs, arthritis occurs in chronic swine erysipelas, there being fibrosis of the joint capsule and tendon sheaths. Fibrosis of joints in lambs is sometimes found to result from infection with *Erysipelothrix rhusiopathiæ*, the causal organism of swine erysipelas. Joint-ill in lambs, due to a streptococcal or staphylococcal infection, takes the form of a suppurative arthritis ; staphylococcal arthritis may be a clinical sign of tick pyæmia.

In some general diseases a diffuse involvement of the locomotor system is present ; it may not be possible to determine the exact site of pain. Thus in equine influenza the animal is stiff, resents being made to move and does so with obvious pain, but an examination will not reveal any point of maximum intensity of pain. Similarly in the dog an acute febrile disease is encountered that is characterised by diffuse pain and subsequently acute endocarditis.

FEET.—In the larger animals, particularly the horse, difficulty in movement may be due to inflammation of the laminar matrix of the hoof, *i.e.* laminitis. Laminitis arises from various causes. In mares laminitis is a serious complication of retention of the fœtal membranes and septic metritis. Laminitis may develop as a sequel to gastric impaction or simple overloading of the stomach, and it frequently occurs in cases of superpurgation. The extreme pain in the feet makes the animal adopt a posture with the hind feet placed forward under the abdomen in order to carry as much weight as possible, the forelegs being extended forward so that the minimum weight is borne on them. The animal is extremely unwilling to move, as any movement necessarily increases the weight carried by the acutely inflamed fore feet. The extreme pain and immobility is accompanied by a sharp rise in temperature and acceleration of pulse and respiration. It is necessary to differentiate between the immobility due to laminitis and that due to other causes, *e.g.* tetanus.

While in any animal an examination of the foot is required in cases of lameness, in the cloven-hoofed animals this examination is of especial importance in view of the possibility that lameness may be due to foot and mouth disease. In any outbreak of enzootic lameness in cattle, sheep or pigs, the feet must be carefully examined for lesions of foot and mouth disease and a general clinical examination of the animal, or animals, made. The skin of the interdigital space, coronary band and bulbs of the heel is inspected for signs of inflammation and vesication. The skin of the coronary band and bulbs of the heel should be subjected to firm digital pressure, in order to reveal any vesicles that may be hidden from inspection. The hooves are inspected for signs of separation around the coronary band. Vesication is common in cattle and sheep, but in pigs a partial separation of the hooves around and below the coronary band gives the appearance known as " thimbling." In any of the cloven-hoofed animals complete separation of the hoof may be due to foot and mouth disease.

In cattle " foul of the foot," associated with *Fusiformis necrophorus*, is a condition associated with extending necrosis of connective tissue and bone. The infection appears to gain entrance at the interdigital space. The condition is extremely painful and loss of condition is rapid. The nature of the lesion and the absence of lesions in the mouth are points of distinction between foul of the foot and foot and mouth disease.

In sheep foot rot causes a separation of the horn from the underlying tissues ; this separation is the result of infection spreading under the sole. The condition is contagious and a high proportion of the flock may be affected. In severe cases the feet are so painful that the sheep may rest on its knees when grazing. The condition is distinguished from foot and mouth disease by the fact that it is the horny part of the foot that is diseased, not the skin.

In pigs lameness may develop as a result of the horn of the sole being worn thin by the abrasive action of recently laid cement floors. Inspection of the feet will enable this condition to be differentiated from foot and mouth disease.

CHAPTER XIII

ALLERGIC REACTIONS

General Principles

Tuberculin Tests :—The Single Intradermal Test—The Comparative Test—The Single Intradermal Comparative Test—The Double Intradermal Comparative Test—The Ophthalmic Test—The Cutaneous Test—The Subcutaneous Test

Mallein Tests :—The Intradermopalpebral Test—The Subcutaneous Test—The Ophthalmic Test

Johnin Test

GENERAL PRINCIPLES

AN exact definition of allergy is rendered difficult owing to the present imperfect comprehension of the precise relationship between allergy, anaphylaxis and immunity. In its widest sense the term allergy is used to indicate a condition of exaggerated or unusual sensitivity to a specific substance that is innocuous or inert when administered in a similar manner to the majority of the normal animals of the same species. In the restricted sense of the term when used to describe the allergic reactions used for diagnostic purposes in veterinary medicine, allergy implies a state of supersensitiveness to the products of infecting organisms on the part of an animal suffering from the specific disease concerned, e.g. sensitivity to tuberculin in tuberculosis and to mallein in glanders.

Though it may be argued that the altered reactivity of the body towards the infecting organism and its products should be considered as part of the phenomena associated with the development of immunity, certain points of distinction can be drawn between immunity and allergy. Under certain conditions an animal may be both allergic and immune to a specific infective agent ; if the animal is desensitised it still remains immune. Desensitisation can be achieved by the repeated administration of small doses of the substance to which the animal is allergic. Desensitisation has an important bearing on the efficacy of the repeated use of allergic tests in cases of doubt. The exact difference between allergy and anaphylaxis is difficult to define. In anaphylaxis as in allergy a state of hypersensitiveness is developed by the animal to a particular substance, but anaphylaxis can be transferred passively to an animal if the circulating antibody is present in the transferred blood ; further, immunity can be transferred passively from one animal to another. It follows that the allergic state that has developed in the individual animal

278

is a response on the part of the tissues to the provocation of a specific infective agent. Since allergy is highly specific it is possible to achieve a high standard of efficiency in differential diagnosis by the application of suitable allergic tests.

In the application of allergic tests for diagnostic purposes the material used is the product of the growth of the specific infective agent plus the disintegration products of the organisms freed from infective organisms ; it is, therefore, incapable of transmitting infection and in a non-infected animal is perfectly innocuous.

In the case of allied infections and variants of any given infection, a certain inter-relationship exists in allergic reaction whereby the degree of specificity is somewhat reduced ; this has led to certain difficulties in the application and interpretation of allergic tests, especially in the differential diagnosis of bovine tuberculosis. It has become evident that as the potency of the agent used in the application of an allergic test increases there is a proportionate decrease in specificity, so it is necessary in the production of the diagnostic agent for the manufacturer to endeavour to achieve a reasonable balance between potency and specificity. Actually it has not been found possible to produce a tuberculin of a potency sufficient to cause a reaction in all animals infected with bovine tuber-culosis which will not cause a reaction in animals sensitised with the other acid-fast organisms causing avian tuberculosis and Johne's disease. It is this group allergy that made it necessary to introduce the comparative test with mammalian and avian tuberculin.

It will readily be appreciated that in allergic tests an accuracy approaching 100 per cent. cannot be expected, but a standard of accuracy sufficiently high for all reasonable practical purposes can be obtained provided the variable factors are realised and allowance made for them. Allergic tests are utilised for two purposes : for the purpose of detecting subclinical infections and carrier animals with a view to eradication of the disease, and in differential diagnosis. The allergic tests used in veterinary medicine are : tuberculin tests, principally applied to cattle, pigs and poultry ; mallein tests, applied only to horses, asses and mules ; and Johnin test, to cattle.

In any allergic reaction there are three variable factors, the diagnostic agent, the individual applying the test and the animal to which the test is being applied. The production of the diagnostic agent can be so con-trolled that a substance of nearly constant potency and specificity can regularly be produced. If the technique of the test is standardised, gross variations in results should not occur, but minor deviations must inevitably appear.

Allergic reactions may be so applied that they provoke either a general reaction or a local reaction or both. Formerly procedures causing a general reaction were in common use, but today tests depending on a local reaction are favoured as they have advantages that will be mentioned in the description of the individual tests.

TUBERCULIN TESTS

It cannot be too strongly emphasised that no single tuberculin test ever demonstrated that an animal was free from tuberculosis. Only when an animal has failed to react to repeated tuberculin tests and has been kept in an environment free from tuberculous infection can it be stated that it is, as far as can be known, free from tuberculosis.

In the preparation of tuberculin *Mycobacterium tuberculosis* is grown under suitable conditions ; the products of the growth and the disintegration products of the organisms are separated from the organisms and suitably concentrated. From time to time various modifications in the methods of producing tuberculin have been made. One of the earliest changes was the introduction of synthetic media to replace the original media of animal origin, as it was thought that a number of non-specific reactions were due to the animal protein contained in the final product. Different methods of concentration of the product have been employed, such as evaporation by heat and precipitation with various salts. It is now considered that the highest standard of accuracy can be achieved with the purified protein derivative tuberculin known as P.P.D. A great advantage of P.P.D. is that it can be issued from the laboratory at a standard potency without undue difficulty, as with the large batches produced at a time the potency tests required are fewer than with other tuberculins and the adjustment of potency is simpler.

It will be obvious from what has been said concerning desensitisation of an allergic animal that repeated testing may well produce a state of desensitisation whereby an animal fails to react to an allergic test. To obviate this risk a general rule may be laid down that second and subsequent tests should not take place until at least sixty days have elapsed since the immediately preceding test. As allergy is essentially a tissue reaction it will be seen that an animal in an advanced stage of the disease may no longer possess the capacity to react to the provocation of the specific antigen ; these cases are less important than they at first sight appear, since it is usually possible to detect disease of such an advanced character by clinical examination. When a number of reactors are found on testing a herd it is essential that a thorough clinical examination of all the animals, but particularly the adults, should be made, as the reactors may have been infected by an animal of the type mentioned which, while infective, no longer possesses the capacity to react to the injection of tuberculin.

It is also important that a clinical examination of the herd be carried out in association with tuberculin testing as it is by this means that diseases interfering with the interpretation of the test are detected, for instance Johne's disease and so-called skin tuberculosis.

It is necessary to emphasise that a positive tuberculin test (*i.e.* the animal is a reactor) does not provide any indication of the site and extent of the disease, nor does the severity of the reaction provide information on these points. Indeed the most violent reaction is usually seen in an animal that has not been tested previously but has been infected for a sufficient length of time for it fully to develop the capacity to react.

The time required by an animal to develop the capacity to react has an important bearing on the application of the test. This period of time is comparable to an incubation period. It has been shown that the capacity to react develops in a period of time varying from as little as five days to as long as fifty-six days ; the great majority of cases have become reactors within thirty days of the time of infection. It has been claimed that under certain ill-defined circumstances the development of the capacity to react may be delayed for as much as six months ; evidence in support of this hypothesis is not at all convincing ; indeed the mass of experience gained in the eradication of tuberculosis from dairy herds by means of the tuberculin test refutes the hypothesis. The period of sixty days postulated as desirable between two tests has, therefore, the merit that if the animal was newly infected at the time of the first test it should have fully developed the capacity to react by the time the second test is applied, and the desensitisation caused by the first test should have passed away.

The tuberculin tests regularly applied in veterinary practice today are the intradermal tests. The subcutaneous and ophthalmic tests are now seldom used. The test most widely employed in Great Britain is the single comparative intradermal test.

INTRADERMAL TUBERCULIN TESTS

When intradermal tuberculin testing of cattle was introduced to Great Britain in 1925 the double intradermal method was employed using a heat-concentrated tuberculin prepared on media containing animal protein. This was replaced by synthetic medium tuberculin concentrated by a method of precipitation. Finally there was produced purified protein derivative tuberculin which has the advantages of possessing a high degree of specificity and because of its method of production can be readily standardised to maintain a constant and adequate potency.

In 1947 the single intradermal comparative tuberculin test, using purified protein derivative tuberculin, was adopted as the standard test for cattle in Great Britain.

APPARATUS AND TECHNIQUE

In order to make an intradermal injection the syringe used must be capable of withstanding a not inconsiderable pressure. The two most frequent sites of leakage in syringes are at the junction of the butt of the needle with the barrel of the syringe, and between the piston and the walls

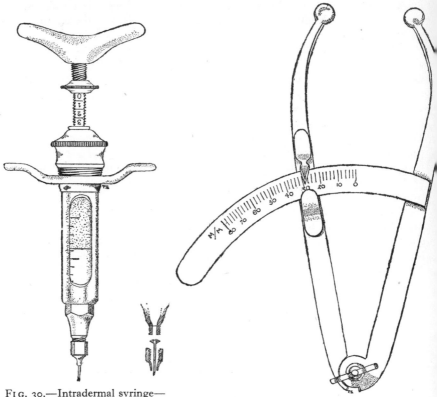

FIG. 30.—Intradermal syringe—
dental type.

FIG. 31.—Hinged callipers.

of the barrel of the syringe. A convenient way of testing the syringe is to fill it with water, then insert the needle into a cork; it should be possible to force water through between the fibres of the cork without the syringe leaking anywhere. The precise type of syringe is to some extent a matter of personal preference, a favourite being the dental type of syringe fitted with a graduated plunger and stop that permits accurate measurement of the dose of tuberculin; the needle is attached by a butt fitted with a screw thread adapted to fit a thread cut on the nozzle of the syringe barrel. The McLintock preset syringe is fitted with a ratchet operating on the notched stem of the plunger. Pressure on a lever depresses the plunger sufficiently to deliver 0·1 c.c. of tuberculin. When the lever is released the ratchet moves up one notch and the syringe is immediately preset to deliver the next dose. Whatever type of syringe is employed the needle must be short, of small diameter and sharp.

In order to measure the skin callipers are required. These may be of the hinged type with a graduated quadrant on which the thickness of the skin can be read off, or the callipers may be of the sliding type used by engineers, the scale being marked along the edge of the sliding portion.

The site of the test is in the middle third of the neck, approximately midway between its upper and lower borders. The hair should be clipped from an area of about one square inch covering the point where it is intended to apply the test.

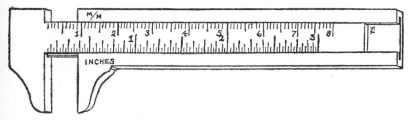

FIG. 32.—Sliding callipers.

A fold of skin including the clipped area is picked up between the forefinger and thumb of one hand and measured with the callipers held in the other hand. The thickness of the fold of skin is recorded in millimetres. It will be realised that the measurement recorded is that of two thicknesses of skin as well as some subcutaneous tissue. With practice it is possible to measure the fold of skin consistently so that the measurements made during the test represent a true indication of the variation in thickness of the skin. Though two individuals may not record the same measurement for a fold of skin, it should be found that if the skins of a large number of animals are measured, any difference in the measurements obtained is consistent ; this difference is not of any significance since the measurements in any test are of comparative and not absolute significance.

The injection of tuberculin is made into the thickness of the skin that has just been measured, with a short dental needle inserted obliquely. Appreciable force is necessary to introduce the tuberculin between the layers of the skin. If very little pressure is required the possibility of a subcutaneous injection should be suspected. When using the McLintock syringe the difference in pressure required to inject the tuberculin correctly is not, due to the mechanics of the syringe, appreciably different from that required to expel some tuberculin into the air. Care must therefore be taken that the tuberculin is in fact introduced into the thickness of the skin. If the injection has been made intradermally the dose of tuberculin can be felt as a small firm pea-like nodule ; this is probably best felt if the skin is allowed to lie flat against the side of the neck and the site of injection is gently stroked with the tip of the forefinger.

THE SINGLE INTRADERMAL TEST

The single intradermal test may be applied to the skin of the neck, or the caudal fold. As the single intradermal test only requires two visits, the first to make the injection and the second, seventy-two hours after the first, to read the reaction, it is a test that takes up the minimum of time and labour.

CATTLE.—THE SKIN TEST.—The test is applied in the skin of the neck as described, the dose of tuberculin being 0·1 c.c. The reaction is read seventy-two hours after the time of injection.

Intradermal tests depend on the development in a tuberculous animal (*i.e.* a reactor) of a necrotising-inflammatory reaction.

In a negative reaction the site of injection should be marked by no more than a very small sharply circumscribed nodule. Any swelling showing signs of diffuseness should be regarded as a positive reaction. On this account great care must be taken when examining the reaction that traces of œdema are detected, this being done both by palpation and by inspection. A small plaque-like swelling can often best be detected by inspection as the swelling shows up against the background formed by the area of skin that was clipped. Pain and heat are detected by palpation.

It has been found, if a tuberculin of uniform potency is used in testing a large number of animals, that the increase in skin measurement in non-reacting animals does not exceed a figure that can be quite accurately assessed for that particular tuberculin. It was shown that with P.P.D. tuberculins prepared by the laboratory of the Ministry of Agriculture and Fisheries, an increase in skin thickness of not more than 2 mm. indicated a negative reaction, whereas an increase of 4 mm. or more indicated a positive reaction, increases falling between these two measurements constitute a doubtful reaction.

Though change in skin thickness represents the only method of measuring the result of a test, the test should not be interpreted solely on measurement, but in addition the nature of any swelling must be taken into account and a record made of its character. Any swelling which shows œdema must be regarded as positive.

CATTLE.—THE CAUDAL FOLD TEST.—In order that the injection of tuberculin may be made properly it is of vital importance that the animal be adequately restrained, as the tissue into which the injection is made is highly sensitive and introduction of the needle may be resented vigorously. If the animal proves unduly fractious, hobbles should be used ; for this purpose a strap may be applied above the hocks in the same way as for restraining a cow that kicks when she is being milked.

It is necessary to cleanse the skin of the caudal fold prior to making the injection ; for this purpose the skin is wiped over with a swab damped with 50 per cent. methylated spirit. The caudal fold on one side is rolled from below the tail with one hand ; the syringe with the needle attached is held in the other hand, and the needle is introduced into the skin in such a way that the needle passes along the side of the caudal fold just beneath the surface of the skin. The needle can be seen in this position and when the tuberculin is introduced it is visible as a minute bleb under the skin. Owing to the delicacy of the skin tissue in the caudal fold, the dose must not exceed $\frac{1}{20}$th c.c. (0·05 c.c.), as a larger dose may cause sufficient tissue damage to provoke a traumatic inflammatory reaction that will interfere with the interpretation of the test reaction. The reaction is examined at the 72nd hour after the injection of tuberculin. The other caudal fold serves as a control.

The positive reaction consists of a painful œdematous swelling varying in size from a hazel-nut to a pigeon's egg. The swelling develops slowly, first appearing about twenty-four hours after injection and gradually increasing in size, reaching its maximum between the 48th and 72nd hour. The swelling is persistent and takes several days to disappear. In non-pigmented skins the reaction may be seen to consist of a central hæmorrhagic focus surrounded by a zone of intense hyperæmia. It may be noticed that the caudal lymphatic glands are enlarged. If the caudal fold test has to be repeated in sixty days the opposite fold should be used for the re-test. The caudal fold test is only applicable to cattle.

Single Intradermal Test in Other Animals

Pigs.—Disease in pigs may be caused by either the bovine or the avian strain of the tubercle bacillus. The simultaneous use of avian and mammalian tuberculin, one on the right and the other on the left ear enables the veterinary surgeon to determine the type of infection. This will enable him to advise on eradication or control.

Luke (1953) suggested that where only detection of infection is required a single injection of mixed avian and mammalian could be used.

The dose of tuberculin for single intradermal tests in the pig is 0·1 c.c. and the site of injection is the skin on the anterior part back of the ear.

A positive reaction consists of a prominent œdematous swelling that in non-pigmented skins is seen to consist of a hæmorrhagic focus surrounded by a zone of intense congestion. The reaction develops slowly and persists for some days.

Horse.—The technique of the single intradermal test is the same in horses as in cattle, but as the skin of the horse's neck is much thinner than in cattle care is required to ensure that the injection is truly intradermal. It has been found that when a group of apparently healthy horses were subjected to a tuberculin test a number reacted and in none of them were lesions of tuberculosis found on post-mortem examination. Holth (1949) pointed out that from a review of the literature on tuberculin tests in the horse it was evident that occasionally the test fails in markedly tuberculous horses and that a great many normal horses give a positive reaction.

Dog.—The single intradermal test has not proved satisfactory in the dog.

Poultry.—The test used for the detection of tuberculous infection in poultry is the single intradermal test. Into the lower border of one wattle of the fowl 0·1 c.c. of avian P.P.D. tuberculin is injected. The other wattle serves as a control. The equipment used for cattle is suitable for the tuberculin testing of cattle.

The bird is held securely by an assistant, usually close to his left side, the right hand firmly grasping the comb in order to restrain the head. The left wattle is thus presented to the operator, who grasps it between the thumb and the forefinger of one hand, manipulating the syringe with his other hand. The needle is inserted longitudinally into the lateral aspect of the dermis as close to the lower edge of the border of the wattle as possible and the tuberculin is injected into the tissues. If the inoculation has been performed correctly a small bleb, or a small, diffuse, but nevertheless observable raised area, lighter in colour than the rest of the wattle, is seen. The bird is then returned to the pen, and after a lapse of forty-eight hours the reaction to the test is examined.

The presence of tuberculous infection is indicated by swelling of the injected wattle, which commences about the 24th hour and persists to the 72nd hour, sometimes even for as long as five days. Transient swellings may occur but rapidly subside and are not apparent at the 48th hour ; these are of no significance, and if the reactions are not inspected until the 48th hour will cause the interpreter no trouble.

The swellings caused by positive reactions vary in individual birds ; some are small and only slightly œdematous, but may be observed easily if the injected wattle is compared with the uninjected one which has been left as a control, when the difference in size will be noticeable ; others show an increase in size and thickness of the wattle from four to five times the normal. Varying amounts of heat and pain are manifest. In extremely sensitive birds the œdema may spread from the wattle to adjacent tissues, particularly overlying the pharynx, and may even on occasion involve the control wattle. Doubtful reactions, i.e. persistent small swellings with little œdema, pain or heat, are sometimes encountered and these should be interpreted in the light of the operator's knowledge of the existence of infection in the flock. If birds showing such reactions are allowed to remain in the flock they should be re-tested in one month's time.

On rare occasions it may be found that in some fowls the wattles are so small as to be useless for the test. In these instances alternative sites such as the side of the comb, or a point on the line of junction of skin and mucosa at the side of the cloaca, may be used for the injection. The former is probably the more satisfactory, but neither site gives as accurate results as the wattle.

The tuberculin test will detect the majority of infected birds, especially in the early stages of the disease. A small number of birds, however, in which infection is generalised, fail to react to the test. These birds are usually unthrifty or emaciated, but in some instances may be in excellent condition. Before testing a flock of birds, all underweight and unthrifty birds should be removed. Those infected birds which were in good condition but failed to react to the tuberculin test will usually have lost weight by the time the next test is applied. Repeated testing of a flock is necessary if ultimate eradication is desired.

Tuberculin testing of other birds such as turkeys and ducks has been performed, but the results appear to be less reliable.

The sites have been, in turkeys, the wattle, the snood, the skin, either at the edge or in the centre of the wing web, and the mucosa of the cloaca ; and in ducks the sites selected have been the skin of the neck, the junction of skin and mucosa around the cloaca, and the web of the foot. The ophthalmic test has also been tried in ducks, but with little success.

THE COMPARATIVE TEST

With the introduction of potent mammalian tuberculin in 1940 fewer infected cattle were missed in testing. Unfortunately this more potent tuberculin was less specific and careful post-mortem and bacteriological examination of many reactors failed to reveal lesions due to the bovine type of the tubercle bacillus. It was found that animals with an increase in skin thickness of less than 5 mm. were not infected with bovine tuberculosis. By the simultaneous use of avian and mammalian tuberculin it was possible to detect the animals reacting to mammalian tuberculin but not infected with bovine tuberculosis. Cattle infected with bovine tuberculosis are said to have a *specific infection* and those not so infected but sensitised by some other means are said to have a *non-specific infection*. This simultaneous use of avian and mammalian tuberculin to detect specific and non-specific infection is the basis of the comparative tuberculin test.

Non-specific reaction in cattle to mammalian tuberculin may be due to infection by avian, human or murine type of *Mycobacterium tuberculosis* or by Johne bacillus, or may be due to so-called skin tuberculosis. It is possible that a short period of sensitivity exists in animals temporarily invaded by non-pathogenic acid-fast bacteria.

In the case of avian tuberculosis and Johne's disease the reaction to mammalian tuberculin is less than to avian tuberculin. Human and murine type of infection do not produce progressive disease in cattle, but the reaction to mammalian tuberculin exceeds that to avian tuberculin. Experimentally the sensitivity to murine type remains for about seven months decreasing slowly during that time. Cattle with lesions of so-called skin tuberculosis often show a greater reaction to mammalian than than to avian tuberculin but over a period of some weeks or months the response tends to equalise or indeed come to a stage when the avian reaction exceeds the mammalian.

The comparative test has been used by the Animal Health Division of the Ministry of Agriculture and Fisheries since 1940 and is the basis of the successful campaign to eradicate bovine tuberculosis from cattle in Great Britain. Smith (1955) in a survey of test charts from a large number of herds found approximately 38 per cent. of all cattle tested reacted non-specifically. In the majority of herds this was attributed to avian tuberculosis from fowls or wild birds or to non-clinical Johne's disease.

The basis of the comparative test is the simultaneous application of an intradermal test at two points of the skin, using at one point mammalian tuberculin and at the other avian tuberculin. When the comparative test was first introduced the injection of mammalian tuberculin was made on one side of the neck and the avian tuberculin was injected into a precisely similar position on the opposite side of the neck. It was found in practice that it was difficult to carry out the test satisfactorily when the injections were made on opposite sides of the body. As equally comparable results can be obtained, if care is exercised in locating the sites of injection, the test is now carried out by making the two injections on the same side of the neck. The Animal Health Division of the Ministry of Agriculture and Fisheries established that suitable areas of similar sensitivity can be obtained if the injections are made in the middle third of the neck, both being on a line drawn parallel to the spine of the scapula, the upper site being about four inches below the crest of the neck and the lower site about five inches below the upper. It has been found most satisfactory to adopt the plan of always using the upper site for avian tuberculin and the lower site for mammalian tuberculin.

When first introduced the comparative test was applied by the double intradermal method, *i.e.* the test was a double intradermal comparative test. Comparison between the double intradermal comparative test and the single intradermal comparative test carried out by the Animal Health Division of the Ministry of Agriculture and Fisheries showed no significant variation in their efficacy. Both tests have a margin of error and neither test showed itself capable of detecting all those infected animals which had not been detected by the other test.

Following these comparisons the single intradermal comparative test was adopted in 1947 by the Animal Health Division of the Ministry of Agriculture and Fisheries as their official tuberculin test under the Attested Herds Scheme.

THE SINGLE INTRADERMAL COMPARATIVE TUBERCULIN TEST

The single intradermal comparative tuberculin test is applied to the skin of the neck, using avian tuberculin and mammalian tuberculin. Both sites should be in the middle third of the neck on a line parallel to the spine of the scapula. The upper site used for avian tuberculin should be at least four inches below the crest and the lower site used for mammalian tuberculin should be five inches below the upper. In young cattle in which there is not room to separate the two sites sufficiently on one side of the neck, one injection may be made on each side of the neck.

For this test purified protein derivative tuberculin is used, the mammalian tuberculin contains 2·0 mgs. of purified protein derivative per c.c. and the avian tuberculin contains 0·5 mg. per c.c., these strengths of tuberculin being used for all tests.

In order to avoid confusion mammalian tuberculin is supplied in bottles labelled in blue and avian tuberculin is coloured red and is supplied in bottles with a red label.

The dose of tuberculin in all cases is 0·1 c.c. In the herd test one post-injection observation is made at the 72nd hour ; in re-testing inconclusive reactors an additional observation may be made if thought necessary at the 96th hour. The selected sites are clipped. The fold of skin at each site is then measured with callipers and the measurement recorded in millimetres. The dose (0·1 c.c.) of tuberculin, avian in the upper site and mammalian in the lower site, is then injected intradermally. If the injection has been made properly a small pea-like swelling is felt at the site of injection ; it is essential that steps be taken to ensure that the injection has been made correctly. If there are any doubts injections should be made on the opposite side of the neck in similar sites.

The reactions are read at the 72nd hour, and the skin thickness being again measured and recorded, and the reaction is examined for signs of œdema. For record purposes the Animal Health Division of the Ministry of Agriculture and Fisheries classify the character of the swelling as circumscribed (C), slight œdema (S.O.), diffuse œdema (D.O.), and extensive œdema (E.O.).

It has been determined that in this test using tuberculins of the strength stated no swelling should be regarded as negative that shows an increase of more than 2 mm. ; swellings of 3 mm. increase should be regarded as doubtful and swellings of 4 mm. or more increase should be regarded

T

as positive. Any swelling showing œdema should be regarded as positive.

The term *doubtful* is applied to the interpretation of an individual reaction whether to avian or mammalian tuberculin when the reaction is neither negative nor positive.

The term *inconclusive* is used when the comparison between the reactions to the two tuberculins does not permit a definite decision as to the significance of the comparative test.

Interpretation of the Single Intradermal Comparative Tuberculin Test

A clinical examination of the herd will have shown the presence of any animals suffering from clinically recognisable forms of tuberculosis. The same examination will have revealed the presence of clinical cases of Johne's disease and of animals affected with so-called skin tuberculosis. This clinical examination is thus of importance in assessing the background of the herd in relation to specific and non-specific infection. A survey of the results of the tuberculin tests will show if there is a proportion of animals showing reactions to the avian tuberculin only or a proportion showing a definite reaction to avian tuberculin and a much less definite reaction to mammalian tuberculin ; reactions of these two types indicating the presence in the herd of non-specific infection such as avian tuberculosis, Johne's disease or so-called skin tuberculosis.

The reactions in individual animals are interpreted against the background provided by the knowledge that non-specific infection is either present or absent from the herd. With this knowledge the following bases of interpretation should be adopted :—

(1) Animals showing a negative reaction to both tests are retained in the herd.

(2) Animals showing a positive or doubtful reaction to avian tuberculin and a negative reaction to mammalian tuberculin are retained in the herd.

(3) Any animal giving a doubtful reaction to mammalian tuberculin and a negative reaction to avian tuberculin should be re-tested.

(4) Any animal showing a positive or doubtful reaction to avian tuberculin and a positive or doubtful reaction to mammalian tuberculin, provided the increase in skin measurement to mammalian tuberculin is not more than 4 mm. greater than the increase in measurement to avian tuberculin should be :—

    retained, if non-specific infection is established

    re-tested, if non-specific infection is not established.

(5) Animals giving a positive reaction to mammalian tuberculin and a negative reaction to avian tuberculin when the increase to mammalian tuberculin does not exceed the avian increase by more than 6 mm. should be :—

re-tested, if non-specific infection is established
removed, if non-specific infection is not established.

(6) Animals which give a positive reaction to mammalian tuberculin and a positive or doubtful reaction to avian tuberculin when the increase to mammalian tuberculin is 5 or 6 mm. greater than the increase to avian tuberculin should be :—

re-tested, if non-specific infection is established
removed, if non-specific infection is not established.

(7) In all tests animals showing a positive reaction to mammalian tuberculin and a positive, doubtful or negative reaction to avian tuberculin should be removed when the increase to mammalian tuberculin is more than 6 mm. greater than the increase to avian tuberculin.

There are certain instances where the circumstances prevailing in the herd indicate the need for a more stringent interpretation of the test. For instance while there may be evidence of non-specific infection in the herd there may also be so many reactions to mammalian tuberculin alone or because a clinical case of tuberculosis may have been found there can be no doubt that mammalian tuberculosis is present along with non-specific infection. In such a herd the test should be interpreted as if non-specific infection was not present in the herd.

In some herds the animals have been maintained in self-contained groups ; there may be a preponderance of mammalian reactors amongst the adult stock necessitating interpretation of the test as though non-specific infection was not present, but in the young stock the absence of mammalian reactors justifies interpretation of the test on the basis that non-specific infection is present.

In herds where there is evidence of non-specific infection other than skin tuberculosis it may be that the only evidence of the presence of bovine tuberculosis is in one or two animals that give reactions just bringing them into the category for removal, i.e. a mammalian reaction 7 or 8 mm. more than the avian. In such cases it is justifiable to re-test before removing them from the herd.

Skin tuberculosis (so-called) is to be regarded as evidence of non-specific infection and animals giving reactions which normally would justify their removal from the herd may be re-tested if lesions of skin tuberculosis are found on them. If there is evidence of skin tuberculosis in the herd even those animals which show no detectable lesions may be re-tested.

In certain cases it may be found that an animal gives a marked increase in skin measurement to both tuberculins with either a small excess in the mammalian measurement or an equal response to both tuberculins ; even though non-specific infection is established in the herd it may be advisable to re-test such an animal.

RE-TESTS.—All animals which it is decided to re-test because of an inconclusive result in the interpretation of the comparative test should be isolated. The re-test is not carried out until at least thirty days have elapsed. The test is applied to the opposite side of the neck, the results, if necessary, being read at the 96th hour as well as the 72nd hour.

If bovine infection is demonstrated in the herd the reactors are isolated with a view to their removal from the herd ; a re-test of the herd is carried out sixty days after the effective separation of the reactors from the rest of the herd. The object of this 60-day re-test is to detect any recently infected animals that had not developed sensitivity at the time of the previous test. The period of sixty days is the shortest time that must elapse between the two tests.

PIGS.—The comparative tuberculin test is not used as such in pigs, but the combined use of avian and mammalian tuberculins is used to determine with which of these two types a pig is infected. The technique of this test is described on page 285.

THE DOUBLE INTRADERMAL TUBERCULIN TEST

CATTLE.—Prior to the adoption of the single intradermal test described on page 284, the method used entailed re-injection of the original site with a further 0·1 c.c. of tuberculin forty-eight hours after the first, skin measurements being made before each injection. The test was interpreted at the 72nd hour after the first injection. Three visits were therefore required. Experiment and field experience has shown that the method has no advantage over the single intradermal test which is of course less laborious and expensive. In the course of eradication schemes many more cattle can be tested in any given period of time by the single method without material loss of accuracy.

Interpretation of the double intradermal test is in the same basis as for the single intradermal test.

Kerr, Lamont and McGirr (1946 and 1949) however suggested that the double intradermal test with an interval of seven days between the injections had advantages. These workers also submitted evidence that there may be a period of reduced sensitivity to tuberculin at parturition due to the loss of sensitivity bodies in the colostrum.

PIG.—The double intradermal test was applied to the skin on the back of the pig's ear. In the pig the single intradermal test on the skin of the ear is usually found quite adequate.

DOG AND CAT.—The double intradermal test has failed to elicit a reaction in known tuberculous animals.

THE DOUBLE INTRADERMAL COMPARATIVE TEST

The injections, measurements and examination of the reactions for both the avian and mammalian tests are carried out in precisely the same manner as that described for the double intradermal test with mammalian tuberculin. The tuberculins used for the double intradermal comparative test are mammalian 2·0 mg. per c.c. and avian 0·5 mg. per c.c. Interpretation of the test is based on the principles described for the interpretation of the single intradermal comparative test.

REFERENCES

ANON. (1947). " A Comparison between the Double Intradermal Comparative Test and the Single Intradermal Comparative Test." *Vet. Record*, vol. lix, pp. 95-97.

HOLTH, H. (1949). " The Tuberculin Reaction in the Horse." *Nord. Vet. Med.*, vol. i, pp. 581-600.

KERR, W. R., LAMONT, H. G., and McGIRR, J. L. (1949). " Further Studies on Tuberculin Sensitivity in the Bovine." *Vet. Record*, vol. lxi, pp. 466-475.

LAMONT, H. G. (1947). " Tuberculin Testing." *Vet. Record*, vol. lix, pp. 407-409.

LUKE, D. (1953). " The Intradermal Tuberculin Test in the Pig." *Vet. Record*, vol. lxv, pp. 533-535.

SMITH, A. W. (1956). Fellowship Thesis lodged in Royal College of Veterinary Surgeons, London. p. 24 *et seq.*

OPHTHALMIC TEST

This test consists of the instillation of a few drops of tuberculin into the conjunctival sac. A positive reaction is constituted by the development of a purulent conjunctivitis. The reaction usually develops in twenty-four hours. The ophthalmic test has not been found reliable.

THE CUTANEOUS TEST

The cutaneous test usually attributed to von Pirquet consists of inoculating an area of skin by scarifying it through a film of tuberculin. A reaction is indicated by the area becoming congested, œdematus and painful ; in some cases pus-formation occurs. The cutaneous test is not dependable.

THE SUBCUTANEOUS TEST

CATTLE.—The subcutaneous tuberculin test depends on the provocation of a general thermal reaction in infected animals sensitised to tuberculin. The animal's temperature is taken before the dose of tuberculin is injected subcutaneously. The pre-injection temperature must not exceed 103° F., but preferably should not exceed 102° F. The dose of dilute (*i.e.* subcutaneous) tuberculin is usually 3 c.c. for cows and 4 c.c. for bulls. Commencing at the 9th hour after injection the animal's temperature is taken every three hours until the 18th hour.

Interpretation of the test is based on the thermal reaction but very often the reacting animal can be spotted by its appearance of general malaise.

A positive reaction consists of a rise in temperature to 104° F., or more, but a sustained progressive rise in temperature should also be considered a positive reaction.

A doubtful reaction consists of a rise in temperature to 103° F., but under 104° F., or a sudden or irregular rise in temperature of less than 2° F.

A negative reaction is one in which the temperature does not rise above 103° F. or in which the increase in temperature is less than 1° F.

Apart from the fact that the application of the subcutaneous tuberculin test to large numbers of cattle is laborious and time-consuming there are many technical advantages in the intradermal tests which have almost entirely replaced the subcutaneous test.

HORSE.—The subcutaneous tuberculin test has been found to be unreliable in horses because of the high proportion of false positive reactions obtained by it.

OTHER ANIMALS.—The subcutaneous tuberculin test is not satisfactory in pigs, dogs and cats.

MALLEIN TESTS

The mallein test is the principal aid in the differential diagnosis of suspected cases of glanders; it also forms the basis of the control and eradication of glanders. Glanders was eradicated in the British Isles by means of the mallein test. During the war 1914-18 the efficiency of horse transport would have been seriously undermined if glanders had become enzootic, but by regular use of the mallein test the disease was kept under firm control. Mallein is prepared from cultures of *Pfeifferella mallei*, the causal organism of glanders. Three types of mallein test exist, namely the Intradermopalpebral, the Subcutaneous and the Ophthalmic. The intradermopalpebral is the most suitable and most convenient test to apply to large numbers of animals under field conditions.

The Intradermopalpebral Test

This test consists of the injection of o·1 c.c. of mallein into the thickness of the skin of the lower eyelid. The same type of syringe as is employed for intradermal tuberculin tests will be found suitable for intradermal mallein tests. The mallein used for this test is prepared by diluting one part of crude concentrated mallein with three parts of o·5 per cent. solution of phenol. Before applying the test the animal's eye must be inspected to see that it is free from any sign of conjunctivitis.

A twitch is applied to the horse's nose and the animal held firmly by a reliable assistant. The left eye is the one preferably used by a right-handed person, but if a retest is being carried out the other eye must be used. The skin of the lower eyelid is tensed by stretching it with the fingers of the left hand, exerting traction in a downward direction. The needle attached to the loaded syringe is introduced very obliquely into the skin at a point about ½ inch below the palpebral margin ; the needle can be seen running under the surface of the skin. The intradermal injection of mallein produces a small, firm nodule that can readily be seen. If the presence of this nodule cannot be determined the injection has probably been made subcutaneously. The reaction develops comparatively slowly and reaches its height between the 24th and 36th hour ; a positive reaction persists for three or four days before declining. The reaction is examined at the 24th, 36th and 48th hour after injection, but if only one examination is convenient this should be made at the 48th hour.

INTERPRETATION.—A positive reaction is seen to consist of a voluminous diffuse œdema of the eyelid causing complete closure of the eye, with an intense conjunctivitis producing a considerable quantity of muco-purulent discharge that escapes from between the eyelids. A doubtful reaction consists of some pouching of the eyelid. A negative reaction consists of a firm swelling at the site of injection of the mallein. Some œdema of the lower eyelid may develop after the injection has been made: in non-reacting animals this disappears in about twelve hours or more.

The intradermopalpebral mallein test has been proved to be sensitive. The positive reaction is distinct and easily appreciated. The test can be applied to animals in a febrile condition. It can be applied to horses out-of-doors. There is no need for the animals to be kept off work while being tested. A large number of animals can be efficiently tested by one individual.

The Subcutaneous Test

The subcutaneous mallein test provokes both a local and a general reaction ; both of these must be considered when interpreting the result of a test. The animals must be kept housed throughout the period of the test. The mallein employed in the subcutaneous test is a dilute mallein consisting of one part of crude mallein and nine parts of diluent fluid.

The animal's temperature is taken twenty-four hours before the commencement of the test and again immediately before the injection of mallein. The temperature thus recorded should not exceed 102° F. The site of the injection is the middle third of the neck, half-way between its upper and lower borders. The dose of mallein is usually 1 c.c. The temperature is taken at the 9th, 12th, 15th and 18th hours after the injection of mallein ; and if the temperature is rising at the 18th hour and has not attained a height that justifies the condemnation of the animal as a reactor, the temperature must also be taken at the 21st and, if necessary, again at the 24th hour. The local reaction is examined when the temperatures are being taken and again at the 48th hour after the injection of mallein.

INTERPRETATION.—In assessing the result of a subcutaneous mallein test consideration must be given to both the local and the general systemic reaction. If the general reaction, as shown by elevation of the temperature, is pronounced the reaction may be considered positive ; if, however, the elevation of temperature is such that the reaction would be considered doubtful, a definite local reaction would justify the decision that the animal is a positive reactor. Consideration of the interpretation of the following combinations of local and thermal reaction will assist interpretation of the test.

Positive Reactions.—A rise of temperature to 104° F. or over, irrespective of the extent of the local reaction.

A rise of temperature to 103° F. or over if the local swelling is pronounced, *i.e.* if it is four inches or more in diameter.

Doubtful Reactions.—A rise of temperature to between 102° F. and 103° F. without any definite local reaction.

A rise of temperature to between 102° F. and 103° F. if the local swelling is less than three inches.

Negative Reactions.—A rise of temperature of less than 1° F. and no definite local swelling. A non-specific local reaction may develop at the site of the test a few hours after injection ; this disappears in from twelve to twenty-four hours, and will not be present when the local reaction is examined at the 48th hour. Some difficulty may arise in assessing the significance of different combinations of the two forms of reaction ; in any case of an indefinite reaction the animal should be isolated and retested.

THE OPHTHALMIC TEST

The ophthalmic test is principally used as a check test along with one of the other mallein tests.

This test consists of the instillation into the conjunctival sac of 3 or 4 drops of concentrated mallein by means of an eye-dropper or syringe with a graduated plunger. The eye must be examined prior to the application of the test to ensure that no conjunctivitis is present.

A positive reaction consists of the development of a purulent conjunctivitis that reaches its maximum height in twenty-four hours, and persists for a day or two thereafter. There is a pronounced œdema of the eyelids and the animal may show signs of photophobia.

In a negative reaction the eye remains normal; there is a little exudate at the inner canthus due to the response of the conjunctiva to the introduction of a foreign substance.

REPETITION OF MALLEIN TESTS

Mallein tests are sometimes repeated at short intervals; this procedure tends to produce indefinite reactions due to the desensitisation that necessarily follows any test. In the horse allergy appears to develop rather more rapidly than in cattle and is, if anything, more pronounced. There is evidence that the repetition of mallein tests at intervals of thirty days does not produce undue desensitisation.

It will be appreciated that under field conditions in wartime it may not be possible to wait as long as a month before applying a retest; in these circumstances the interval may be reduced to fourteen days, and has on occasion been reduced to as little as seven days, though there are obvious objections to repeated retesting at so short an interval.

JOHNIN TEST

The Johnin test has been used in the differential diagnosis of cases of clinical disease and in the detection of subclinical cases of Johne's disease. Johnin is prepared from cultures of *Mycobacterium paratuberculosis* (bacillus of Johne's disease). Though considerable progress has been made in the production of a Johnin of adequate potency and satisfactory specificity, the test has not yet attained a high degree of accuracy. This would appear to be due, at least in part, to the failure of infected animals to develop a pronounced degree of allergy. Infection with Johne's disease does not cause destruction of tissue cells to the same extent as tuberculosis or glanders, but on the contrary causes proliferation of the intestinal epithelium with thickening and corrugation of the mucous membrane. It may be that this essential difference in the pathology of the disease is the explanation of the inadequacy of the allergic response. In Johne's disease there appears to be a lack of specificity in the allergy developed, as cases of Johne's disease are found to give a reaction to both mammalian and avian tuberculin, though the reaction is not so pronounced as when the animal is infected with either bovine or avian tuberculosis. The testing of cattle for Johne's disease is therefore complicated if the herd is infected with either bovine or avian tuberculosis.

It may be that a comparative test using tuberculin and Johnin will provide a solution of this difficulty, but the results to date have been disappointing.

The only Johnin test now employed is the intradermal, and P.P.D. Johnin is in use. The technique is the same as for the intradermal tuberculin test, the dose for each injection being 0·1 c.c. The local reaction with the Johnin test in infected animals is not so pronounced as those produced by a tuberculin test, but the criteria by which a Johnin reaction is judged are similar to those detailed for the tuberculin test.

In suspected clinical cases of Johne's disease the microscopic examination of the fæces for *Mycobacterium paratuberculosis* will give a higher standard of accuracy than the Johnin test. It has been shown that the causal organism can be demonstrated in the fæces by microscopic methods in a high proportion of clinical cases of Johne's disease. Alternatively the complement-fixation test described on page 332 may be used, bearing in mind the limitations in the application and interpretation of this test.

CHAPTER XIV

COLLECTION OF MATERIAL
FOR LABORATORY EXAMINATION

Urine—Blood—Milk—Fæces—Pus—Liver Biopsy

URINE

SAMPLES of urine should always be placed in clean bottles. Bottles that have contained cosmetic preparations or soft drinks unless very thoroughly cleaned may contain traces of aromatic compounds or pigments that give conflicting results with some of the tests used in urine analysis. Even very minute traces of synthetic detergents can interfere with the tests for bile salts. If they have been used to clean a bottle thorough and repeated rinsing must be carried out to remove all traces of the detergent.

Samples of urine may be collected in a suitable receptacle when the patient is passing urine or in those animals in which it is practical a catheter specimen may be obtained. Samples of urine collected off the floor are liable to contain a proportion of extraneous matter that may interfere with urine analysis.

HORSE.—Horses in stables living a life governed by routine urinate at fairly regular intervals ; an observant animal attendant will notice the horse's habits and can usually secure a sample of urine with little difficulty. If this cannot be done it will be necessary to pass the catheter. In mares digital dilatation of the urethral orifice is often sufficient to induce micturition. Alternatively a catheter can be passed.

CATTLE AND SHEEP.—In male cattle the frequency of micturition usually makes it possible to obtain a sample of urine in the course of a very few hours. If the receptacle used to collect the urine is of plastic material the animal is not disturbed in the act by the sound of urine striking the vessel. In male sheep less accustomed to handling it may be difficult to approach the sheep without disturbing it and so causing it to cease micturition. Catheterisation of male cattle and sheep is not practicable.

In dairy cows, under a regular system of management, urination is performed with remarkable regularity and little difficulty is experienced in collecting samples. Digital stimulation of the lower labial commissure may induce micturition. If necessary a catheter may be used to obtain a sample of urine from a cow. Catheterisation is the only convenient method of obtaining a sample of urine from a ewe.

Dog.—In some cases in both dogs and bitches a specimen of urine can on occasion be collected in a receptacle such as a small basin if available to catch the urine as it is being passed. On the whole the most satisfactory way of obtaining urine samples in both dogs and bitches is to pass the catheter. In the dog catheterisation presents no substantial difficulty. In the bitch it is necessary to use a vaginal speculum and an illuminated speculum is of great assistance in seeing where to introduce the catheter.

If a sample of urine is to be examined microscopically by dark ground illumination it should be examined as soon as possible after collection. Living motile *Leptospira canicola* can be detected in urine by this method up to twenty-four hours after collection if the temperature of the urine is raised to blood heat. If examination of the urine is likely to be unduly delayed, the specimen should be buffered to control the damage to leptospiræ by the normally acid urine. Dilute alkali should be added to the urine until it is amphoteric or very slightly alkaline to litmus.

CATS.—The only satisfactory method of collecting urine from either male or female cats is catheterisation.

BLOOD

It is of the utmost importance that the clinician collecting blood samples for laboratory investigation should realise that the method of dealing with the sample on collection is governed by the particular examination required. In general the methods may be divided into two main categories (i) the blood is allowed to clot and (ii) clotting of the blood is prevented. There are several methods by which clotting can be prevented, and selection of a particular method is dependent on the examinations to be carried out in the laboratory. A sample of blood in which clotting has been prevented by one method making it suitable for one type of laboratory examination may not be suitable for another type of laboratory examination. Whatever the form of anticoagulant used, the blood sample should never be shaken vigorously but should be gently rotated between the palms of the hands to disperse the anticoagulant and facilitate its solution. The laboratory examinations carried out on samples of blood as an aid to clinical diagnosis can be divided into three main sections, viz. serological hæmatological and biochemical. In the serological group only one type of sample is required ; in the hæmatological group two types of sample may be required ; but in the biochemical group the method of dealing with the sample after collection varies according to the examination required and no single type of sample is suitable for all the examinations in regular use.

SEROLOGICAL EXAMINATION.—The serological examinations most frequently required as an aid to clinical diagnosis are agglutination tests and complement-fixation tests, less commonly tests for the presence of anti-toxin are needed. For all these tests it is serum that is required. The sample most often provided for this purpose is one of clotted blood. The sample of blood is collected into a clean sterile bottle and allowed to clot. For most purposes five cubic centimetres of blood is sufficient. If the blood is to be sent some distance by post or other method entailing handling, the sample should be allowed to stand until a firm clot is formed. If there is any reason to fear that transit of the sample may be delayed especially in warm weather it may be wise to separate the serum before dispatching the sample. This avoids the arrival of a hæmolysed sample of blood at the laboratory. A convenient method of separating the serum is to allow the blood sample to clot and when separation has taken place the serum is aspirated with a sterile syringe and needle and transferred to a clean sterile bottle. If it is intended to use this method it will be found helpful to withdraw rather more than 5 c.c. of blood—if this is possible—so that withdrawal of the serum can be achieved without disturbing the clot.

HÆMATOLOGICAL EXAMINATION

For a complete hæmatological examination the laboratory require a blood smear made on a clean microscope slide and a sample of unclotted blood. The sample of unclotted blood must be available for examination within a few hours' collection. If delivery of the samples is likely to be delayed overnight or longer it is probably best if a good blood smear fixed in methyl alcohol is the material supplied to the laboratory. The choice of anticoagulant for samples intended for hæmatological work is governed by the need to use a compound that causes the minimum of damage or distortion to the blood cells. For this purpose the anticoagulant of Heller and Paul has been found the most satisfactory. This consists of 1·2 gramme of ammonium oxalate and 0·8 gramme of potassium oxalate is dissolved in 100 ml. of distilled water. Into each sample bottle there is placed 0·2 ml. of this solution. The bottles are then dried off in an oven, excessive heating being avoided. The quantity of anticoagulant is sufficient to prevent the coagulation of 2 ml. of blood.

REFERENCE

HELLER, V. G., and PAUL, H. (1934). *J. Lab. Clin. Med.*, vol. xix, p. 777.

BIOCHEMICAL EXAMINATION

A clotted sample of blood is required for the estimation of calcium, magnesium, inorganic phosphate, transaminase and cholinesterase. A clotted sample of blood is also required for the estimation of lead, but the blood should be collected into special bottles made from lead free glass. These can be obtained from the laboratory concerned.

For biochemical purposes potassium oxalate alone is used as an anti-coagulant. Two mg. of potassium oxalate is sufficient for each 4 c.c. of blood. If there is likely to be any delay between taking the blood sample and the estimation of blood sugar, sodium fluoride at the rate of 1 mg. for each c.c. of blood should be added to prevent glycolysis.

The bottles are prepared in the same way as described above by making a solution adding an aliquot part to each bottle and drying off with a moderate degree of heat. Neither ammonium oxalate nor sodium fluoride should be used in the collection of blood samples for urea estimations since these substances interfere with the chemical processes entailed.

As a general rule 5 c.c. of blood is sufficient for any one biochemical estimation.

If blood copper estimations are required special polythene bottles must be obtained from the laboratory carrying out the analyses and their instructions regarding the method of samples must be observed.

It is useful to review the uses that can be made of the various types of blood samples described.

CLOTTED BLOOD.—Serological investigations, Biochemical Estimations of Calcium Magnesium, Inorganic Phosphate, Transaminase and Cholinesterase.

UNCLOTTED BLOOD.—With ammonium and potassium oxalate as an anticoagulant hæmatological examination : With potassium oxalate alone as an anticoagulant blood urea estimations : With potassium oxalate and sodium fluoride blood sugar estimations.

The ketone content of blood can be estimated on serum or on unclotted blood using potassium oxalate as an anticoagulant ; sodium fluoride does not interfere with ketone estimations.

TECHNIQUE OF BLOOD SAMPLING

All samples are obtained by venepuncture, the choice of vein being governed by the availability of a particular vein according to the species. It is most important that thoroughly sharp needles should be used and the usual precautions must be taken of sterilising the needle by boiling and of disinfecting the skin over the vein.

HORSE.—The animal should be restrained by the application of a twitch to the nose. The jugular vein is distended either by digital pressure or a cord round the neck is drawn tight so as to exert pressure on a rolled bandage placed in the jugular furrow. A needle two inches long and with a diameter of ten or twelve in the standard wire gauge is used. A piece of rubber tubing two or three inches long attached to the bulb of the needle facilitates control of the blood flow. The needle is inserted into the vein with the point directed towards the head. When the sample has been collected, pressure on the vein must be released before withdrawing the needle otherwise subcutaneous leakage may occur.

CATTLE.—The animal should be restrained with the head raised so that the neck is extended. In smaller animals restraint by gripping the nose between finger and thumb may suffice, but in larger animals bull holders applied to the nostrils are necessary. In bulls the ring in the nose is used. In cattle the jugular vein can be distended with a cord alone drawn tight round the neck. An alternative site in cows and heifers is the mammary vein. The technique of puncturing the vein and withdrawing blood is the same as in the horse.

SHEEP.—If the wool is removed from the neck over the jugular furrow blood can be withdrawn from the jugular vein as in cattle. A needle $1\frac{1}{2}$ inches long and diameter size 20 in the standard wire gauge is used. An alternative site is the recurrent tarsal (*saphena parva*) vein, the technique being the same as that described below for dogs.

PIG.—In pigs samples of blood can be withdrawn from the cranial vena cava. This is possible because the external jugular veins join to form the cranial vena cava just within the arch formed by the first ribs. Small pigs are restrained on their backs, with the head extended, restraint being made easier if the pig is placed in a V-shaped wooden trough. The needle, at least $1\frac{1}{2}$ inches long and size 20 is inserted at a point about one inch from the point of the sternum on a line joining it to the base of the ear on the side selected. The needle is directed inwards backwards and downwards. Larger pigs are restrained by a rope looped round the snout, the pig tending to pull back against the rope so tensing the neck. A needle 2 to $2\frac{1}{2}$ inches long is required but it is undesirable to use a needle of bore wider than size 20. In a site similar to that described in small pigs the needle is directed inwards backwards and upwards. Immediately the vena cava is penetrated blood flows freely.

An alternative method in pigs is to use the dorsal vein of the ear. The vein is distended by an assistant grasping the base of the ear. A needle one inch long and of diameter between 10 and 20 according to the size of the vein is used. It is usually found convenient to draw the blood into a 5 or 10 c.c. syringe, the blood being gently discharged from the syringe into the collecting bottle. In very small pigs an incision is made with a sharp scalpel into the vein near the edge of the ear and the blood is allowed to flow directly into the collecting bottle. As a rule when pressure on the base of the ear is relaxed the flow of blood ceases. If necessary a pad of gauze may be fixed over the incision with adhesive plaster.

DOG.—There are two sites available in the dog. First the recurrent tarsal (*saphena parva*) vein where it curves over the lateral aspect of the tibia and the gastrocnemius tendon. When using this vein the animal is laid on its side and the upper hind leg is grasped firmly just below the stifle, pressure being exerted on the posterior part of the limb so that the vein is compressed. The second site is the cephalic vein in the forearm. The animal is held in a prone position with forelegs extended towards the operator. The foreleg from which blood is to be withdrawn is grasped around the elbow joint and firmly compressed. A needle one inch long and size 20 is used. The use of a syringe to collect the blood will be found an advantage.

CATS.—The most common practice is to withdraw blood from the cephalic vein in cats. The technique is the same as described in dogs.

MILK

For the purposes of clinical diagnosis milk samples are required for two purposes, (1) for bacteriological examination and (2) for ketone examination. Samples required for the chemical demonstration of ketone bodies can be withdrawn from the udder into a clean bottle without any special precautions. Milk samples required for bacteriological examination must be obtained in such a way that gross external contamination is avoided.

It is preferable that the bottle used should have a wide neck and a ground glass stopper. The bottle must be clean and sterile. The udder and teats are cleansed of gross dirt and then wiped with some non-irritant antiseptic which evaporates readily. For this purpose 70 per cent. alcohol is very suitable. Obviously, the operator's hands should be thoroughly washed before withdrawing the sample. If possible the stream of milk should be directed into the centre of the neck of the bottle so that there is no film of milk between stopper and neck. As a general rule, unless the quantity of secretion in the udder is very scanty, the first few jets of secretion expelled from the teat should be discarded. Samples of milk required for the demonstration of *Mycobacterium tuberculosis* should consist of, or include, some of the strippings from the udder.

Milk samples must reach the laboratory with the minimum of delay, especially in warm weather. In order to prevent souring and clotting in transit in warm weather a preservative may be added to the sample, but it is preferable to aim at prompt delivery without using a preservative. One part of a 5 per cent. solution of boric acid to ten parts of milk will prevent souring and clotting but does not interfere with cultural or biological examination. Borax at a concentration of 2 per cent. in milk has been found useful as a preservative for milk samples destined for biological examination in guinea pigs for the presence of tubercle bacilli. A few drops of 40 per cent. solution of formaldehyde will prevent souring and clotting but renders the sample useless for cultural and biological examination.

SKIN SCRAPINGS

The methods employed in preparing skin scrapings are described in the chapter dealing with examination of the skin. (See p. 232).

FÆCES

Specimens of fæces may be required for bacteriological examination for the demonstration of evidence of helminthiasis and in some instances for biochemical examination, as for instance, for the presence of blood or in dogs for evidence of pancreatic deficiency.

Specimens for bacteriological examination may be lifted with a sterile spatula from recently passed fæces. The specimen should be taken from the centre of the mass so as to avoid contamination from the floor. The sample is transferred to a clean and preferably sterile container; a tin with a tight-fitting lid, a bottle with a wide mouth or a plastic jar with a screw on lid are all equally suitable. If recently passed fæces are not available, a sample may be taken from the rectum, manually in the larger animals and by digital manipulation in the smaller animals.

If fæces are required solely for the purpose of establishing the presence or absence of helminthiasis by the demonstration of eggs or larvæ a representative sample of any fæcal mass will suffice.

Where an egg count is desired this can be carried out on an isolated sample of fæces and this is the usual procedure in sheep where a few pellets of fæces are removed from the rectum by drawing them out with the forefinger. In some instances it may be desirable to obtain a more representative sample, as for instance, in estimating the helminth burden in horses. Then the fæces passed in a twenty-four hour period should be collected, thoroughly mixed and a representative sample taken from the whole. At least 2 grammes of fæces are required for worm egg counts. If, however, the fæces are abnormally fluid a much larger sample is required to allow for the high water content.

It is desirable that fæces samples should be placed in impervious containers with tight-fitting lids or stoppers. Fluid or semi-fluid fæces in the usual form of pill box lose a high proportion of the water content to the fabric of the box leaving a layer of soft material adhering to the surface.

Fæces for biochemical examination must be collected in such a way that contamination with extraneous matter is avoided. A glass or plastic container is preferable to a tin. If examination of the fæces for lead is required the fæces must be placed in a glass or plastic container. Traces of lead from glass are so small as to be unimportant in relation to the lead content of fæces.

PERITONEAL AND PLEURITIC FLUID

The methods of obtaining specimens of peritoneal and pleuritic fluid are described in the chapters dealing with the examination of the abdomen and chest. (See pp. 41 and 103), and the special method of obtaining peritoneal fluid in suspected cases of anthrax in pigs is described on p. 324

Most frequently peritoneal or pleuritic fluids are examined bacteriologically. The examination may be made microscopically, culturally or biologically. Whatever examination is intended the fluid must be collected with aseptic precautions and placed in a clean sterile container.

Pus

Specimens of pus are collected for bacteriological examination. If microscopic examination of a stained smear is thought likely to suffice it is only necessary to make a smear with a sterile platinum loop on a clean slide. The smear is allowed to dry, and, if packed for transit should be so placed that the surface of the smear is protected. Specimens of pus may be taken with a sterile swab, from which smears can be made or material obtained for cultural examination. If the purulent material is fluid and plentiful it may be collected directly into a sterile tube or bottle, or a quantity may be drawn up into a sterile syringe and discharged into a sterile tube or bottle. Thick viscid pus may be collected in a sterile swab or may be scraped up with a sterile knife.

Liver Biopsy

Samples of liver tissue for either chemical analysis or histological examination can be obtained in both adult cattle and sheep by means of a trocar and cannula passed into the substance of the liver where it lies close under the costal arch on the right side.

The trocar and cannula should have a total length of from 18 to 20 cm. with an external diameter of from 5 to 8 mm. The point of the trocar must be sharp and the penetrant end of the cannula should be ground to give a cutting edge.

In cattle the site is the intercostal space between the 11th and 12th ribs on the right side at a point 6 to 8 inches from the top of the spinous processes of the corresponding vertebrae. The animal is therefore restrained with its left side against some firm support such as a gate. An area of skin including the site is clipped, shaved if thought fit, and disinfected. The skin and underlying tissue are then infiltrated with a suitable local anæsthetic. A small incision is made through the skin at the site of puncture. The trocar and cannula are then introduced in a downward and slightly forward direction. Comparatively little resistance is felt when passing through the tissues overlying the liver, but when the liver is reached the resistance is felt to increase and passage into the liver substance gives a feeling of " crunching." When this point is reached the trocar is withdrawn and the cannula is pushed in into the liver substance for distance of $2\frac{1}{2}$ to 3 inches (6 to 7 cms.). The tip of the cannula is then moved slightly to free the end of the core of liver substance. It may be possible to withdraw the cannula with the core inside it by closing the free end of the cannula by pressing with a finger. It has been found more convenient to attach a 20 cc. syringe to the free end of the cannula and by withdrawing the plunger to exert negative pressure on the core of liver. The syringe should be so adapted that it is possible to fix the plunger in the withdrawn position to maintain the vacuum ; this can be done by boring two or three holes in the stem of the plunger into one of which a pin can be inserted, when the syringe and cannula can be withdrawn. The core of liver is expelled from the cannula by exerting positive pressure with the syringe.

In sheep the site of puncture is in the upper third of the ninth inter-costal space. A cannula 18 cm. long and 5 mm. external diameter is suitable for the purpose. Otherwise the technique is similar to that described for cattle, though it will be found more convenient to carry out the operation on a sheep laid on a table on its left side.

CHAPTER XV

CLINICAL CHEMISTRY

URINE ANALYSIS

INTRODUCTION

THE following system of urine analysis consists of qualitative tests that are simple in application. The system has been found satisfactory in that it is sufficiently comprehensive without being unduly laborious. It is possible to carry out all the tests described if two ounces of urine are available. If two ounces cannot be collected at one time, aggregation of urine collected at more than one time is permissible. The practitioner may prefer to carry out a complete routine examination of a specimen of urine, or it may be that the clinical examination has suggested certain possibilities that can be refuted or confirmed by urine analysis and therefore only the tests applicable in these circumstances are employed. There are good grounds for supporting the contention that as a general rule it is preferable to carry out a complete routine examination of each specimen of urine.

A routine examination of urine includes the following : Specific Gravity, Reaction, Protein, Bile Pigment, Bile salts, Blood Pigment, Sugar, Ketone Bodies, and in dog's urine Indican. If protein is found the deposits from the urine are examined with a view to showing additional evidence of the site and nature of a possible inflammatory lesion in the urinary system. If tests for blood pigment are positive a distinction must be drawn between hæmoglobinuria and hæmaturia.

The application and interpretation of urine analysis are discussed in Chapter XIX.

SPECIFIC GRAVITY

The specific gravity is estimated with a hydrometer possessing a range from 1·000 to 1·060. If the quantity is too small to float the hydrometer the volume can be increased by adding to the urine an accurately measured proportion of distilled water ; the specific gravity of the diluted urine is estimated and the specific gravity of the original sample computed.

REACTION

The reaction is conveniently determined by the use of red and blue litmus paper. (*Acid turns litmus red, alkali turns litmus blue.*)

If an estimate of the *p*H is desired this can be secured by using first a universal colour indicator (*e.g.* the B.D.H. Universal Indicator) and then a colour indicator of a more restricted range according to the results of the first test. Test papers are available in place of test fluids. Within limits these colour reagents give a reasonably accurate estimate of the *p*H of urine.

PROTEIN

Tests for protein can only be performed satisfactorily if the urine is clear ; if turbid the specimen must be filtered.

HEAT PLUS ACIDULATION.—The upper part of a column of urine in a test-tube is boiled ; a few drops of 3 per cent. acetic acid are added and boiling repeated. Coagulation of protein will render the contents of the upper part of the tube cloudy. The comparison of the boiled and unboiled portions of urine is necessary if the opacity due to very small quantities of protein is to be detected. Acidulation is necessary to avoid errors due to the precipitation of earthy phosphates by boiling alone. This test is suitable for the urine of any of the domestic animals. In the urine of horses and cattle the addition of acid may cause some evolution of gas if carbonates are present.

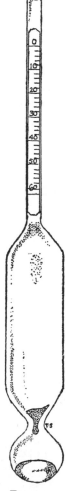

FIG. 33.—
Hydrometer.

COLD NITRIC ACID.—Concentrated nitric acid is run down the side of a test-tube containing urine so that a layer of acid is formed underneath the urine. At the junction of the acid and urine a white ring forms if protein is present. A crystalline layer may develop between the acid and concentrated urine ; this is not indicative of protein, the ring formed with protein being fluffy in character. The nitric acid test is of no value in testing the urine of the herbivora, owing to intense pigment formation that results from the reaction between the nitric acid and organic sulphur compounds in the urine, masking the white ring of the protein reaction.

The nitric acid test is considered capable of detecting protein in as low a concentration as 0·2 per cent., but there are possible fallacies due to the formation of a white layer with compounds other than protein.

SALICYL-SULPHONIC ACID TEST.—For this test a 20 per cent. aqueous solution of salicyl-sulphonic acid is used. This solution has a higher specific gravity than that of most samples of urine. It is, therefore, most satisfactory to place a small quantity of the solution in the bottom of a test-tube—preferably a small test-tube—and then the urine is layered on to the top of the salicyl-sulphonic acid solution. The presence of protein is indicated by the development of a white ring at the junction of the two fluids, and mixing the two fluids then produces a white opalescence throughout the fluid which persists. The test is extremely sensitive and is capable of detecting as little as 5 to 10 mg. of protein per 100 ml. of urine.

ALBUSTIX.*—The test material consists of a paper strip impregnated at one end with an inert base containing tetrabromophenol blue buffered to pH.3 with a citrate buffer. This test may be performed in turbid urine without filtration. The "albustix" will react to protein with a urine pH range of 5.2 to 7.5. The paper strip is immersed in urine and if protein is present a change in colour from yellow through green to blue takes place. The amount of colour change depends on the concentration of protein in the urine. A range of colours is provided as a basis for comparison with a view to assessing the amount of protein present.

This test has been found satisfactory with two exceptions. It is not applicable to cat's urine and false reactions may be obtained with stale dog urine.

BILE

BILE PIGMENT

FOUCHET'S TEST.—For Fouchet's test two solutions are required :—

1. A 10 per cent. solution of barium chloride
2. Fouchet's Reagent—

Trichloracetic acid	25 grammes
Distilled water . . .	100 c.c.
10 per cent. ferric chloride . .	10 c.c.

If alkaline, the urine should be acidified with acetic acid. To approximately 10 c.c. of urine 5 c.c. of the barium chloride solution are added. The solutions are mixed and filtered. The filter paper is unfolded and laid flat on a dry filter paper. One drop of Fouchet's reagent is allowed

* Ames Company.

to fall on the precipitate. The appearance of a green or blue colour indicates the presence of bile pigments. The test is sensitive and has been found useful in the testing of dog's urine.

ICTOTEST.*—Five drops of urine are placed on a special thick asbestos-cellulose fibre mat. A tablet containing a stable diazo dye, sulpho-salicylic acid and sodium bicarbonate is placed on the mat moistened with urine. Two drops of water, not necessarily distilled water, are allowed to flow over the surface of the tablet. If bilirubin is present a purple colour develops on the mat around the tablet. Colour developing after half a minute is ignored.

The " ictotest " is less time-consuming than Fouchet's test but it may be more difficult to read the colour reaction.

BILE SALTS

HAY'S SULPHUR TEST.—The presence of bile salts reduces the surface tension of the urine, so that flowers of sulphur sprinkled on the surface of a column of urine sink to the bottom. With normal urine the sulphur remains floating on the surface. The slightest trace of a synthetic detergent may cause a false positive with this test.

BLOOD PIGMENT AND BLOOD

BENZIDINE TEST.—As much benzidine base as will form a saturated solution is dissolved in 2 c.c. of glacial acetic acid in a test-tube ; to this is added an equal volume of hydrogen peroxide. Then 2 c.c. of the urine are added and mixed. The appearance of a blue colour indicates the presence of blood pigment. If the urine is added drop by drop the test becomes semi-quantitative giving an approximate indication of the degree of concentration of blood pigment in the urine.

GUAIACUM TEST.—To about 2 c.c. of urine there is added five drops of freshly prepared tincture of guaiacum and then 10 per cent. ozonic alcohol is slowly added, until a blue or green colour develops or a definite excess has been added without any colour appearing. (Ozonic alcohol is prepared by mixing 10 parts of 20 vol. hydrogen peroxide with 90 parts of alcohol). The disadvantages of this test are that both reagents must be fresh, and the test carried out with old stale reagents is useless.

OCCULTEST.*—A drop of urine is placed on a piece of Whatman No. 1 filter paper and a tablet, containing orthotolidine, strontium peroxide, calcium acetate, tartaric acid and sodium bicarbonate, is placed in the centre of the paper. Two drops of water—not necessarily distilled water—are allowed to flow over the tablet. A blue colour develops around the tablet within two minutes if blood is present in the urine. Any colour appearing after two minutes is disregarded. The colour results

* Ames Company.

from the oxidation of orthotolidine due to the peroxidase activity of hæmoglobin.

As it is important to draw a distinction between blood pigment and blood this should always be done when a positive reaction to the test for blood pigment is obtained. If the quantity of blood in the urine is substantial it will settle out from the urine as a layer easily visible to the naked eye. Placing the sample of urine in a glass cylinder with a conical bottom will facilitate the detection of this separation. If the quantity of blood is small the distinction can only be achieved if the blood cells are spun down in a centrifuge and a smear for microscopic examination made from the deposits thus obtained.

SPECTROSCOPIC TEST.—The most accurate test for hæmoglobin is the spectroscopic test as the spectrum of oxyhæmoglobin can be readily identified.

SUGAR

Organismal growth may destroy sugar in urine. The tests for sugar (reducing substances) are, therefore, best applied to fresh urine. If there is likely to be any undue delay in carrying out the tests the sample of urine, while still fresh, should be boiled to destroy any organisms in it.

BENEDICT'S TEST.—For Benedict's test only one solution is required, the formula being :

Copper sulphate	17·3 grammes
Sodium citrate . . .	173·0 ,,
Anhydrous sodium carbonate . .	100·0 ,,
Water	to 1000 c.c.

The copper sulphate is dissolved in 100 c.c. of water and the sodium citrate and anhydrous sodium carbonate in 600 c.c. of water. The copper sulphate solution is added slowly to the alkaline solution and the volume is made up to 1000 c.c. with water. The reagent so made is stable and will keep indefinitely.

To 5 c.c. of Benedict's reagent in a test-tube there are added 0·5 c.c. of urine. The tube is immersed in a bath of boiling water for ten minutes. A positive test for reducing substance is given when a red, yellow or green colour develops and when, on standing, a definite coloured precipitate is formed. A green colour with no precipitate is not a positive reaction. If there is no reduction of copper with heat but a faint precipitate forms on cooling, there is only a faint trace of reducing substance present. If reduction is marked and takes place quickly, there are substantial amounts of reducing substances present. The degree of reduction and speed with which it occurs provides a rough guide to the amount of reducing substance present. Like any other qualitative test, Benedict's test is not specific for glucose (sugar) ; it only indicates the presence of a reducing substance. If necessary, the results of a positive test may be checked by means of the fermentation test.

FEHLING'S TEST.—For Fehling's test two solutions are required ; they are :

No. I solution—

Copper sulphate	.	.	.	34·64 grammes
Distilled water .	.	.	.	500 c.c.

No. II solution—

Sodium potassium tartrate .	.	.	180 grammes
Caustic soda	.	.	.	70 ,,
Distilled water .	.	.	.	500 c.c.

Immediately prior to use, equal quantities of No. I and No. II solutions are mixed and boiled ; a clear brilliant-blue solution should result. A quantity of urine equal to that formed by the mixture of No. I and No. II solutions is boiled and the hot urine is poured into the hot Fehling's solution. If appreciable quantities (*i.e.* 1 per cent. or more) of sugar are present there results an immediate precipitate of yellow copper oxide. If no precipitate occurs the whole resulting solution is brought to the boil. Should a yellow precipitate still not appear it may be taken that no appreciable quantity of sugar is present. Prolonged boiling must be avoided, as this may produce fallacies, the most frequent being that due to the presence of glycuronic acid.

If albumin is present in the urine this must be removed by boiling and filtering before applying Fehling's test.

CLINISTIX.*—One end of a paper strip is impregnated with the enzyme glucose-oxidase, orthotolidine and peroxidase. When dipped in urine and withdrawn any glucose present is oxidised in the air in the presence of the enzyme with the production of gluconic acid and hydrogen peroxide. The hydrogen peroxide then reacts with the orthotolidine in the presence of the peroxidase to produce a blue colour.

The " clinistix " being a test for glucose is more reliable in detecting a true glycosuria than other tests, such as Benedicts, which are essentially tests for reducing substances. The bottle holding the clinistix must be tightly closed to prevent deterioration of the enzyme.

CLINITEST.*—The " clinitest " tablets contain copper sulphate, sodium hydroxide, citric acid and sodium carbonate. When a tablet is dissolved in five drops of urine diluted with ten drops of water heat is generated by the sodium hydroxide going into solution, then by neutralisation of a part of it by citric acid reduction of the copper takes place if reducing substances are present. The cuprous oxide produced gives green, yellow

* Ames Company.

or orange colours similar to Benedict's test.   By comparing the resulting colour with a chart the clinitest reaction can be used as a rough quantitative test.

FERMENTATION TEST.—In view of the possibility of the fallacies that may arise with Benedict's test, Fehling's test and Nylander's test, it is always well to check the results of these tests, when positive, with a fermentation test.   The fermentation test is the most accurate test for sugar, and has the additional advantage that it is possible to differentiate between lactose and glucose.   Lactose is not fermented by yeast, but reduces Benedict's, Fehling's and Nylander's solutions.   Appreciable quantities of lactose are found in the urine of pregnant and lactating animals.   In a primiparous animal lactose appears in the urine as soon as the functional activity of the mammary gland commences.

The fermentation test is carried out with baker's yeast, which should be washed with distilled water to remove any traces of sugar.   The urine used for the test should be boiled to drive off any gas that may be in solution and to destroy any organisms that may be present.   Three tubes are so set up that any gas evolved from the contents will be collected in the upper part of the tube.   To the contents of each of the tubes a small quantity of yeast is added.   It will be found convenient to mix the yeast with the urine before filling the tubes.   The first tube contains normal urine ; in this tube no gas should be evolved, indicating that there is no admixture of glucose with the yeast.   A second tube is set up with normal urine to which glucose has been added ; in this tube gas should be evolved, indicating that the yeast is active.   In the third tube is placed the suspected urine ; evolution of gas indicates the presence of glucose. An additional refinement is to put up a fourth tube containing washed yeast and distilled water ; no gas should be evolved in this tube ; if gas is evolved the yeast has not been washed properly.   Special fermentation tubes are obtainable, but if they are not available a test-tube containing the urine can be inverted in a beaker.   In order to facilitate fermentation the tubes must be kept in a warm room.

INDICAN

JAFFE'S TEST.—A few drops of chloroform are added to some urine in a test-tube ; this is thoroughly shaken and then there is added a quantity of concentrated hydrochloric acid equal to that of the urine.   A dilute solution of bleaching powder is added drop by drop and the tube is gently shaken.   The presence of indican is shown by the development of a blue-violet colour.   The density of the colour is proportional to the amount of indican present.   The colour can be removed by the addition of excess of bleaching powder solution.   If only small quantities of indican are present the colour may make only a fleeting appearance, appearing and disappearing after the addition of only one drop of bleaching powder solution.

KETONES

ROTHERA'S TEST (MODIFIED).—The modified Rothera's reagent consists of :—

Ammonium sulphate	. . .	100 grammes
Sodium carbonate anhydrous	. .	50 ,,
Sodium nitro-prusside	. . .	3 ,,

Half an inch of the powdered reagent is placed in a dry test-tube. The urine is carefully run into the test-tube to form a layer above the reagent. Without mixing, the tube is set aside for a few minutes. The development of a permanganate colour indicates the presence of the ketone bodies, diacetic acid and acetone. This test is also effective when applied to milk. Milk gives a more accurate indication of the blood level of ketones, than urine in which ketones are concentrated.

ACETEST.*—The special tablet used for this test contains sodium nitro-prusside, disodium phosphate and lactose. A tablet is placed on a clean white surface and one drop of urine is allowed to fall on it. If the reaction is positive a purple colour develops within thirty seconds, and the intensity of the colour is proportional to the concentration of ketone bodies. This test does not appear to have any advantages over the modified Rothera's test, beyond the convenience of a ready prepared tablet. The colour reaction with positive urine is less brilliant than with Rothera's test and the reaction with milk containing ketone bodies is not always clear.

GERHARDT'S TEST.—Ferric chloride test for diacetic acid. A dilute solution of perchloride of iron is added drop by drop to some urine in a test-tube for as long as any precipitate of phosphate of iron continues to form. The urine is then filtered. To the filtrate is added a drop or two more of the ferric chloride solution. If diacetic acid is present a reddish-brown colour develops. Fallacies may occur if the animal has been receiving coal-tar antipyretics, salicylates or some other drugs, but these do not give a permanganate colour with Rothera's test. Gerhardt's test is much less sensitive than Rothera's test.

GLYCURONIC ACID

TOLLEN'S TEST.—This test will only be performed when it is desired to determine the efficiency of the liver's detoxicating function, an absence of glycuronates indicating an abnormal liver function.

To 20 c.c. of urine, 5 c.c. of 10 per cent. solution of basic lead acetate are added, and the resulting solution is filtered. Into a test-tube 10 c.c.

* Ames Company.

of the filtrate are measured, and to this are added 5 c.c. of concentrated hydrochloric acid and 1 c.c. of a 1 per cent. alcoholic solution of naphthoresorcin. The tube is heated in a boiling water bath for fifteen minutes. The tube is cooled under running water. When cold 2 c.c. of ether are added and the tube inverted several times. The ethereal layer assumes a purple tinge if glycuronates are present; their presence is not indicated by a red colour.

DEPOSITS

The deposits may be obtained by allowing a sample of urine to stand in a conical glass jar for twenty-four hours. The deposits can be obtained more rapidly by means of either a hand or an electric centrifuge. Smears are made from the deposit on a glass slide and are fixed by gentle heat. For general routine purposes staining with methylene blue is satisfactory, but special staining methods will be required to demonstrate organisms and blood cells. As the deposits in urine are chiefly of significance in the differential diagnosis of urinary disease a detailed description of their identification is given in the chapter dealing with the urinary system (Chapter VI).

BLOOD ANALYSIS

Quantitative analysis for various blood constituents provides information that in some instances may be of material assistance in differential diagnosis. The majority if not all of the methods employed in blood analysis require the facilities of a chemical laboratory. The following details of blood chemistry are therefore limited to a description of the material required, the principles of the technique employed, and the significance of the results obtained. While blood chemistry in research embraces a large number of substances, the assistance that can be obtained in diagnosis and differential diagnosis in clinical practice is virtually limited to the quantitative estimation of sugar, urea, calcium, magnesium, inorganic phosphate, bilirubin and transaminase.

The application and interpretation of blood analysis are discussed in Chapter XIX. For further details of the laboratory methods employed reference should be made to standard works in clinical chemistry as for instance, Harrison, G. A., *Chemical Methods in Clinical Chemistry*, 4th Edition, 1947, J. & A. Churchill, Ltd., London.

SUGAR

At least 2 ml. of unclotted blood is required for sugar estimations. The blood proteins are precipitated and the precipitate is removed by filtration. A measured volume of the filtrate is treated with a copper reagent and heat, a precipitate of cuprous oxide being formed. The cuprous oxide is then dissolved in a chromogenic reagent. The intensity of colour produced by the unknown is compared colorimetrically with that produced by known standard solutions of sugar.

UREA

One ml. of unclotted blood is required for urea estimation. The principle involved in urea estimations is that the urea in blood is converted into ammonium carbonate by means of the ferment " urease," the amount of ammonium carbonate formed being directly proportional to the amount of urea. A controlled alkaline solution of the iodides of mercury and potassium is used to produce a colour reaction with the ammonium carbonate. This colour reaction is read colorimetrically against the colour produced by standard solutions of ammonium sulphate.

CALCIUM

For blood calcium estimation a sample of clotted blood should be furnished to the laboratory, 5 ml. being sufficient. There are a number of methods in use for determining blood calcium.

MAGNESIUM

For blood magnesium estimation a sample of clotted blood is required, 5 ml. being sufficient. In its most severe form acute blood magnesium deficiency is characterised by a very brief illness so that the animal may not be seen until it is either moribund or dead. It is necessary to emphasise that samples of blood obtained shortly before or after death are useless for magnesium estimations.

INORGANIC PHOSPHATE

For organic phosphate estimation a sample of clotted blood is required, 5 ml. being sufficient.

BILIRUBIN

VAN DEN BERGH TEST.—Five ml. of unclotted blood is required for the Van den Bergh test.

The principle of the Van den Bergh test is that when a diazonium salt in acid solution is added to a solution of conjugated bilirubin (chole-bilirubin, *i.e.* bilirubin that has been acted on by the liver cells to produce bilirubin glycuronate) an immediate direct reaction takes place with the formation of a purple compound azo-bilirubin. The diazonium compound is formed by mixing a solution of sulphanilic acid in hydrochloric acid with sodium nitrite.

TECHNIQUE OF DIRECT TEST

Diazo Reagent

A. Sulphanilic Acid   1 gramme
   Concentrated Hydrochloric Acid   15 ml.
   Distilled Water   to 1,000 ml.
   (This solution keeps well.)

B. Sodium Nitrite   0·5 gramme
   Distilled Water   to 100 ml.
   (This solution slowly oxidises ; it should be renewed monthly.)

25 ml. of solution A are mixed with 0·75 ml. of solution B, or proportionately smaller quantities. The diazo reagent thus made will keep for one day only.

To 1 ml. of serum or plasma add 0·5 ml. of diazo reagent. Watch for colour change and note the time taken for it to develop. If the reaction is immediate the change in colour to bluish-violet begins at once and reaches its maximum in from ten to thirty seconds. If no colour change occurs within fifteen minutes the reaction is regarded as being negative.

QUANTITATIVE TEST.—The quantitative Van den Bergh test provides a means of measuring the intensity of jaundice.

The principle of the quantitative test is that the intensity of the colour due to azo-bilirubin is directly proportional to the concentration of bilirubin in the serum. As a standard for comparison with the serum in the colorimeter a solution of anhydrous cobaltous sulphate is used in place of the solution of ferri-thiocyanate previously employed. It is sometimes found difficult to secure satisfactory matching of the two solutions in the colorimeter owing to differences in tone.

With this method it is possible to express the results in terms of milligrammes of bilirubin per 100 c.c. of blood.

TRANSAMINASE

Two ml. of serum is required for transaminase estimations. It is usual to estimate both glutamic-pyruvic transaminase (G.P.T.) and glutamic-oxalo-acetic transaminase (G.O.T.).

REFERENCES

KING, J. (1958). *J. Med. Lab. Tech.* vol. xv, pp. 17-22.
KING, J. (1960). *J. Med. Lab. Tech.* vol. xvii, pp. 1-19.

COPPER

As mentioned in Chapter XIV, blood for copper estimation should be collected in special polythene bottles according to the directions of the laboratory concerned.

Copper estimations on liver biopsy specimens are a more satisfactory method of estimating the copper status of an animal than blood copper estimations.

COBALT

It is doubtful if blood cobalt estimations are of any value in clinical diagnosis.

FÆCES

PANCREATIC DEFICIENCY IN DOGS

Apart from an examination of fæces for occult blood (see p. 50) for worm eggs and larvæ (see Chapter XVII) and for bacteriological purposes, fæces from dogs are examined for evidence of pancreatic deficiency. The examination falls into three parts. In the first the fæces are examined microscopically with a view to determining whether or not the fats have been emulsified. Sometimes it is possible to see with the naked eye globules of unemulsified fat in the fæces. Secondly a smear of the fæces is examined microscopically to see whether muscle fibres in the diet have been digested. And thirdly the trypsin content of the fæces is estimated. An emulsion of the fæces is rendered slightly alkaline. Drops of serial dilutions are placed on a strip of undeveloped photographic film which is placed in an incubator providing a temperature of 37° C. Digestion of the emulsion takes place in about half-an-hour and the degree of activity can be estimated by the weakest dilution causing digestion.

TOXICOLOGICAL INVESTIGATIONS

LEAD

In the living animal the lead content of blood and fæces is estimated with a view to assisting diagnosis. In the dead animal the most useful tissue for lead estimation is the kidney since lead that has been absorbed is excreted by the kidney and during excretion is concentrated in that organ. The liver is another tissue in which absorbed lead accumulates. The ingesta are also useful. In cattle lead can be recovered from the wall of the abomasum in severe cases of acute lead poisoning. (If available samples of foodstuffs, paint or other material that could be a source of lead poisoning should be sent for analysis.)

FLUORINE

Analysis for the estimation of fluorine content is usually restricted to material from cattle and sheep. This analysis can be carried out in a sample of urine ; for this purpose not less than four ounces should be provided. Analysis to estimate the fluorine storage in tissues is usually conducted on a sample of bone. In cattle and the living animal the terminal vertebra of the tail is a suitable tissue and can conveniently be removed. Samples of herbage and other foodstuffs can be analysed for their fluorine content.

ORGANO-PHOSPHORUS COMPOUNDS

The organo-phosphorus insecticides inhibit cholinesterase the enzyme that hydrolyses acetylcholine. The effect then produced is one of overactivity of the parasympathetic system.

Laboratory demonstration of a fall in blood cholinesterase level will provide supporting evidence of poisoning by organo-phosphorus insecticides. The principle underlying blood cholinesterase estimation is the production of acetic acid by the interaction between acetyl choline and the cholinesterase present in the sample.

The amount of acetic acid produced is estimated colorimetrically using bromothymol blue as an indicator or chromogenic agent.

BRACKEN

Bracken poisoning in horses is caused by a thermo-labile anti-thiamine factor. In consequence there is a reduction in the blood thiamine content in clinical cases of bracken poisoning in horses. If the clinical findings are not conclusive a sample of clotted blood may be provided for blood thiamine estimation.

Bracken poisoning in cattle is associated with a toxic factor causing bone marrow damage. This results in a leucopoenia and thrombocytopoenia ; these can be demonstrated in samples of blood.

For further details of the diagnosis of various forms of poisoning reference should be made to a standard text-book on veterinary toxicology such as Garner, R. J., *Veterinary Toxicology*. Baillière, Tindall & Cox, London. 1957.

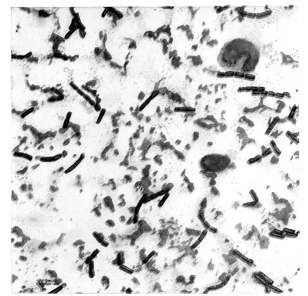

FIG. 34.—Anthrax bacilli in blood smear stained polychrome methylene blue. × 1000.

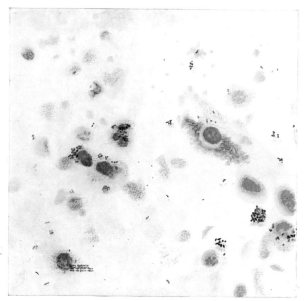

FIG. 35.—*Brucella abortus* smear from cotyledon stained differential Carbo-Fuchsin. × 1000.

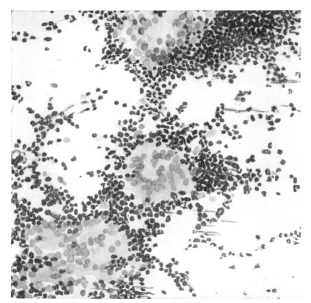

FIG. 36.—Tuberculous mastitis deposit, cell groups, stained Ziehl-Neelsen (low power).

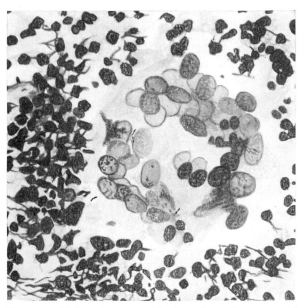

FIG. 37.—Tuberculous mastitis deposit, cell groups and tubercle bacilli, stained Ziehl-Neelsen. × 1000.

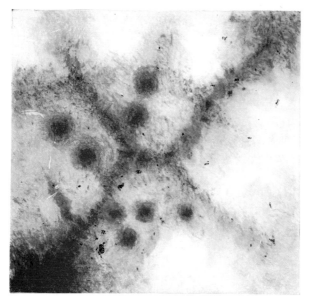

Fig. 38.—Johne's bacilli in fæces, stained Ziehl-Neelsen. × 1000.

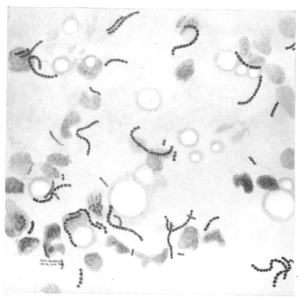

Fig. 39.—Streptococcal mastitis, smear of incubated milk, stained Newman. × 1000.

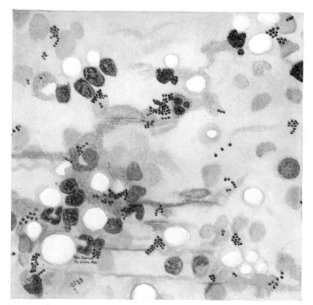

FIG. 40.—Staphylococcal mastitis, smear of incubated milk, stained Newman. × 1000.

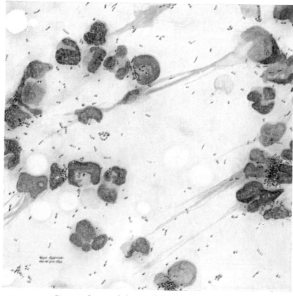

FIG. 41.—Corynebacterial mastitis, smear of incubated milk, stained Newman. × 1000.

CHAPTER XVI

CLINICAL BACTERIOLOGY

Staining methods : Methylene Blue—Gram—Ziehl-Neelsen—Newman —Stain for *Brucella abortus*
Examination for *B. anthracis*—*M. tuberculosis*—*M. paratuberculosis*— Mastitis organisms—*Brucella abortus*—*Coccidia*—*Leptospiræ* in Urine —*Salmonella* in Fæces
Agglutination Tests for Contagious Bovine Abortion—Salmonellosis— Leptospirosis—Bacillary White Diarrhœa—Actinobacillosis
Complement-Fixation Tests for Johne's Disease—Foot-and-Mouth Disease—Canine Contagious Hepatitis
Hæmagglutination Inhibition Test for Fowl Pest

STAINING METHODS

LÖFFLER'S METHYLENE BLUE.—Löffler's methylene blue solution contains :—

Saturated solution of methylene blue in alcohol . . . . 30 c.c.
1/10,000 solution of caustic potash in water . 100 c.c.

(*Note.*—A 1/10,000 solution of caustic potash is made by adding 1 c.c. of 1 per cent. solution of caustic potash to 99 c.c. of water.)

Technique.—The slide is flooded with the stain, which is allowed to act for three minutes or longer ; the stain is then washed off with water.

POLYCHROME METHYLENE BLUE.—Löffler's methylene blue solution slowly assumes polychrome characters ; this process of " ripening " may take twelve months to complete. Polychrome methylene blue may be prepared more rapidly by dissolving 1 gramme of methylene blue powder in 100 c.c. of 0·5 per cent. solution of bicarbonate of soda ; the solution is gently heated and filtered when cold. In the process of ripening new violet compounds are formed by oxidation ; this takes place more rapidly in an alkaline solution of methylene blue than in Löffler's solution.

Technique.—The technique of staining with polychrome methylene blue is the same as with Löffler's stain. In preparing blood films for the demonstration of *Bacillus anthracis* the film is allowed to dry in the air and the slide is then passed through a flame two or three times.

GRAM'S STAIN

For routine staining the following solutions have been found to give the most reliable results.

Solution A. Methyl Violet.—
Methyl violet 6 B Powder . . . 0·5 gramme
Distilled water . . . . . 100 c.c.

The methyl violet is dissolved in the water and the solution filtered. The filtered solution will keep indefinitely but should be filtered again before use.

Solution B. Iodine.—

Iodine crystals .	. . .	1 gramme
Potassium iodide	. .	2 grammes
Distilled water .	. . .	100 c.c.

Solution C. Dilute Carbol Fuchsin.—

Ziehl-Neelsen's carbol fuchsin	.	1 part
Distilled water .	. . .	9 parts

Technique.—The fixed preparation on the slide is flooded with the methyl violet solution, which is allowed to act for 2-3 minutes. The excess stain is poured off the slide. With the slide held at a slant the iodine solution is poured down it so that the methyl violet is washed away by the iodine. The iodine is then allowed to act for one minute. Again holding the slide at a slant the iodine is washed off with absolute alcohol or methylated spirits ; the application of spirit being continued until no further colour comes from the main mass of the preparation. The degree of discoloration is most easily seen if the slide is held over a white sink or some other suitable white background. Colour emerging from any very thick portions of the preparation should be ignored, and so should colour appearing at the edges of the film. Some practice is necessary to avoid excessive decolorisation. The preparation is now thoroughly washed in water. The dilute carbol fuchsin is applied as a counter-stain for 15 seconds. The counter-stain is removed by washing in water, and the slide allowed to drain or is dried with fluffless blotting paper.

If Gram's staining method is properly carried out, Gram-positive organisms and fibrin are stained a deep violet colour by the methyl violet, and Gram-negative organisms, together with the nuclei and protoplasm of pus cells and tissue cells are stained a pink colour by the counter-stain. The Gram-positive and Gram-negative organisms of veterinary importance are :—

Gram-positive	*Gram-negative*
Actinomyces	Actinobacillus
Erysipelothrix	Pfeifferella mallei
Corynebacterium	Pseudomonas
Streptococci	Proteus
Staphylococci	Fusiformis
Bacillus anthracis and spore-bearing aerobes	Salmonella
	Brucella
Clostridium tetani	Coliform organisms
,, welchii	Pasteurella
,, septique	
,, chauvœi	
and other clostridia	

ZIEHL-NEELSEN'S STAIN

Ziehl-Neelsen's method of staining is used to demonstrate the presence of acid-fast organisms. The solutions required for this method are :—

Ziehl-Neelsen's Carbol Fuchsin (strong).—
Basic fuchsin powder . . . . 1 gramme
Absolute alcohol . . . . . 10 c.c.
5 per cent. aqueous solution of carbolic
acid . . . . 100 c.c.

The basic fuchsin is dissolved in the alcohol and this solution is added to the carbolic acid solution.

Decolourising Agents.—
Either 20 per cent. aqueous solution of sulphuric acid ;
or 3 per cent. solution of hydrochloric acid in absolute alcohol ;
or 1 per cent. solution of sulphuric acid in absolute alcohol.

Counter-stain.—Löffler's methylene blue.

Technique.—The strong solution of carbol fuchsin is poured on to the slide through a filter paper to remove any granules of stain. The slide should be flooded with stain. The slide is then gently heated with a flame until steam rises. The hot stain is allowed to act for five minutes, the heating process being repeated as often as may be required, if necessary more stain being added to prevent the surface becoming dry. The preparation is washed in water and decolourised by flooding with one of the acid solutions which is allowed to act for about one minute, and is then removed by washing. The process of using the acid solution and washing is repeated until the preparation assumes a faint pink colour. (If acid alone has been used as a decolourising agent the preparation may now be treated with absolute alcohol or methylated spirits for 2-3 minutes.) The preparation is thoroughly washed in water and counter-stained with Löffler's methylene blue for ½-3 minutes according to the thickness of the smear or tissue on the slide. The counter-stain is washed off and the preparation drained, or dried with fluffless blotting paper.

NEWMAN'S STAIN

Newman's stain contains :—

Methylene blue powder . . . . 1·2 grammes
95 per cent. ethyl alcohol . . . 54 c.c.
Tetrachlorethane . . . . . 40 c.c.
Glacial acetic acid . . . . 6 c.c.

The methylene blue is thoroughly dissolved in the alcohol and the other ingredients are then added.

(Xylol or chloroform may be substituted for the tetrachlorethane, when the stain will give equally good results.)

Technique.—Newman's stain is used to demonstrate the organisms, other than *Mycobacterium tuberculosis*, present in cases of mastitis. The smear made from the milk requires to be freshly prepared. The smear is allowed to dry and is then immersed in Newman's staining solution for 5 minutes. The staining solution fixes the preparation, extracts the fat and stains simultaneously. After the period of immersion the preparation is thoroughly washed and allowed to drain and dry in the air.

DIFFERENTIAL STAIN FOR THE DEMONSTRATION OF *Brucella abortus*
SOLUTIONS required :—

  A. Dilute Carbol Fuchsin (as in Gram's stain)—
       Ziehl-Neelsen's carbol fuchsin   .   . 1 part
       Distilled water   .   .   .   .   . 9 parts
  B. Acetic Acid—
       ½ per cent. solution in distilled water.
  C. Löffler's Methylene Blue.

Technique.—The slide is flooded with the dilute carbol fuchsin and this is allowed to stain for 15 minutes. The slide is then immersed in the ½ per cent. acetic acid solution, or the solution is poured down the slide held at a slant. The acid must not be allowed to act for more than ten seconds. The proper use of the acid is necessary for differentiation. The preparation is washed thoroughly, counter-stained with Löffler's methylene blue for one minute, rinsed free of stain and dried.

EXAMINATION FOR ANTHRAX BACILLI

In cattle and sheep films are prepared with blood taken from an ear vein that has been incised ; after the blood has been obtained the incision on the ear should be sealed by searing with a piece of iron heated to a dull red heat. The blood film, which should be of moderate thickness, is allowed to dry on the slide and then the slide is held three times in a flame, with the film upwards, for one second. The effect of this method of fixing is to cause some disintegration of the bacillary capsules. The fixing of the film by heat must not be overdone or the film is fixed too completely and disintegration of the capsules does not occur. As in anthrax in the horse, bacilli may be present in the blood, it is well to examine a blood film in suspected cases. In the pig bacilli are not usually present in the blood in sufficient numbers for them to be demonstrated microscopically. In the acute intestinal form of anthrax in pigs death may take place very rapidly without invasion of the blood stream by anthrax bacilli. When the intestinal lesion has been sufficiently severe to cause death there is usually peritonitis. If a small incision is made through the abdominal wall and a sterile swab is introduced into the peritoneal cavity organisms can usually be recovered in smears made from the peritoneal fluid thus obtained. If œdematous swellings of the throat are present in horses, pigs or dogs, organisms may be found in smears made from the œdematous fluid, but the organisms may only be present in the fluid in very small numbers. In these cases anthrax bacilli will be found more readily in smears made from the cut surface of the freshly incised regional lymphatic gland. The addition of a drop of blood to a smear made from œdematous fluid or the cut surface of a lymphatic gland appears to assist the capsular staining reaction.

Films for the demonstration of anthrax bacilli are stained with polychrome methylene blue. Anthrax bacilli are large bacilli with sharply cut or slightly concave ends ; these are disposed singly, in pairs or in short chains. In a film prepared and stained as described there is an amorphous or granular material scattered between the bacilli, stained violet or reddish purple. This material is the capsule disintegrated by the method of imperfect fixation. In some cases the colour reaction is sufficiently pronounced to be recognised by the naked eye. This staining reaction is of great assistance in distinguishing anthrax bacilli from putrefactive organisms that may be present in blood films. Putrefactive organisms frequently occur in long chains and may show centrally located spores. Sporulation of anthrax bacilli does not occur in the body of an animal.

The name of McFadyean is associated with this method of staining anthrax bacilli, the colour phenomenon being known as the McFadyean reaction. McFadyean pointed out that it is not necessary to use an alkaline polychrome methylene blue to obtain this reaction, and stated that it can be obtained with a simple aqueous solution of methylene blue. He attributed the staining reaction to the traces of methylene azure which are almost always present in methylene blue.

EXAMINATION FOR TUBERCLE BACILLI

SPUTUM.—The sputum is spread on the slide with the blade of a sterile scalpel ; organisms are more likely to be found in a thick viscid portion of sputum than in clear mucoid material. The film is fixed by heat. Films of sputum are stained by Ziehl-Neelsen's method and examined microscopically. The presence of acid-fast organisms in a smear of sputum, if taken in conjunction with symptoms and clinical signs of tuberculosis, is dependable evidence of the existence of tuberculosis of the respiratory tract. Failure to demonstrate tubercle bacilli in a smear of sputum does not eliminate the possibility of tuberculosis, as the organisms are not necessarily present in every portion of the expectorate.

PLEURAL OR PERITONEAL FLUID.—In suspected cases of tuberculosis in dogs and cats with either pleural or peritoneal effusion fluid should be withdrawn by paracentesis. This fluid must be spun in a centrifuge and smears made from the deposit, these being stained by Ziehl-Neelsen's method. In these cases tubercle bacilli may not be present in the fluid in sufficient numbers for them to be found by microscopic examination of stained smears. It may therefore be necessary to resort to biological methods.

MILK.—The sample of milk is spun in an electric centrifuge for three minutes at 2000 revolutions, or in a hand centrifuge for six minutes at 1000 revolutions per minute. The cream is removed from the top of the centrifuge tube and the supernatant fluid poured off. Some of the deposit is removed with a platinum loop—previously sterilised by heating to red heat in a flame—and a thin smear is made on a glass slide. The film is allowed to dry in air and fixed by gentle heat. Before staining milk smears it is advisable to " defat " them to facilitate the staining. This is done by flooding the slide with a solution composed of equal parts of ether and absolute alcohol, which is allowed to act for thirty seconds ; the slide is then washed in water and the staining process carried out. Films of the deposit of milk for the demonstration of tubercle bacilli are stained by Ziehl-Neelsen's method.

Before examining the milk smear with an oil-immersion lens for tubercle bacilli, the preparation should be inspected with the low power ($\frac{1}{2}$ inch objective) for the presence of cell groups. The cells which form these groups are the so-called epithelioid cells ; these are larger than the other cells found in the sediment from milk. They stain lightly with the counter-stain, but show a number of darker nuclear areas scattered throughout the cell. It is a characteristic peculiarity of the deposit from tuberculous milk that these epithelioid cells are arranged in groups. Matthews described these groups as occurring in three fairly distinct types. In the round cell group the cells are arranged in a circle. In a cell mass the cells are closely packed together piled on each other. In a loose cell group the cells, though aggregated together, are not in close contact with one another. Any preparation of tuberculous milk may contain cell groups of one or all these types. In addition to being characteristic of tuberculous milk these cell groups are of importance in that tubercle bacilli are very frequently found within or around them. Tubercle bacilli are more commonly found in connection with the round cell group or the cell mass than in connection with the loose cell group. It would appear that the likelihood of finding tubercle bacilli in a microscopic field is directly proportional to the number of epithelioid cells present. When stained with Ziehl-Neelsen's method, tubercle bacilli appear as slender straight rods stained a light red colour ; they are disposed singly, in pairs, or in groups like a bundle of faggots. Cellular or other elements in the smear are stained blue with the counter-stain. The final criterion of the absence of tubercle bacilli in a sample of milk is a negative biological test.

URINE.—Urine is thoroughly spun in the centrifuge, and films are made from the deposit.

FÆCES.—The direct microscopic examination of stained smears of fæces is of little or no use in the detection of tubercle bacilli owing to the difficulty of distinguishing between the various acid-fast organisms. If it is desirable to ascertain whether tubercle bacilli are present in the fæces, a sample should be forwarded to a bacteriological laboratory.

EXAMINATION FOR JOHNE'S BACILLUS

The sample of fæces is passed through a fine wire gauze sieve to remove grosser vegetable particles. The fæces are centrifuged for 15 minutes at 1000 revolutions and smears made from the deposit. The smears are stained by Ziehl-Neelsen's method. The organisms (*Mycobacterium paratuberculosis* or Johne's bacillus) form clumps or groups of short acid-fast organisms. Organisms can be demonstrated microscopically from fæcal preparations in a high proportion of clinical cases of Johne's disease, but the method is not infallible. Smears may be made from material obtained by scraping the mucous membrane of a suspected portion of bowel discovered during the course of a post-mortem examination.

EXAMINATION FOR MASTITIS ORGANISMS

Smears may be made from the deposits obtained by centrifuging fresh samples of milk. The best results are obtained when the sample of milk is incubated for 18 hours at 37° C. (98·6° F.). If an incubator is not available, satisfactory results will be obtained if the sample of milk is kept in a dark warm place where the temperature is reasonably constant. When incubated the sample of milk is thoroughly shaken and two or three loopfuls of the whole milk are smeared thinly on to a slide. If individual samples have been taken from the four quarters of the udder, a slide may be divided into four by means of transverse lines drawn with a grease pencil ; the smears from each of the four quarters are then made on the same slide. The smear is allowed to dry and is stained with Newman's stain.

Bacteria and cells are stained blue by Newman's stain, the diagnosis being made on the morphology of the organisms present. Long and short chained streptococci, with varying numbers of polymorphonuclear cells, indicates streptococcal mastitis ; the number of cells present indicates the severity of the inflammatory reaction. Grape-like clusters of cocci with numerous polymorphs indicates staphylococcal mastitis.

Clumps of small bacilli or cocco-bacilli, usually in large numbers with numerous polymorphonuclear cells, indicates a *Corynebacterium pyogenes* infection.

This method of staining milk smears is useful for ascertaining the organisms present in cases of mastitis, especially in acute cases. Diagnosis of the bacterial cause of the mastitis makes it possible to select suitable treatment. The method is one that can readily be applied in veterinary practice, facilitating the early adoption of appropriate treatment. The method has the advantage that it reduces the time and labour required to the simple procedure of making the smear and immersing it in the staining fluid.

EXAMINATION FOR *Brucella Abortus*

Smears are made from vaginal discharge, from the fresh surface of a cotyledon, or from the foetal stomach content. The smear is fixed by heat and stained with dilute carbol fuchsin, differential decolorisation is carried out with ½ per cent. acetic acid, and the preparation is counter-stained with Löffler's methylene blue. *Brucella abortus* organisms are stained red by this method, and may be identified by their small size and their appearance in groups usually in appreciable numbers. Other organisms are stained by the counter-stain.

COCCIDIOSIS

The diagnosis of coccidiosis in cattle, sheep, rabbits and poultry is based on the demonstration of oöcysts in the fæces. The mere demonstration of oöcysts in the fæces does not justify a diagnosis of coccidiosis. When associated with disease the oöcysts are present in the fæces in large numbers and this finding should be considered in relation to the clinical signs. This may be done by making direct smears or by a concentration method such as Sheather's sugar flotation method described in Chapter XVII.

The examination should be made with the high power (⅛ inch objective) of the microscope.

The oöcysts in cattle measure 13-28 μ by 12-20 μ; in rabbits they are rather smaller, and in sheep and poultry they are rather longer.

During the course of a post-mortem examination, scrapings may be made from the intestinal mucous membrane with a view to demonstrating oöcysts, smears being made from the material thus obtained.

LEPTOSPIRÆ IN URINE

During the acute phase of canine infection with *Leptospira canicola* the organisms can be demonstrated in the urine in a high proportion of cases. They are usually present in sufficient numbers that microscopic examination by dark-ground illumination of a drop of urine makes it possible to reveal the freely motile segmented organisms. Demonstration of the organisms in films stained with Indian ink has failed to give satisfactory results.

SALMONELLA IN FÆCES

The identification of Salmonella in the fæces of any of the domestic animals requires the facilities provided in an adequately equipped bacteriological laboratory. It has been shown that Salmonellosis in cattle is prevalent in many parts of Great Britain and that the disease also occurs in other species.

AGGLUTINATION TESTS

Since some days must elapse before agglutinins are formed an agglutination test will not assist differential diagnosis in the early stages of acute infections. During the course of disease the formation of agglutinins producing a rising titre provides a method of confirming a tentative diagnosis where it has not been possible to demonstrate the causal organism. Agglutination tests are a valuable method of diagnosis in chronic disease and also in the detection of carrier animals the removal of which is desired in order to eradicate a source of infection. Agglutination tests used regularly in veterinary diagnosis are those concerned with contagious bovine abortion, salmonellosis, leptospirosis and bacillary white diarrhœa. In carrying out agglutination tests the laboratory uses serum from the blood sample supplied ; this must be free from contaminating organisms and hæmoglobin. The sample of blood should therefore be withdrawn from the vein with due regard to asepsis and should be allowed to form a firm clot before being despatched to the laboratory.

CONTAGIOUS BOVINE ABORTION

The agglutination test against *Brucella abortus* is employed to detect infected animals regardless of whether they have actually aborted. Following the act of normal parturition or of abortion agglutinins may be absent from the blood for a month or even longer so in these circumstances a negative agglutination is not of diagnostic significance. A single negative agglutination test is not necessarily significant since the animal may have been recently infected and agglutinins may not yet be present in the blood.

In the interpretation of the agglutination test for contagious abortion if there is no agglutination or agglutination at a titre of 1 in 10 but not above, the animal is considered to have passed the test. If agglutination occurs at a titre of 1 in 20 but not above the result is considered indefinite and the animal should be retested. If agglutination occurs at a titre of 1 in 40 or over the animal has failed the test. This interpretation applies in Great Britain using the standard antigen there available and may be varied in the future as it has been in the past. Retests in recently calved or aborted animals should be delayed for a month ; in other animals the interval may be reduced if the prevailing circumstances appear to render this desirable.

Whey can be used for an agglutination test, which is conducted in the same way as with serum. As antibodies are concentrated in the colostrum the whey agglutination test will give higher titres shortly before and soon after parturition than in mid-lactation.

The Milk Ring test is used as screening test to detect infected herds. It is a sensitive test that can be applied to a sample of milk obtained from the bulked produce of the herd.

Stained antigen is mixed in a tube with the milk and incubated for half an hour. The brucella are clumped by agglutinins if present and the clumps are brought up by the fat globules to form a coloured ring above the remainder of the milk.

SALMONELLOSIS

The agglutination test is employed to detect carrier adult animals. Field (1948) has shown that young cattle recovered from an attack of Salmonellosis do not continue to harbour the organisms, and agglutinins are lost from the blood. Adult cattle recovering from the disease and those which have passed through a subclinical attack harbour the organisms and agglutinins persist in their blood.

Further work is required before the criteria for interpretation of the agglutination test can be defined exactly. Some laboratories regard agglutination at a titre of higher than 1 in 80 as indicative of a past infection. Field (1948) stated that in normal adult cattle the flagellar agglutination titre is not usually higher than 1 in 160 and the somatic titre than 1 in 40. He suggests that the clearest results are obtained by using the flagellar antigen and that a flagellar titre greater than 1 in 320 can be taken as evidence that the animal is a carrier.

LEPTOSPIROSIS

The agglutination tests against *Leptospira canicola* and *Leptospira icterohæmorrhagiæ* can be used to detect those animals that have passed through an attack of either of these diseases ; in the case of acute illness a rising titre over a period of seven days indicates the presence of leptospirosis and renders possible a differentiation between the two species mentioned and also between other species of leptospiræ.

McIntyre and Stuart (1949) have shown that during the invasive stage of the illness due to infection with *Leptospira canicola* the agglutination titre rises from nothing to 1 in 1000. In the primary renal stage the agglutination titre reaches 1 in 10,000 or there is a distinct rise in titre between successive examinations at a week's interval. In the secondary renal stage of the disease the agglutination titre may attain a dilution of 1 in 3000. Following recovery the agglutination titre gradually falls over a period of several months, until a comparatively low level, such as 1 in 30, is reached ; this low level may persist for several years if not for the rest of the dog's life.

Similarly in infections with *Leptospira icterohæmorrhagiæ* the agglutination titre rises and then falls.

In any form of leptospirosis acute illness may terminate in death before there has been time for the substantial production of agglutinins.

BACILLARY WHITE DIARRHŒA

The agglutination test is employed to detect carrier hens that are capable of transmitting infection through the egg to the chick. Two forms of the test are used, the tube test carried out in a laboratory and the rapid plate test carried out in the field (see Chapter XXI).

ACTINOBACILLOSIS

The agglutination test has been employed to assist in the differential diagnosis of actinobacillosis involving thoracic and abdominal organs in cattle. Due to antigenic variation among strains of *Actinobacillus lignieresi*, difficulties have been encountered in the clinical application of the test, but there are hopes that these may be overcome.

REFERENCES

BRENNAN, A. D. J. (1953). "Anthrax with Special Reference to the Recent Outbreaks." *Vet. Record*, vol. lxv, pp. 255-258.
FIELD, H. I. (1948). "A Survey of Bovine Salmonellosis in Mid and West Wales." *Vet. J.*, vol. xiv, pp. 251-266, 294-302 and 323-339.
McINTYRE, W. I. M., and STUART, R. D. (1949). "Canine Leptospirosis." *Vet. Record*, vol. lxi, pp. 411-414.
MATTHEWS, H. T. (1931). "The Microscopic Examination of Milk for Tubercle Cell Groups." *Vet. Record*, vol. xliii, No. 15, pp. 403-405.
ROWLANDS, W. T., and FIELD, H. I. (1943). "The Examination of Milk Samples for Mastitis." *Vet. Record*, vol. lv, No. 52, pp. 495-497.

BIBLIOGRAPHY

MACKIE, T. J., and McCARTNEY, J. E. (1960). Ed : Cruickshank, R. *Handbook of Bacteriology*. E. & S. Livingstone, Edinburgh.

COMPLEMENT FIXATION TESTS

As a means of assisting diagnosis in the living animal the complement fixation test is carried out on serum. The blood sample should be obtained from the vein with due regard to asepsis and should be allowed to clot before being dispatched to the laboratory.

JOHNE'S DISEASE

The possible value of the complement fixation test for the diagnosis of Johne's disease has been under investigation for several years. Hole (1952), reporting his observations, said that in animals free from tuberculosis the test had proved a valuable aid in the confirmation of the disease in suspected cases. Even in cases where examination of fæces for the bacilli of Johne's disease has proved negative, positive results with the complement fixation test have subsequently been justified. Hopes that the complement fixation test would prove a reasonably accurate method of detecting animals suffering from a sub-clinical infection have not been realised. It is known that a considerable interval elapses between infection and the development of a serological response ; this was thought to be as long as nine months, but experience has shown that the serological response may not develop until the animal becomes clinically affected. Passive transfer of antibodies from an infected cow may give rise to a transitory serological reaction in a calf, but Hole (1952) reports only encountering such reactions in calves less than nine months old.

FOOT AND MOUTH DISEASE

The workers at the Foot and Mouth Disease Research Institute at Pirbright have perfected a method of using the complement fixation test, both as a means of showing the presence of foot and mouth virus and as a means of determining the immunological types of virus strains.

CANINE CONTAGIOUS HEPATITIS

The complement fixation test has been used in the diagnosis of canine contagious hepatitis, but there are a number of difficulties in its application. The test may be applied to tissues and body fluids removed from a dog which has died. For satisfactory results, these materials should reach the laboratory within 24 hours of death. The complement fixation test can be applied to blood removed from living animals but is of little value during the time of the acute clinical illness as the antibody content of the serum has not had time to develop. Samples taken two to four weeks after the phase of acute illness may, by means of the complement fixation test, show that the dog had suffered from the disease. If the disease is thought to exist in a kennel, the demonstration of high complement fixation titres, in apparently normal dogs, would indicate that the animals had passed through a subclinical attack of the disease. It is also possible that carrier animals might be detected by the complement fixation test but the difficulty then would be to distinguish between carrier and convalescent animals.

REFERENCES

Johne's Disease

HOLE, N. H. (1952). "Johne's Disease. Present-Day Diagnosis and a Preliminary Note on an Investigation into the Value of a Serological Method." *Vet. Record*, vol. lxiv, pp. 601-603.

Foot and Mouth Disease

Agricultural Research Council (1952). Foot and Mouth Disease Research. Interim Report. Research Institute, Pirbright. H.M.S.O., London.

Canine Contagious Hepatitis

HODGMAN, S. F. J., and LARIN, N. M. (1953). "Diagnosis of Canine Virus Hepatitis." *Vet. Record*, vol. lxv, pp. 447-450.
LARIN, N. M. (1951). "Studies on the Agent of Canine Virus Hepatitis. Complement Fixation and Precipitin Tests." *J. Hyg.*, vol. xlix, pp. 410-426.

HÆMAGGLUTINATION INHIBITION TEST

The virus of Fowl Pest (Newcastle disease or avian pneumo-encephalitis), when mixed with washed blood cells, causes them to clump or agglutinate. If the serum from fowls convalescent from Fowl Pest is added to the mixture of virus and washed red blood cells, the clumping or agglutination is prevented. This hæmagglutination inhibition is not caused by serum from healthy birds or by serum from birds suffering from any other disease. For convenience of description the test is often referred to as the H.I. test. The property of inhibiting agglutination is developed in the serum of infected fowls about 48 hours after the appearance of clinical signs. Its concentration in the serum increases slowly during the next two days and thereafter increases rapidly to reach a maximum greatly in excess of the original value.

REFERENCE

Handbook on Poultry Diseases. N.V.M.A. Publication No. 15. Second Edition, 1948. British Veterinary Association, London.

IDENTIFICATION OF BACTERIAL TOXINS

In the enterotoxæmic diseases of sheep identification of the specific clostridial toxin may be required before a definite diagnosis can be established. The material required by the laboratory for this investigation is intestinal contents. These should be removed from the intestine to a suitable container and a small quantity of chloroform added to control destruction of the toxin. The filtrate of such material is used to inoculate small laboratory animals some of which have been protected with specific anti-toxin. It is then possible to determine which specific anti-toxin protected against a challenging injection of unknown toxin. Positive results must obviously depend on survival of the particular toxin in the intestinal contents.

IDENTIFICATION OF VIRUS INFECTIONS

The identification of specific virus infections can be carried out in three ways. As already mentioned when a suitable technique is available the complement fixation test may be used. Experimental inoculation of susceptible animals with a view to producing the specific disease may be employed. This is dependent on obtaining suitable infective material. In some diseases the causal virus is present in the blood at the height of the febrile reaction, e.g. louping ill and distemper. In others the causal virus can be recovered from local lesions, e.g. the fluid from vesicles or fresh epithelium from the surface of vesicles in foot and mouth disease or material from the lesions of orf (contagious pustular dermatitis) if removed before they have become grossly contaminated with secondary invaders. The presence of antibodies may be demonstrated in the serum of convalescent or recovered animals. If the identification of a virus infection is required it is desirable to consult the laboratory concerned as to the material required and the methods of collection and transport.

CHAPTER XVII

CLINICAL HELMINTHOLOGY

Fæces :—Macroscopic Examination—Microscopic Examination—Direct
Smears—Concentration Methods—Egg-Counting Technique—Ex-
amination of Larvæ
Identification of Eggs and Larvæ—Interpretation of Worm-egg Counts
Examination of Sputum—Post-Mortem Examination for Helminth
Parasites—Pathogenicity Table

EXAMINATION OF FÆCES

I. Naked Eye Examination

DIRECT examination of the fæces by the naked eye will reveal the presence
of tape-worm segments. If diarrhœa is present the segments are more
easily seen ; in doubtful cases a purgative will expel the segments in
greater numbers and these are readily seen in contrast to the fluid fæces.
It is only occasionally that round worms are seen in the fæces ; very
heavy round worm infestations may be present in any of the domestic
animals without any worms being seen in the fæces. In *Oxyuris* infestation in the horse the ovigerous female or dead females that have laid
their eggs may be seen in the fæces. As the ovigerous *Oxyuris* female
attaches herself to the skin of the perineum to lay her eggs, diagnosis of
Oxyuris infestation is established by an inspection of the perineum.

II. Direct or Simple Smear

Though this is the simplest and quickest method of examining fæces
microscopically for the presence of worm eggs or larvæ, it cannot be
depended on to detect small infestations except in the case of those
species that are very prolific in their egg laying capacity. It is probable
that any infestation with *Hæmonchus contortus* that is sufficiently heavy
to cause illness can be detected by a direct smear.

In the pig, dog and cat the direct smear may be used to demonstrate
the presence of ascarid eggs. The finding of even one egg is sufficient
to establish infestation with this parasite, but no estimate as to the severity
of the infestation can be based on the number of eggs present in the
smear. Further, the absence of an infestation is not established by
negative findings in a direct smear.

Though the larvae of worms parasitic in the respiratory tract are
coughed up into the pharynx, swallowed and passed through the alimentary canal, they are not likely to be sufficiently numerous in the fæces

335

for them to be detected in direct smears of fæces. The technique described on page 322 should be used for this purpose.

TECHNIQUE.—The direct smear is made by mixing a small portion of fæces with a drop of water on a slide until a uniform suspension is secured. Any large pieces of solid matter must be removed. The film of fæcal suspension is covered with a cover-slip and examined with the low power of a microscope (⅔-inch objective).

III. CONCENTRATION METHODS

If direct smears do not reveal any eggs one of the following concentration methods may be employed to determine the presence of infestations not sufficiently heavy to ensure eggs being found by direct smear.

EXAMINATION OF SEDIMENT.—A representative sample of fæces about the size of a walnut is thoroughly mixed with water to form a suspension ; this is passed through a fine wire sieve into a 100 c.c. cylinder. The cylinder is filled with water, well shaken and allowed to stand for thirty minutes. The supernatant fluid is poured off ; the cylinder is again filled with water, well shaken and allowed to stand for thirty minutes. The process is repeated a third time. After the supernatant fluid has been poured off some of the sediment is drawn into a pipette and transferred to a slide. A coverslip is placed on the sediment and the preparation examined with a ⅔-inch objective. The method is the most convenient one for the demonstration of fluke eggs.

FLOTATION METHOD.—In this method the eggs are floated to the top of a column of fluid, the density of which is sufficiently high to ensure rapid flotation of the eggs ; for this purpose a saturated solution of sodium chloride or a solution containing 1 lb. of cane sugar in 12 fluid ounces of water may be used. One part of fæces is made into a uniform suspension with ten parts of the flotation liquid ; the suspension is passed through a fine wire gauze sieve and placed in a tall glass cylinder. This is allowed to stand for from fifteen minutes to half an hour. A cover-slip is then lowered on to the top of the column of liquid so that it just touches the surface of the fluid and the upper layer is removed with the cover-slip. To do this the cover-slip may be held in a pair of forceps, or a small cylinder of plasticine may be used to form a " handle " attached to the upper side of the cover-slip. The cover-slip with the hanging drop of fluid is lowered on to a glass slide and the preparation is examined microscopically.

REFERENCE

SHEATHER, A. L. (1924). " The Detection of Worm Eggs and Protozoa in the Fæces of Animals." *Vet. Record*, vol. iv, No. 26, pp. 552-555.

IV. Egg-counting Technique

The Gordon-Whitlock Technique (Modified).—Though devised for the examination of sheep fæces, this method has been found satisfactory for egg-counting in samples of fæces from all species of animals. The method is not, however, suitable for the demonstration of fluke eggs, which are of too high a specific gravity to rise in the suspending fluid.

Apparatus required :

Simple balance to weigh 2 grammes of fæces.
Measuring cylinder of at least 60 c.c. capacity.
Saturated solution of sodium chloride.
Fine wire gauze sieve.
Evaporating dish large enough to contain sieve and 60 c.c. of fluid.
Spoon.
Blunt pipette (8 mm. bore) with rubber teat.
Gordon-Whitlock Special Egg-counting slide as described on page 338.

Technique :

Two grammes of fæces are weighed and placed in the sieve which is sitting in the evaporating dish. With the measuring cylinder 60 c.c. of the saturated salt solution are measured. Half of this quantity is poured over the fæces and with the spoon the fæces are macerated through the sieve to form a suspension in the dish. Any residue left in the sieve is washed with the remainder of the salt solution, the washings passing into the dish. The special counting slide is prepared by breathing on it so that the surfaces are moistened and filling of the chambers is facilitated. The fæcal suspension is thoroughly stirred with the spoon and without delay the pipette is filled and one chamber of the special slide charged with suspension. The residue in the pipette is discarded, the suspension re-stirred, and the pipette again filled to charge the second chamber.

The slide is placed on the mechanical stage of a microscope and using a $\frac{2}{3}$-inch objective one corner of the etched lines of one chamber is focussed. The eggs rise in the salt solution and come to lie against the under surface of the glass slide forming the top of the counting chamber. With the mechanical stage the slide is moved up and down the columns formed by the etched lines. All eggs seen are counted and if necessary differentiated. The process is repeated with the second chamber and the total number of eggs seen in both chambers is noted.

Calculation :

The counting chamber has a depth of 1·5 mm. The area covered by the etched lines on the surface of each chamber is 1 sq. cm. So the volume

Y

of fluid in which eggs are counted in each chamber is 0·15 c.c.   The total volume of fluid in which eggs were counted in both chambers is then 0·3 c.c.

$$\text{0·3 c.c. contains } X \text{ eggs}$$

$$\text{60 c.c. contain } \frac{X \times 60}{0·3}$$

But the eggs counted were derived from 2 grammes of fæces

$$\therefore \text{ 1 gramme of fæces contains } \frac{X \times 60}{0·3 \times 2} = X \times 100$$

So the number of eggs per gramme of fæces is calculated by multiplying by 100 the total number of eggs counted in both chambers.

It will be realised that each egg counted alters the final count by 100, which means that allowing for any errors in technique the count is only accurate to the nearest 100 eggs per gramme.

The Special Slide.—The special slide with counting chambers is made by mounting on an ordinary glass slide strips of glass 1·5 mm. thick ; on these is mounted a glass slide on the under-side of which an area of 1 sq. cm. has been ruled, for each counting chamber, the area

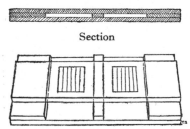

Section

FIG. 42.—The Gordon-Whitlock Special Counting Slide.

being divided by transverse lines to facilitate counting of the eggs.   Canada balsam is a convenient mounting fluid.   The special slides are cleaned in cold running water ; immediately after use excess water is shaken off and the slides allowed to dry standing on their edge.   Hot water must not be used nor must the slides be dried by heat.

REFERENCE

GORDON, H. McL., and WHITLOCK, H. V. (1939).   " A New Technique for Counting Nematode Eggs in Sheep Fæces." *Journal of the Council for Scientific and Industrial Research. Australia,* vol. xii, No. 1, pp. 50-52.

STOLL'S METHOD (MODIFIED).—Three grammes of the fæces are weighed; these are shaken up in a bottle with 42 c.c. of water; glass beads are placed in the bottle to facilitate dispersion of the fæces. When the fæcal suspension is uniform it is poured through a sieve into a clean porcelain basin. With a special measuring pipette (the Macdonald pipette) 0·15 c.c. of the fluid is removed and delivered on to the surface of a slide and covered with a cover-slip. All the eggs are counted—to do this a mechanical stage is required. One egg in the preparation examined microscopically is considered to be equivalent to 100 eggs per gramme of fæces. This method may be used for counting all types of helminth eggs.

REFERENCE

STOLL, N. R. (1930). " On Methods of Counting Nematode Ova in Sheep Dung." *Parasitology*, vol. xxii, pp. 116-136.

DE RIVAS'S METHOD FOR THE DETECTION OF EGGS.—Where infestations are suspected as being slight, de Rivas's technique may be useful, particularly for the fæces of pigs, dogs and cats. Though recommended for fluke eggs it is not entirely satisfactory in the case of fæces from herbivorous animals.

One gramme of fæces is thoroughly broken down with 10 c.c. or half a centrifuge tubeful of 5 per cent. acetic acid. The resulting mixture is then passed through a fine wire-gauze sieve. The solution is placed in a centrifuge tube and an equal quantity of ether is added. The centrifuge tube and its contents are then thoroughly shaken till emulsification occurs. The tube is immediately spun in a centrifuge for one minute at 2500 revolutions per minute. The tube will be found to contain an upper layer of ethereal extract, a plug of fæcal debris, a clear column of acetic acid solution and at the bottom of the tube a small quantity of deposit. The ethereal layer is poured off, the plug of fæcal debris loosened and floated out of the tube with the acetic acid solution. The deposit is broken down with the minimum required quantity of water and removed with a pipette, the whole quantity being placed in a glass slide covered with a cover-slip and examined. The total number of eggs represents the majority of the eggs present in one gramme of fæces—a certain number of eggs will inevitably not reach the final preparation on the slide. The ethereal layer may be used to test for occult blood.

REFERENCE

DE RIVAS, D. (1928). " An Efficient and Rapid Method of Concentration for the Detection of Ova and Cysts of Intestinal Parasites." *Amer. Journ. Trop. Med.*, vol. viii, pp. 63-72.

COUNTING OF FLUKE EGGS

In the absence of accurate information regarding the relationship between the number of fluke eggs in the fæces and the number of flukes present in the liver, enumeration of liver fluke eggs in the fæces is not practised in the clinical diagnosis of fascioliasis in cattle and sheep the presence or absence of fluke eggs being determined by a sedimentation technique.

A method for counting fluke eggs in the fæces was described by Olsen (1946).

REFERENCE

OLSEN, O. W. (1946). " Common Liver Fluke in Sheep." *Amer. Journ. Vet. Res.*, vol. vii, pp. 358-364.

EXAMINATION OF LARVÆ

BÆRMAN TECHNIQUE (MODIFIED).—This method is used for the demonstration of the larvæ of lung worms in cattle and sheep and for the demonstration of the larvæ of intestinal helminths in any animal. A glass funnel 20 cm. in diameter at the top is fitted with a rubber tube and metal clip and is fixed in a vertical stand. A piece of wire gauze is folded to form a sieve within the upper part of the funnel, or a small round sieve that will fit into the funnel is placed in position. A few pellets of fæces are placed in the sieve and the funnel filled up with warm water (40° C.) until the fæces are covered, warm water stimulating movement of the larvæ. The preparation is allowed to stand in a warm room for two or three hours. The larvæ swim out from the fæces and sink through the water to the bottom of the funnel. Samples of the fluid in the bottom of the funnel are withdrawn into watch-glasses and the larvæ examined microscopically.

REFERENCE

SPREHN, C. E. W. (1932). *Lehrbuch der Helminthologie*, pp. 170 *et seq.*

IDENTIFICATION OF EGGS AND LARVÆ

Owing to the similarity in appearance of the eggs passed by the various intestinal parasites, it is not often possible positively to identify the parasites from which eggs in the fæces have originated, but very useful information is obtained if the general classes of the parasites infesting the host can be identified. The recognition of the various types of eggs will be much assisted by a study of the illustrations accompanying this section. The following are the essential details of the eggs and larvæ of the more common parasites of the domestic animals.

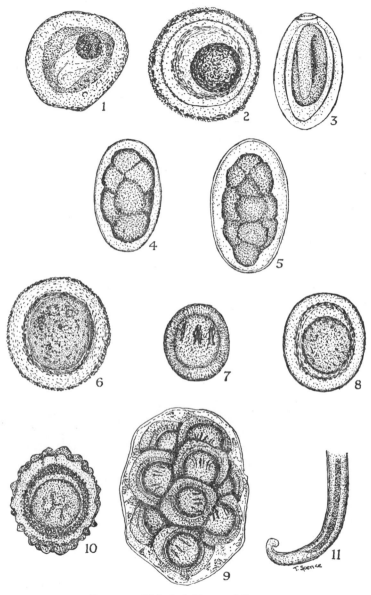

FIG. 43.—Helminth Eggs and Larvæ.

1. *Anoplocephala perfoliata.*   2. *Ascaris equorum.*   3. *Oxyuris equi.*
4. Strongylus spp.   5. Trichonema spp.
6. *Toxocara canis.*   7. Tænia spp.   8. *Toxascaris leonina.*
9. *Dipylidium caninum* egg capsules.
10. *Ascaris lumbricoides.*   11. Metastrongylus larva.
× 350 (approx.)

HORSE

Ascaris equorum.—Eggs round, brownish in colour, thick double contour shell with pitted surface, 90-100 μ in diameter.

Strongylus spp.—Eggs oval, thin-shelled, eggs segmented when laid 70-85 μ by 40-47 μ.

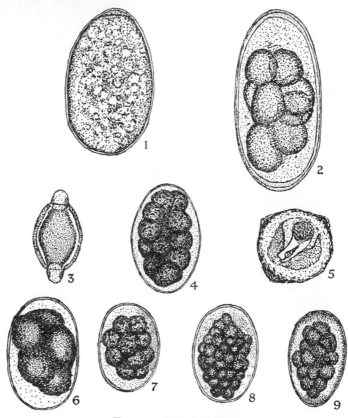

FIG. 44.—Helminth Eggs.

1. *Fasciola hepatica.*	2. Nematodirus spp.
3. *Trichuris ovis.*	4. *Chabertia ovina.*	5. *Moniezia expansa.*
6. *Bunostomum trigonocephalum.*	7. *Hæmonchus contortus.*
8. Ostertaga spp.	9. Trichostrongylus spp.

× 350 (approx.).

Smaller Strongylid Parasites.—Eggs indistinguishable from Strongylus eggs, but those of some species are appreciably larger.

Oxyuris equi.—Eggs are oval and elongated, slightly flattened on one side—*i.e.* the eggs are asymmetrical—and provided with an operculum, their size being about 90 μ by 42 μ.

Strongyloides westeri.—Eggs small, thin-shelled, already containing fully developed larva when passed in the fæces, 40-52 μ by 32-40 μ.

Anoplocephala perfoliata.—Eggs have a pyriform apparatus and are 50-60 μ in diameter.

CATTLE

Fasciola hepatica.—Eggs oval, thin-shelled, operculated, yellowish in colour and measure 130-150 μ by 63-90 μ.

The typical trichostrongyle egg is oval, thin-shelled, contains a segmented embryo of 16-32 cells and measures 75-95 μ by 40-50 μ. This description applies to the eggs of Hæmonchus, Ostertagia, Trichostrongylus, Cooperia, Bunostomum, Chabertia and Oesophagostomum species, all of which occur commonly in ruminants.

Moniezia expansa.—Eggs triangular in section, contain a pyriform apparatus and measure 56-67 μ in diameter.

Dictyocaulus viviparus.—The first-stage larva seen in the fæces is 0·3 mm. long, has no anterior knob like the larvæ of *Dictyocaulus filaria* in sheep fæces ; the intestinal cells of the larvæ contain numerous granules of a brown colour.

SHEEP

Fasciola hepatica.—As in cattle.

Hæmonchus contortus.
Trichostrongylus spp.
Ostertagia spp.
Cooperia spp.
Bunostomum (Mondontus) trigonocephalum.
Chabertia spp.
Oesophagostum species

These strongyloid parasites all produce thin-shelled, oval, segmented eggs as described above.

Trichuris ovis.—The eggs are barrel-shaped with a transparent plug at either end ; the embryo is unsegmented in eggs in fresh fæces ; they measure 70-80 μ by 30-42 μ.

Nematodirus spp.—Eggs relatively large, 150-230 μ by 80-110 μ, being the largest eggs found in sheep fæces ; embryo partially segmented in eggs in fresh fæces.

Moniezia expansa.—As in cattle.

Dictyocaulus filaria.—The eggs when laid in the lungs contain fully formed larvæ ; the eggs may hatch in the lungs, but usually hatching takes place during the passage through the alimentary canal, after they have been coughed up and swallowed. The first-stage larva in the fæces is about 0·5 to 0·6 mm. long and carries a small cuticular knob at its anterior end ; the intestinal cells are seen to contain a number of food granules that appear brown in colour.

Protostrongylus rufescens.—The eggs when laid in the lesser bronchioles are unsegmented ; development takes place in the respiratory passages of the host and hatching occurs in the alimentary canal.   The first-stage larva is o·25 to o·30 mm. long.   The tip of the tail of the larva is wavy in outline.   There is no dorsal spine.

Muellerius capillaris.—The eggs when laid are unsegmented and development proceeds as in Protostrongylus.   The larvæ seen in the fæces are o·25 to o·30 mm. long.   The tip of the tail of the larva is wavy in outline and there is a dorsal spine.

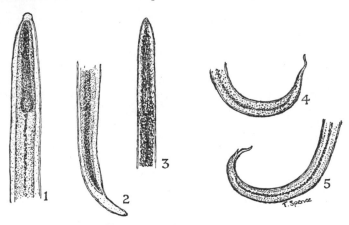

FIG. 45.—Helminth Larvæ.

1. *Dictyocaulus filaria*, anterior end.   3. *Dictyocaulus viviparus.*
2. *Dictyocaulus filaria*, posterior end.   4. *Protostrongylus rufescens.*
5. *Muellerius capillaris.*
× 350 (approx.).

PIG

Ascaris lumbricoides.—The eggs are oval, brownish in colour and have thick double contoured shells ; on the outer surface there are a number of fimbriate projections ; they measure 50-75 μ by 40-50 μ.

Metastrongylus apri.—The eggs are deposited in the bronchi or bronchioles, they are coughed up and swallowed.   The eggs contain a segmented embryo and may hatch soon after being passed in the fæces or may hatch after being swallowed by the intermediate host.

Hyostrongylus rubidus.—The eggs measure about 70 μ by 36 μ, but their identification in the fæces can only be tentative.

Oesophagostomum dentatum.—The eggs measure about 70-74 μ by 40-42 μ, they are thin-shelled oval and segmented.

Diagnosis of infestation by the last two species can only be definitely confirmed by the post-mortem examination of a suspected case.

DOG

Toxocara canis.—The eggs are round with double contoured greenish-brown shells, the surface of these being finely pitted; their diameter is 75·90 μ.

Toxascaris leonina.—The eggs are unpigmented and definitely oval; the shells are double contoured and smooth. Egg-laying in both Toxocara and Toxascaris appears to take place in cycles consisting of alternate periods each lasting two or three weeks.

Tænia spp.—The eggs are small, 42 μ in diameter, and are practically never found in fæces. Diagnosis is based on macroscopic identification of the gravid segments in the fæces. While fresh tapeworm segments are easily recognised, shrivelled segments from the perianal region have often to be used to assist diagnosis. In their dry and shrivelled condition these are not easily identified, but if soaked in tepid water they soon recover their form and can be recognised. This " reconstitution " makes it possible to distinguish between the segments of Tænia and Dipylidium, a distinction that is of importance because of the different intermediate hosts involved. If infestation with Dipylidium is established it will be necessary to supplement anthelmintic treatment with an attack on the ecto-parasite intermediate host.

Dipylidium caninum.—The gravid segments are oval in outline, resembling cucumber seeds; there are two genital pores, one on each side of the segment. The eggs are not free but are contained in capsules, each of which may enclose as many as twenty eggs. These egg capsules can be identified microscopically in preparations made from the fæces; frequently they are found in simple smears.

Filaroides osleri (Oslerus osleri).—The larvæ can be demonstrated in either sputum or fæces. These larvae closely resemble those of *Muellerius capillaris* (Fig. 45). The adult parasites cause lesions in the mucous membrane of the lower part of the trachea and bronchi.

CAT

Toxascaris leonina.—Eggs as in the dog.

Toxocara mystax.—Eggs similar to *T. canis.*

Tænia tæniæformis (T. crassicolis).—The eggs are similar to those of the canine species of Tænia. The gravid segments have a rounded and a flattened end, causing the segment to be bell-shaped. The head and hooks (scolex) are much larger than those of other species of tænia.

INTERPRETATION OF WORM-EGG COUNTS

The demonstration of helminth eggs in the fæces is evidence of the presence of parasitism, but if an estimate of the measure of the infestation is desired, one of the methods that gives an indication of the number of eggs per gramme of fæces must be utilised. Some of these methods give only an arbitrary figure, but either Stoll's method or that of Gordon and Whitlock give a reasonably accurate indication of the number of eggs. However accurate the method of computing the number of eggs may be, it must be remembered that there are a number of uncontrolled variables that materially influence the significance of the results obtained by estimating the number of eggs per gramme of fæces. These variables include the number of ovigerous females in proportion to the whole infestation, the regularity of egg-laying by the females, the egg-laying capacities of the various species, the season of the year, and the bulk and water content of the fæces. To a considerable extent the effects of these variable factors in diagnosis can be avoided if the results of the fæcal examination are interpreted in conjunction with the history, symptoms and clinical signs of the case. It is well to emphasise that a diagnosis of clinical helminthiasis cannot with accuracy be based solely on the results of an examination of the fæces for worm eggs. The extent to which alimentary parasitism is responsible for disease is dependent to a large extent on the nutritional level at which the animal is kept. A well-fed sheep may be found to harbour double the number of parasites present in an ill-nourished sheep clearly suffering from the effects of clinical helminthiasis. Many horses in good condition but destroyed for some reason other than illness are found to harbour large numbers of parasitic helminths. Young animals are as a rule more susceptible to the effects of helminthiasis than older animals. There is also evidence that animals possess in a varying degree immunity to alimentary parasites, and in those animals with a marked degree of immunity parasitic infestation does not readily occur. Other animals appear to possess considerable powers of resistance to the effects of even gross parasitism. When allowance has been made for all these factors an attempt may be made to draw a line that will delineate the measure of infestation that cannot exist without disturbance of health. Many workers have given estimates of the numbers of eggs per gramme of fæces that may be considered as positively indicating helminthiasis as the cause of disease. Alimentary parasitism is practically never due to infestations with only one species of parasite, but is due to a mixed infestation; the exceptions are ascarid infestations in the pig, dog and cat, tape-worm infestations of dogs and cats, and liver-fluke infestations in cattle and sheep. As it is not practicable to distinguish between the eggs of all the different parasites, the total worm-egg count depicts the composite parasitic picture. The following estimates of the relation of egg counts to disease serve as a guide, but the figures should not be regarded as having absolute precision.

EQUINE STRONGYLOSIS.—Mild infestation probably causing no clinical signs, 500 eggs per gramme of fæces. Moderate infestation possibly causing clinical signs, 800-1000 eggs per gramme of fæces.

Severe infestation probably causing marked clinical signs, 1500-2500 eggs per gramme of fæces.

PARASITIC GASTRO-ENTERITIS IN CATTLE.—Clinical signs have been noted where the egg count was between 300 and 600 eggs per gramme, but in severe cases much higher figures than these have been recorded.

PARASITIC GASTRO-ENTERITIS IN SHEEP.—Clinical signs indicative of severe infestation are found to coincide with 2000-6000 eggs per gramme of fæces, but severe infestation with *Hæmonchus contortus* in lambs may be found to be associated with counts as high as 10,000 per gramme of fæces owing to prolific egg-laying capacities of this parasite.

NEMATODIRIASIS IN LAMBS.—Diarrhœa in lambs infested with *Nematodirus battus* may be seen in association with an egg count of 500 e.p.g. Death may take place in association with an egg count of 1000 to 1500 e.p.g.

Death from nematodiriasis may take place in lambs before eggs are detectable in the fæces, when a very heavy larval infection has been acquired ; in these circumstances diagnosis can only be established by post-mortem examination. If lambs survive the critical stages during which high egg counts are obtained it may be found the egg count drops to a figure below 500 e.p.g.

FASCIOLIASIS IN CATTLE.—Signs of disease develop in association with a fæcal count of 100-200 eggs per gramme.

FASCIOLIASIS IN SHEEP.—The figure for sheep is higher than in cattle, being in the neighbourhood of 300-600 eggs per gramme of fæces.

REFERENCE

TAYLOR, E. L. (1939). " The Diagnosis of Helminthiasis by Means of Egg Counts." *Vet. Record*, vol. li, No. 29, pp. 895-898.

In connection with the significance of worm-egg counts the following estimates of the egg-laying capacities of parasitic helminths of the sheep have been made by Ross and Gordon.

Hæmonchus contortus.—5000-10,000 eggs per day per female.

Ostertagia spp. and *Trichostrongylus spp.*—One-tenth to one-fifth capacity of *Hæmonchus contortus.*

Nematodirus filicollis.—One-fortieth to one-hundredth capacity of *Hæmonchus contortus.*

The same workers have computed the number of helminths likely to produce clinical signs of disease in sheep.

H. contortus.—500 parasites will cause illness, but probably at least 1000 parasites are present in fatal cases.

Ostertagia circumcincta.—Death is not likely to occur unless the infestation exceeds 8000 parasites.

Trichostrongylus spp.—Probably 10,000 or more parasites are required to cause death.

Chabertia ovina.—An infestation of 100 parasites is considered to be a heavy one.

EXAMINATION OF SPUTUM

Examination of sputum and nasal discharge is sometimes performed in cattle, sheep and pigs to confirm a tentative diagnosis of parasitic bronchitis, but it will usually be found more satisfactory to examine the fæces for first-stage larvæ. As neither eggs nor larvæ are constantly present in the sputum or nasal discharge, failure to demonstrate them does not negative a tentative diagnosis formed on the symptoms and clinical signs. A smear of the sputum or nasal discharge is made on a glass slide and covered with a cover-slip.

POST-MORTEM EXAMINATION FOR PARASITES

Particularly in the case of sheep but often in young cattle too, the most satisfactory method of confirming a diagnosis of helminthiasis is a post-mortem examination of a dead animal if available. The veterinary clinician may not feel that it is necessary to count the number of parasites in the alimentary tract, being content to form an estimate as to whether they are few in number, comparatively numerous, or present in great number. Many of the parasites of the alimentary tract can be seen by a naked-eye inspection of the alimentary mucosa and the ingesta, but some, e.g. *Trichostrongylus*, are sufficiently small to make it necessary that a scraping from the surface of the mucous membrane should be examined under a dissecting microscope, or preferably through the low power of a microscope unless methods such as those to be described are used to separate the parasites from the ingesta.

If a more accurate estimate of the number of parasites is required a method similar to that described by Taylor (1934) should be adopted.

The principle of this method is that all the parasites are collected in a measured volume of fluid and the number present in an aliquot part are counted.

After opening the abdomen in the usual way ligatures are applied to both ends of the three parts of the alimentary canal required, namely the abomasum, the small intestine and the large intestine. These three portions with their contents are then removed separately. Each portion is then opened and its contents emptied into a large vessel containing 2 litres of water or normal saline solution ; the walls of the viscus are then washed with water or physiological saline so that any parasites adherent to the walls are washed into the receiving vessel. The material so collected is then passed through a sieve of about 60 meshes to the inch. It may be necessary to invert the sieve from time to time and clear the mesh by washing it with a jet of water so that the washings fall back among the original material. When screening is completed the volume of fluid is brought up to 4 litres by adding more water or normal

TABLE IV

Sheep Worm Burden Pathogenicity Table

Species of Helminth	PATHOGENIC		LETHAL	
	Young Host	Adult Host	Young Host	Adult Host
Abomasum				
(1) Hæmonchus contortus	500	1000	1500-2500	3000-6000
(2) Ostertagia spp.	3000	6000	9000-15,000	12,000-36,000
(3) Trichostrongylus spp.	4000	8000	12,000-20,000	24,000-48,000
Small Intestine				
(1) Cooperia curticei	4000	8000	12,000-20,000	24,000-48,000
(2) Strongyloides papillosus	4000	8000	12,000-20,000	24,000-48,000
(3) Nematodirus spp.	4000	8000	12,000-20,000	24,000-48,000
(4) Bunostomum trigonocephalum	50	100	150- 250	300- 600
Large Intestine				
(1) Chabertia ovina	100	200	300- 500	600- 1,200
(2) Œsophagostomum venulosum	200	400	600- 1000	1200- 2400
(3) Trichuris ovis	200	400	600- 1000	1200- 2400
Larvæ of above	4000	8000	12,000-20,000	24,000-48,000

With Acknowledgements to the late Dr. D. O. Morgan.

saline. While this solution is being stirred vigorously portions are withdrawn by means of a bulb pipette with a trumpet-shaped end and discharged into a 50 c.c. measuring cylinder until 40 c.c. have been withdrawn. The worms in this fluid are then counted; it is found more convenient to do this in four lots of 10 c.c. To 250 c.c. of water in a shallow glass dish about six inches in diameter and two or three inches deep are added 10 c.c. of the fluid from the measuring cylinder. The larger worms are picked out with a pair of dissecting forceps and the smaller ones sucked into a bulb pipette with a wide end. The sediment that remains in the bottom of the glass dish may be transferred to a watch-glass and examined under a dissecting microscope in order that any worms which have been missed may be picked out. The number of worms counted multiplied by

100 gives the total in the particular portion of the alimentary canal. An alternative method is to allow the alimentary contents to settle to the bottom of the large vessel, pour off the supernatant fluid and count the worms in aliquot parts of the remainder. The total number of worms is computed by multiplying the number counted by the factor relating the aliquot part to the volume of the sediment. The process adopted is carried out with each of the three ligatured portions of the alimentary canal.

If desired a differential count of the species of worms present may be made. Taylor (1935) described a technique for this differential count. After sieving and after removing 40 c.c. for a total count the worms are allowed to settle to the bottom of the large vessel; about 3000 c.c. of the supernatant liquid are then decanted. The remainder is agitated and small samples withdrawn by the trumpet-ended pipette. These are placed on glass microscope slides and covered with a cover-slip. The slide is then examined systematically, each worm being identified, until 50 worms have been counted. The proportion obtained by this differential count is then applied to the total count obtained earlier. For the significance of differential worm counts see sheep worm burden pathogenicity table on page 349.

REFERENCES

TAYLOR, E. L. (1934). " A Method of Estimating the Number of Worms Present in the Fourth Stomach and Small Intestine of Sheep and Cattle for the Definite Diagnosis of Parasitic Gastritis." *Vet. Record*, vol. xlvi (new series xiv), pp. 474-476.

TAYLOR, E. L. (1935). " Differential Enumeration of the Species of Nematodes Associated with Parasitic Gastritis in Sheep and Cattle." *Vet. Record*, vol. xlvii (new series xv), pp. 1511-1514.

BIBLIOGRAPHY

1. MÖNNIG, H. O. (1947). *Veterinary Helminthology and Entomology*, 3rd Edition. Baillière, Tindall & Cox, London.
2. ROSS, I. CLUNIES, and GORDON, H. McL. (1936). *The Internal Parasites and Parasitic Diseases of Sheep*. Angus & Robertson, Sydney.

CHAPTER XVIII

CLINICAL HÆMATOLOGY

Red Blood Cell Picture—Hæmoglobin Estimation—Red Cell Count—
Packed Cell Volume—Erythrocyte Indices—Stained Blood Smear
White Blood Cell Picture—Total White Cell Count—Differential White
Cell Count—Stained Blood Smear
Additional Tests—Platelet Count—Blood Sedimentation Rate

WITH the exception of certain supplementary tests mentioned towards
the end of this Chapter all the examinations can be carried out if a blood
film and a sample of unclotted blood is available. Special requirements
will be mentioned where applicable in dealing with the supplementary
tests.

A routine blood examination usually consists of hæmoglobin estimation, red blood cell count, total white cell count and differential white
cell count. The need for further examinations will be shown either by
the clinical features of the case or by the findings of the routine blood
examination.

RED BLOOD CELL PICTURE

HÆMOGLOBIN ESTIMATION

TALLQVIST METHOD.—This simple test is of use in confirming or
refuting the presence of anæmia, though it is admittedly not possessed
of a high degree of accuracy. A drop of blood taken direct from a vein
or from a sample of unclotted blood is placed on a piece of absorbent
paper. The colour is compared with a colour series representing 100, 90,
80 per cent. and so on of which 100 is equivalent to 13·8 g. of hæmoglobin
per 100 ml. It will be found that with blood from animals the matching
with colour series prepared for human blood is not perfect.

HALDANE METHOD.—Blood hæmolysed with water is mixed with coal
gas and then diluted drop by drop with water until a match with a standard
is achieved. Though the method is sufficiently accurate for clinical work,
it is now chiefly of historical interest because the technique tends to be
tedious and inconvenient.

SAHLI METHOD.—This method depends on the formation of acid
hæmatin by adding 20 c.mm. of blood using a special hæmoglobin pipette
to N/10 hydrochloric acid filled to the 20 mark on the graduated Sahli
tube, following which a standard time of five to ten minutes is allowed
to elapse and the amount of acid hæmatin formed is estimated by comparing
with known standards, using some form of colorimeter or comparator.

ALKALINE HÆMATIN METHOD.—Hæmoglobin derivatives are converted to alkaline hæmatin by the addition of dilute alkali. 0·05 ml. of blood is added to 4·95 ml. of N/10 NaOH and heated in a boiling water bath for four minutes. The mixture is then cooled and matched in a photo-electric colorimeter or visual colorimeter against a known artificial standard similarly treated. In lipæmic blood, turbidity may occur but this can be dispersed by the addition of one or two drops of liquid detergent.

PHOTOMETRIC METHODS.—Various instruments are available which make it possible to achieve a rapid, easy and accurate estimate of the hæmoglobin content of blood. They are chiefly of use in a laboratory dealing with large numbers of samples. An example of this type of instrument is the M.R.C Photometer which depends on a neutral wedge being manipulated to achieve a balanced transmission of light through the unknown and the standard.

HÆMATOCRIT METHOD.—This method is discussed on page 355.

RED CELL COUNT

The red cell count (the erythrocyte count) is carried out on blood diluted to such an extent that the number of cells can conveniently be counted under the microscope. The blood can be diluted by means of a micro-pipette or a bulk dilution method can be used. As a general rule a dilution of 1 in 200 is used.

Dacies' fluid has been found satisfactory for diluting blood for erythrocyte counts as it keeps well and preserves the shape of the red cells. The fluid is prepared by adding 1 ml. of formalin (40 per cent. formaldehyde) to 99 ml. of a 3 per cent. aqueous solution of sodium citrate.

Strong's fluid contains 1 g. sodium citrate, 0·6 g. sodium chloride, 1·0 ml. formalin and 98 ml. of distilled water.

MICRO-PIPETTE METHOD OF DILUTION.—Using the Thoma red count pipette shown in Fig. 46 a sample of blood is obtained direct from a free flowing capillary puncture or from a well mixed sample of blood containing anti-coagulant. The pipette is filled by means of a rubber suction tube. Blood is drawn up until it reaches the 05 (0·5) mark on the stem of the pipette (if the patient is obviously very anæmic blood may be drawn up to the 1 mark). The blood must not pass the mark and no air bubbles must be allowed to enter the pipette. Only the tip of the pipette should be held in the blood sample ; any blood on the outside of the pipette should be carefully removed by wiping with a clean piece of absorbent cloth. The pipette is then filled with the diluting fluid till it reaches the 101 mark above the bulb of the pipette. The contents of the pipette are thoroughly mixed with a twisting or rotating motion for at least three minutes. Mixing is assisted by the bead in the bulb of the pipette which is usually coloured red to distinguish the red count pipette from the white count (*i.e.* leucocyte) pipette. After the pipette is filled and its contents mixed it will be seen that the stem of the pipette is filled with diluting fluid ; the stem contains 1 part of diluting fluid and the bulb 0·5 of blood in 100 of diluting fluid, that is to say the dilution in the bulb is 1 in 200 (1 in 100 if blood was drawn up to the 1 mark). Approximately one-third of the contents of the pipette are now blown out and discarded, the sample in the pipette now being ready to transfer to the counting chamber.

BULK DILUTION METHOD.—Blood is drawn up into a hæmoglobin pipette graduated at one mark for 20 c.mm. (0·02 ml.), the same precautions as described in the micro-pipette method of avoiding air bubbles and of cleaning the outside of the pipette are observed. The contents of the pipette are delivered into a tube containing 4 ml. of diluting fluid ;

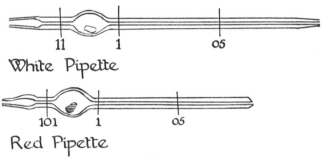

White Pipette

Red Pipette

FIG. 46.—Thoma Pipettes.

the pipette is rinsed out by drawing up the diluting fluid and discharging it into the tube. The tube is stoppered and the contents mixed by rotating the tube for at least three minutes. The pipette is then filled with the diluted blood and used to fill the counting chamber.

The dilution of blood by this method is 1 in 201 and so there is an error of 0·5 per cent. between values estimated by this method compared with those obtained by the micro-pipette method. This minor difference can be ignored as other experimental errors in the technique are greater and in any case the difference is of no clinical significance.

PREPARATION AND FILLING OF THE COUNTING CHAMBER.—It is essential that the counting chamber and the cover-slip are thoroughly clean and free from grease. The cover-slip is placed in position on the empty chamber so that it rests on the raised bars on either side of the troughs ; it should completely cover the ruled area. When the cover-slip is lightly pressed on to the chamber over the ruled area not more than six inference fringes (Newton's rings) should appear. The red cell pipette with freshly mixed blood from which some of the erythrocyte suspension has been expelled is placed with the free end at an angle of approximately 45° to

Z

the chamber so that the fluid flows under the cover-slip by capillary attraction. The ruled area of the chamber must be completely filled; care must be taken that excess fluid does not run into the troughs and that no air bubbles appear under the cover-slip. If any of these faults occur the counting chamber must be emptied, it and the cover-glass cleaned

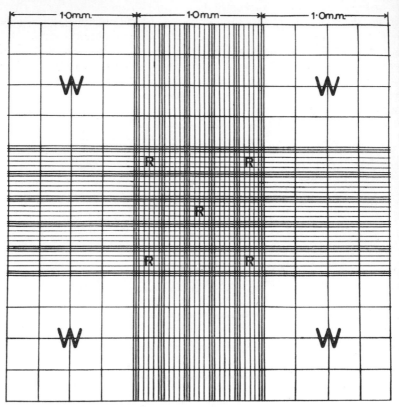

FIG. 47.—Ruled areas of Hæmocytometer Slide.

and dried and the procedure of filling repeated. The counting chamber when satisfactorily filled is allowed to stand for three minutes to allow the erythrocytes to settle. The chamber is placed under the microscope and examined with a $\frac{2}{3}$-in. objective to ensure that there is an even distribution of the cells.

COUNTING PROCEDURE.—The cells are counted with the $\frac{1}{6}$-in. objective. The central area of the counting chamber marked R at its four corners and in the centre on Fig. 47 is 1 sq. mm. and is divided into 25 squares which in turn are divided into 16 smaller squares. The area of each of the small squares is $\frac{1}{400}$ of a sq. m. The depth of the counting chamber is $\frac{1}{10}$ mm. The squares in the central area of the counting chamber are used for the erythrocyte count and the red cells are counted in 5 sets of small squares each containing 16 smaller squares making a total of 80 smaller squares in which the red cells are counted. The following rules should be observed in counting the cells. If a start is made with the top left hand square, those cells which lie within the left hand and upper lines should be counted. Cells touching the right hand or bottom lines should be excluded from the count in that square. This process is repeated until the required number of squares have been counted. In order to attain a reasonable degree of accuracy at least 500 cells must be counted. In cases of anæmia to attain this minimum it may be necessary to count more squares, when it is probably best to count double the number of squares. Alternatively the blood dilution may be limited to 1 in 100.

CALCULATION.—In the improved Neubauer counting chamber each small square$=\frac{1}{400}$ sq. mm. The depth of the counting chamber$=\frac{1}{10}$ mm. The volume represented by one small square$=\frac{1}{4000}$ c.mm. The dilution of the blood is 1 in 200 (or 1 in 100).

Let N represent the number of erythrocytes counted in R small squares :

Then $\dfrac{R}{4000}$ c.mm. of diluted blood (1 in 200) contains N erythrocytes.

∴ 1 c.mm. of undiluted blood contains

$$N \times \frac{4000}{R} \times 200 \text{ erythrocytes.}$$

If the number of small squares counted is 80 as suggested and total of at least 500 cells were counted in them the formula can be simplified :

$$N \times \frac{4000}{80} \times 200 = N \times 10{,}000 \text{ per c.mm.}$$

PACKED CELL VOLUME OR HÆMATOCRIT

The packed cell volume, percentage corpuscular volume, the corpuscular volume or the hæmatocrit to name all the terms applied by hæmatologists to the same measurement is obtained by spinning blood containing anticoagulant in a centrifuge. The effect of this is to deposit the red blood cells in the lower part of the tube, the white blood cells form a thin layer above the red cells and above them is plasma. The anticoagulant used for this purpose is that consisting of potassium and ammonium oxalate as described in Chapter XIV.

WINTROBE METHOD.—For this method Wintrobe's hæmatocrit tubes are used. They hold approximately 1 ml. of blood are closed at one end and graduated along their length in 100 mm. divisions. The tubes are filled from the samples of unclotted blood by means of a Pasteur pipette, filling must be achieved without introducing bubbles into the tubes.

It has been found difficult to achieve an end point beyond which no further packing of the erythrocytes will occur. To overcome this difficulty and achieve a technique that can be used uniformly, the tubes have been spun at a rate of 3000 revolutions per minute and the time fixed for one hour. If large numbers of samples have to be examined this is time consuming and the wear and tear on centrifuges becomes a quite serious source of expense. Cleaning the Wintrobe tubes is tedious and takes up a lot of technician's time. Inevitably there is a considerable breakage rate.

HAWKESLY MICRO-CENTRIFUGE.—This method depends on using capillary tubes which are spun in a high speed centrifuge capable of giving 12,500 revolutions per minute. The head carries twenty-four tubes and the centrifuge is fitted with an automatic timer so that the time of spinning is standardised. Five minutes is found sufficient to give consistent results.

Two types of capillary tubes are available, one is a plain tube for use with blood already containing anticoagulant, the other type contains anticoagulant in the form of heparin. The second type of tube is used when the sample of blood is being taken direct from capillary or vene-puncture. The tubes fill quite easily by capillary attraction. They are discarded after use and the cost of tubes has been found to be less than the cost of replacing Wintrobe tubes apart from the saving in labour costs.

When spinning is completed the tubes are removed from the centrifuge and placed in a special reading scale known as the Micro-hæmatocrit reader which allows the packed cell volume to be recorded as a percentage and an estimate of the total white cell count can also be obtained. Any abnormality of the plasma such as the presence of hæmoglobin or bile pigment can also be noted.

ERYTHROCYTE INDICES

When the hæmoglobin content of the blood is known, a red cell count has been made and the packed cell volume has been determined, it is possible to calculate two indices in relation to the red blood cells that may be useful in determining the nature of particular cases of anæmia.

MEAN CORPUSCULAR HÆMOGLOBIN CONCENTRATION.—The concentration of hæmoglobin constitutes the M.C.H.C. It is calculated :—

$$\text{M.C.H.C.} = \frac{\text{Hæmoglobin in grams per 100 ml.} \times 100}{\text{Packed cell volume as a percentage}}$$

MEAN CORPUSCULAR VOLUME.—The average or mean size of the red blood cells constitutes the M.C.V. and is calculated :—

$$\text{M.C.V. (in cubic microns } c\mu) = \frac{\text{Packed cell volume as percentage} \times 10}{\text{Red cell count in millions per c.mm.}}$$

EXAMINATION OF STAINED BLOOD SMEAR

If anæmia has been detected in the course of estimating the hæmoglobin content and the red cell count it will be desirable to ascertain if there is any evidence of regeneration indicating persistence of bone marrow activity. For this purpose the blood smear to be used in the differential white count is examined for evidence of young or immature erythrocytes. The changes looked for are differences in staining, size and shape.

An easily recognised sign of regenerative changes is that a proportion of the erythrocytes have a bluish tinge (Polychromasia) or that they have a stippled appearance due to purple granules (Punctate basophilia). If the demands on regeneration have been prolonged it may be noticed that there are considerable differences in the size of the erythrocytes from very large to very small (Anisocytosis) similarly there may be noted variation in shape (Poikilocytosis).

Further proof of regeneration can be obtained by making a special preparation to demonstrate the presence of reticulocytes—see additional tests page 360.

WHITE BLOOD CELL PICTURE

TOTAL WHITE CELL COUNT

The principles involved in producing a total white cell count are the same as those used in making a red cell count. An appropriate dilution of the blood is made and in a special slide fitted with a counting chamber the number of white blood cells are counted in a pre-determined volume of diluted blood. The diluting fluid recommended for this purpose is either made by adding 1 ml. of a 1 per cent. solution of gentian violet to 100 ml. of 2 per cent. acetic acid, or 1 per cent hydrochloric acid can be used instead of acetic acid.

MICRO-PIPETTE METHOD.—Using the white pipette shown in Fig. 46 blood from a free flowing capillary puncture or from a well mixed sample containing anticoagulant is drawn up to the 05 (0·5) mark. (If leucopenia is suspected the blood may be drawn up to the mark 1). Precautions in regard to air bubbles and subsequent cleaning of the stem of the pipette are the same as when making a red cell count. The pipette is then filled with the leucocyte diluting fluid to the 11 mark. The dilution attained is 1 in 20 when 05 mark is used and 1 in 10 when 1 mark is used to measure the amount of blood. The contents of the pipette are thoroughly mixed by a twisting or rotating motion and in the process of mixing the erythrocytes will become hæmolysed. The contents of the stem of the pipette are discarded and the counting chamber is filled in the same way as described in doing a red cell count.

BULK DILUTION METHOD.—Blood from a suitable sample is drawn

into a hæmoglobin pipette to the 5 c.mm. (0·05 ml.) mark. Excess blood on the stem is removed by wiping and the contents of the pipette are discharged into a tube containing 0·95 ml. of diluting fluid. The tube is stoppered with a rubber bung and thoroughly mixed for at least three minutes. The counting chamber is then filled with the diluted cell suspension using a pipette as described for the similar technique for counting red blood cells.

COUNTING PROCEDURE.—When filled the chamber is examined under the $\frac{2}{3}$-in. objective of the microscope to make sure that the cells are evenly distributed. The chamber is then allowed to stand on the microscope for at least three minutes to allow the cells to settle. The squares in the four areas marked W on the diagram of the ruled area shown in Fig. 47. are each 1 sq. mm. in area. All the cells in the 1 sq. mm. areas must be counted and at least four squares must be counted, but if less than 120 cells have been recorded more areas should be counted.

CALCULATION.—Each square has an area of 1 sq. mm. and a depth of 0·1 mm. giving a volume of 0·1 c.mm.

Let W=the total number of cells counted in 4 squares

4 squares=0·4 c.mm.

0·4 c.mm. contained W cells

1 c.mm. of diluted blood would contain $\dfrac{W}{0·4}$

But blood was diluted in 20

$\therefore$ 1 c.mm. of blood contained $\dfrac{W \times 20}{0·4}$

$$= W \times 50$$

An alternative method of calculating the total white cell count is to find the average of the total cell content recorded for all squares counted and multiply by 200 to give the number of cells per c.mm. Thus 200 cells counted in eight squares would give $25 \times 200 = 5000$ cells/c.mm. If the total number of cells counted is a multiple of 100, calculation of the percentages of the various types is facilitated and with the percentage thus obtained the absolute figures form the total white count.

DIFFERENTIAL WHITE CELL COUNT

In order to obtain a differential white cell count a blood smear is required. For this purpose a thoroughly clean dry slide is essential. A drop of fresh blood or a drop of recently collected blood containing anti-coagulant is placed towards the end of the slide pretty well in the middle. Another glass slide is held at an angle to that with the drop of blood and drawn towards the blood until it just touches the drop. The second slide is then moved quite briskly along the surface of the first and in doing so the blood is pulled out into a thin film. If the corners of one end of a slide are cut off, the narrowed end will be found useful to spread the film, which will be less than the full width of the slide on which it is made. The " spreader " slide must be thoroughly cleaned before making another film. The smear is allowed to dry in air. (A blood smear made by spreading a drop of blood on a slide with a platinum loop is practically useless for the purpose of a differential count since the distribution of the cells is disturbed and many cells have been damaged so as to be unrecognisable.)

STAINING OF BLOOD FILM.—Leishman's stain is probably the most useful and convenient for routine staining of blood films. The stain can be obtained ready for use. With a teated pipette the prepared slide is covered with undiluted stain. The preparation is left for $\frac{1}{2}$ to 1 minute so that the alcohol in the stain fixes the blood film. Distilled water is then added to the stain on the slide ; ideally the volume of distilled water should be twice the volume of stain used. The diluted stain is left on the slide for 5, 10 or 15 minutes, the time being largely governed by the known activity of the stain. The stain is then washed off with distilled water and the surface flooded with distilled water for a few seconds until the smear appears to have a rose-pink colour. The water is decanted, excess moisture removed with blotting paper and the smear dried in air.

COUNTING TECHNIQUE.—The slide is scanned with the $\frac{2}{3}$-in. objective and area selected where the smear is of uniform thickness and evenly staining. As a general rule identification and counting is carried out with $\frac{1}{12}$-in. oil immersion objective.

There are two main methods of examining the slide. In one, the parallel strip method, the slide is moved in one direction with the mechanical stage until the strip of the selected area has been traversed. The slide is then moved to the side until the next contiguous field is in view. The slide is then moved in the opposite direction to that for examining the first strip. In this way a series of parallel and contiguous strips are examined, the cells identified and counted. At least 200 cells in all must be counted. The need for counting of a larger number may be indicated by the clinical findings of the case or from evidence acquired while counting 200 cells, such as noticeably uneven distribution, an unusual preponderance of one type of cell or the presence of unusual types of cell.

An alternative method of examining the slide is by the battlement or four field meander method. The basis of this method is to examine four areas at the edge of the smear, the areas being defined by the outline of imaginary battlements imposed on the edge of the smear. Fifty cells are counted in each of these four areas giving a total of 200 cells.

The cells can be classified in a number of ways. Elaborate and complicated classifications are of no more help in clinical diagnosis than simple classifications and incidentally the former are much more prone to errors. The following classification has been found convenient and effective.

Neutrophils   Non-lobulated
               Lobulated
Eosinophils
Basophils
Lymphocytes
Monocytes

If a large number of blood samples are being examined it is a convenience to have a board to which are fitted six counters so that as each cell is identified it is recorded on the appropriate machine. Alternatively six columns can be drawn on a sheet of paper and each cell recorded in the appropriate column. In the case of cells that are numerous it is convenient to make the records in blocks of ten.

The classification of neutrophils into non-lobulated and lobulated is necessarily somewhat arbitrary but is based on the extent to which the nucleus has undergone change and is separating into lobules. All neutrophils in which the nucleus is divided into segments although the segments are joined by threads or bands are classified as lobulated. The purpose of the classification is that the non-lobulated neutrophils are young or immature cells, while the lobulated neutrophils are older or mature cells. Non-lobulated neutrophils do not usually exceed 4 to 5 per cent. of the differential count ; if they exceed 7 per cent. there has been some stimulus to neutrophil production.

The characteristics of the various forms of white blood cells are shown in the coloured frontispiece.

ADDITIONAL TESTS

SUPRA-VITAL STAINING FOR RETICULOCYTES.—The technique employed in this test is to apply the blood to the surface of a slide on which there is a dry film of the appropriate stain. The slides are prepared for this purpose by spreading a drop of a saturated solution of brilliant cresyl blue in absolute alcohol on the slide in the same way as a blood film would be made. An even film of stain is essential. The stain is allowed to dry and a supply of such prepared slides can be stored for use when required. A drop of fresh blood from capillary puncture or vene-puncture is placed on the middle of the prepared slide. A cover-slip is placed on the blood and the preparation allowed to sit for at least fifteen minutes. The cover-slip is now slid off the slide drawing the blood out into a thin smear. The smear is dried quickly in warm air. The preparation can then be counterstained with Leishman's stain (see p. 359). Under the microscope the reticulocytes are seen as orange-coloured corpuscles containing a purple network.

CLOTTING TIME

Blood clotting time or coagulation time may be increased by a variety of factors of which perhaps the outstanding is the toxic action of the rat poisons of the warfarin type. The basis of the test employed is that blood from a freshly made puncture is drawn into glass capillary tubes 10-12 inches long and approximately 1 mm. external diameter. One end of the tube is plugged with any suitable substance—plasticine does quite well. The tube is stood upright in water, the temperature of which is maintained at between 37° and 40° C. Starting after half-a-minute a small piece of the tube is broken off. This is repeated every half minute until breaking the tube reveals a thread of fibrin. While this test is obviously of limited accuracy it can show whether the clotting time is say 2-4 minutes or prolonged to 15-20 minutes.

PLATELET COUNT

Platelet or thrombocyte counts are not of much value in clinical diagnosis ; they are of value in the investigation of the nature of disease processes. The technique involved is rather tricky and this may explain the contradictory statements made by different authors as to the presence of a thrombocytopenia in certain diseases of the domesticated animals.

BLOOD SEDIMENTATION RATE

The term blood sedimentation rate implies the rate at which the red blood cells sink when a sample of blood containing anticoagulant is allowed to stand. Here then is another example of double nomenclature for the terms Blood Sedimentation Rate (B.S.R.) and Erythrocyte Sedimentation Rate (E.S.R.) are both applied to the same measurement.

The hæmatocrit tubes of Wintrobe are suitable for this test. They are loaded with blood containing anticoagulant within three hours of its being obtained from the patient. The tube is set upright in a stand and the fall in erythrocytes measured after a standard time which may be fixed at one hour.

CHAPTER XIX

APPLICATION AND INTERPRETATION OF CLINICAL LABORATORY AIDS IN DIAGNOSIS

INTRODUCTION

CLINICAL laboratory methods are used to assist in diagnosis and differential diagnosis of cases of illness in individual animals, but they are also of value in the investigation of disease problems affecting groups of animals. In acute conditions the information obtainable by laboratory investigation may well be available too late to influence any decision as to how the individual sick animal should be treated, and the decision to treat must be taken on the clinical evidence alone. However it may be of considerable value in regard to future policy to know the status of a group of animals and laboratory investigations while not helping the individual sick animal may provide information that will be of material help to any of its fellows when afflicted with the same malady. In less acute conditions an assessment of the group status may give a much clearer picture than would be obtained by studying one animal and a group study may provide the information required to solve a diagnostic problem.

It cannot be too strongly emphasised that clinical laboratory methods are aids to diagnosis and are not short cuts to diagnosis, a comment that also applies to X-ray examinations and electrocardiograph investigations.

This in effect means that the results of laboratory investigations must be interpreted in conjunction with a consideration of the clinical findings. These are available for before contemplating the use of clinical laboratory methods as aids to diagnosis the clinician will have made a thorough clinical examination including the collection of all relevant history. It is in the light of the evidence thus obtained that the clinician has decided to make use of laboratory investigation. It may be he wishes to decide between two possibilities, or he may wish to ascertain the significance of a particular piece of clinical evidence with a view to deciding the next steps necessary in the clinical investigation. In regard to group problems the history of the incident in all its aspects is often of vital significance.

Clinical laboratory methods may reveal deviations from the normal, but very often the abnormality thus shown has no specific diagnostic significance. Thus the demonstration of protein in urine does nothing more than indicate the existence of an abnormality in the urinary system ; by itself it neither indicates where the abnormality is situated nor how severe it may be. Similarly, a sharp increase in the total number of white blood cells with a definite increase in the percentage of neutrophils and the proportion of non-lobulated neutrophils suggests the presence of a reaction to an invasive bacterium, but gives no indication of the site or severity of the lesion. A mild degree of ketosis develops in a relatively short time in a ruminant that is not taking food. This can be demonstrated by testing milk or urine, but the question then arises: Is the ketosis thus demonstrated primary or secondary and is it in effect what might be termed a starvation ketosis? The history and clinical signs may provide the answer but the laboratory alone certainly cannot do so.

In assessing the results of laboratory investigations it is necessary to appreciate that there are quite considerable biological variations in normal animals and these variations must be considered before assuming that a certain measurement is significant of abnormality.

In normal cattle there is a quite considerable diurnal variation in temperature, but under certain conditions such as late pregnancy or hot stuffy buildings the temperature may be very appreciably above the accepted normal range. The normal blood calcium in the domesticated animals is usually stated as being in the range 9-11 mgs./100 ml. but nobody is going to suggest that a figure of 8·5 is of grave significance. Where the variation between the maximum and minimum of the majority of normal animals is small as in the figures for blood calcium it is quite satisfactory to give a range, but in other biological measurements it is found more informative and therefore more satisfactory to state a mean and give the standard deviation around that mean. This method is particularly applicable to blood counts but could with advantage be used more frequently to describe biochemical findings. The standard deviation (S.D.) is expressed as a figure + or — the mean. Thus the total white cell count in thousands in the dog as shown in Table V is 11·3±3·3 (see p. 378). The figure for a very considerable proportion of dogs will fall within the range of 8·0 and 14·6, *i.e.* applying one standard deviation. All but a few very exceptional animals will fall within the range 4·7-17·9, *i.e.* applying two standard deviations. The extreme range to cover all possible individual idiosyncrasies would be 1·4 to 22·2, *i.e.* applying three standard deviations. A total white count of 1400 cells would undoubtedly be regarded by many as indicating a leucopoenia and one of 22,200 as indicating a leucocytosis. The interpretation of such counts on a purely mathematical basis can obviously lead to absurdities, but if the total count is considered in relation to the history and clinical signs on the one hand and the distribution of the white cells as shown by the differential count it will become possible in many cases to arrive at the correct interpretation.

Finally it is well to remember that in the case of an anomalous laboratory result this can be checked. A second sample from the animal may reveal that a temporary abnormality has gone. A repeat of the laboratory process may show up an unsuspected error in technique which may have been human or mechanical in origin.

PART I

CLINICAL CHEMISTRY

URINE ANALYSIS

The type of case in which urine analysis is likely to provide assistance in diagnosis is best appreciated if it is realised that the abnormalities demonstrated by urine analysis fall into two main categories (1) pre-renal and (2) renal and post-renal; changes in specific gravity and reaction occurring in both categories.

Urinary abnormalities can then be classified.

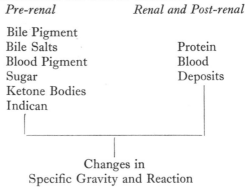

Pre-renal	*Renal and Post-renal*
Bile Pigment	
Bile Salts	Protein
Blood Pigment	Blood
Sugar	Deposits
Ketone Bodies	
Indican	

Changes in
Specific Gravity and Reaction

As a general rule unless the clinical evidence points strongly to some particular condition it is wise to subject samples of urine to a complete methodical examination for the abnormalities mentioned in the classification given above. The results then obtained permit the fullest use to be made of urine analysis as an aid to differential diagnosis.

SPECIFIC GRAVITY.—The specific gravity of the urine in a normal animal is subject to considerable variations according to the balance between fluid intake and the water needs of the body. The range and approximate average figure for normal animals of the various species are as follows :—

Horse	1·020-1·050	average 1.035
Cattle	1·005-1·040	average 1·015
Pig	1·005-1·025	average 1·020
Dog	1·015-1·045	average 1·020

The specific gravity of urine is increased in any condition leading to dehydration. It is increased when the molecular concentration of the urine is increased as occurs in diabetes mellitus in the dog when owing to the presence of sugar in the urine the specific gravity may be as high as 1·060 or even higher. The specific gravity is decreased when the kidneys have lost the power of concentrating urine as is the case in chronic interstitial nephritis in dogs. The specific gravity is very low in diabetes insipidus in horses, a form of polyuria apparently related to impairment of pituitary function.

REACTION.—For ordinary clinical purposes testing of the reaction of urine with litmus paper is sufficient. The reaction may be more accurately determined by means of colour indicators designed to give an indication of the pH of the urine. In cattle the pH of normal urine is between 7·5 and 8·0 ; in dogs it is between 6·0 and 7·0. In relation to litmus the urine of the domestic animals gives the following reactions. In normal herbivorous animals the urine is alkaline, but in dairy cows with a liberal water supply the urine may be very dilute and amphoteric to litmus ; in omnivorous animals such as the pig the reaction depends on the character of the diet ; in carnivorous animals, e.g. dog and cat, the urine is acid.

In herbivorous animals in fever and following abstinence from food for more than a few hours the urine tends to become acid. In acute nephritis in all animals the urine shows an increase in acidity. In diseases associated with a definite measure of ketosis the urine becomes increasingly acid in reaction. In chronic interstitial nephritis in the dog the urine may be so dilute that it is amphoteric to litmus. In cystitis in dogs with bacterial decomposition of the urine the reaction may be markedly alkaline.

PROTEIN.—Protein in urine must be renal or post-renal in origin The problem for the clinician is to assess the significance of proteinuria.

If as ought to be the case the sample of urine has been obtained as a result of the findings of a clinical examination the clinician is in a position to interpret the presence of proteinuria and his interpretation may be greatly assisted if as a result of finding proteinuria an examination for deposits has been made. The relationship of proteinuria to renal disease has been discussed in Chapter VI and mention was made there of transient proteinuria associated with fairly severe febrile reactions.

BILE PIGMENTS.—It is only in urine from dogs and cats that tests for bile pigments have been found reliable. In urine from herbivorous animals the presence of other pigments confuses the reaction.

Small traces of bile pigment are found quite frequently in the urine of normal dogs.

A test for bile pigment in urine is useful in confirming a clinical suspicion of jaundice, but should only be regarded as doing so when the result of the test is definitely positive.

BILE SALTS.—A positive reaction to Hay's sulphur test in conjunction with a positive reaction to a test for bile pigment can be accepted as definite evidence of the presence of bile in urine. (It is necessary to mention again that synthetic detergents used for cleaning the bottle used for the urine sample can give a false positive to Hay's test).

BLOOD PIGMENT AND BLOOD.—When a positive test for blood pigment is obtained it is necessary to determine whether the condition is one of hæmoglobinuria or hæmaturia. If hæmoglobinuria, the urine remains uniformly discoloured, whereas if hæmaturia, a sediment settles out of the urine. If the amount of blood is considerable the sediment of red blood cells is obvious, but if the amount of blood is small it will be necessary to spin some of the urine in a centrifuge tube and examine the deposit. If the condition is one of hæmoglobinuria the source is pre-natal ; if hæmaturia the source is renal or post-renal.

In the disease known as paralytic equine myohæmoglobinuria (Azoturia) the urine contains myohæmoglobin (muscle pigment) which gives a positive reaction to tests for hæmoglobin.

SUGAR.—The presence of glucose in urine usually indicates that the renal threshold for glucose has been exceeded, thereby indicating an abnormally high blood sugar. In the case of lactating animals a certain amount of lactose may be absorbed into the blood stream and excreted in the urine. This is a reducing substance that can be distinguished from glucose by the " clinistix " test or by the fermentation test with yeast.

In diabetes mellitus in the dog the urine usually contains ketones as well as glucose. If no ketones are present in dog's urine containing glucose it is necessary to investigate the case further before accepting a diagnosis of diabetes mellitus. A second sample of urine should be obtained after at least a twenty-four hour interval. If that is still positive for glucose, the presence of a transient glycosuria can be excluded. Then a blood sugar estimation should be carried out to establish that the glycosuria is due to a hyperglycæmia. In a very small proportion of dogs the renal threshold for glucose appears to be unusually low and if the dog has been on a diet with a high proportion of sugar this is reflected by the appearance of glucose in the urine. Fasting for twenty-four hours will in these cases lead to a disappearance of glucose from the urine. In these cases ketones are not present in the urine.

The presence of sugar in the urine has been noted in cases of pulpy kidney and enterotoxæmia in sheep. Whether this is of any diagnostic significance is uncertain, but it would not be a very convenient or practical procedure to attempt to use this observation as an aid to diagnosis of this disease in the field.

INDICAN.—In herbivorous animals indican is normally present in the urine in considerable quantities. A number of compounds are formed in the gut by bacterial action, e.g. indol is formed as a result of the putrefaction of protein ; this process is active in the alimentary canal of horses, cattle, sheep and other herbivores. These compounds are absorbed to some extent and are conjugated in the liver and then excreted in the urine, indol being excreted as indican. Indican is only present in the urine of a normal dog as the very slightest of traces. Definite quantities of indican in dog's urine are usually found to be associated with intestinal stasis or more commonly with putrefaction of the intestinal contents.

KETONES.—In dogs ketonuria is an index of deficient carbohydrate intake or faulty carbohydrate metabolism leading to imperfect oxidation of fats and the consequent presence in the circulation of the lower fatty acids, beta-hydroxybutyric acid, diacetic acid and acetone. In diabetes mellitus in dogs the urine is found to contain glucose and ketone bodies ; there is probably no other disease of dogs in which glycosuria and ketonuria are both present.

Ketosis is encountered in dogs as a post-operative phenomenon associated with liver damage and was more prone to occur when anæsthetics containing a halogen compound were in common use.

In cattle an increase in blood ketones is a feature of the metabolic disturbance or disturbances commonly referred to as ketosis. The cause of this disease or group of diseases is not completely understood and the name ketosis is descriptive of part of the clinical syndrome which includes loss of appetite, suspension of rumination, constipation, loss of milk yield and progressive loss of condition. As the ketone bodies in milk more nearly approximate the blood ketone level, tests for ketones are most satisfactory when applied to milk than urine in which ketones are concentrated and may greatly exceed the blood level.

A mild degree of ketosis develops in cattle when food is withheld or refused, thus ketosis is found in cases of displaced abomasum. In sheep ketosis is encountered in pregnancy toxæmia, in starvation and conditions in which there is a rapid loss of bodily condition.

GLYCURONIC ACID.—The test for glycuronic acid in urine is an example of a test that can be used to determine the efficiency of one function of the liver. This is the power of the liver to conjugate toxic substances as glycuronates which are excreted in the urine.

In herbivorous animals there are normally large amounts of glycuronates in the urine, presumably as a result of the conjugation of substance absorbed from the gut, where bacterial activity is an essential feature of cellulose digestion.

In dogs glycuronates are not normally present in the urine, but if the animal is given a drug like aspirin by mouth or camphor in oil by intramuscular injection, the aspirin or camphor is conjugated in the liver as a glycuronate and excreted in the urine. The absence of glycuronates in the urine after the administration of aspirin or camphor would indicate suppression of this liver function. Unfortunately as long as even a small amount of liver tissue continues to function glycuronates are formed. So like some other liver function tests this one has not been found of much practical value.

BLOOD ANALYSES

As far as the individual animal is concerned blood analysis with a view to estimating the proportion of particular compounds is largely confined to estimations of sugar, urea, bilirubin and transaminase and it is in the dog that these quantitative estimations have proved of most assistance in diagnosis.

In cattle and sheep calcium and magnesium estimations are unlikely to be of any value in regard to the individual affected animal as treatment to be effective must be applied immediately, so the clinician cannot await the outcome of a blood analysis. On the other hand it may be of great help to the clinician to know the calcium and magnesium status of the animals in a herd and so he may take blood samples with a view to determining the blood levels of these mineral elements with a view to guiding him in regard to future cases.

The significance of blood analyses will now be discussed in detail in relation to the elements mentioned in Chapter XV.

SUGAR.—In dogs the blood sugar level normally lies within the range of 80-100 mg./100 ml. The renal threshold for glucose in the dog is of the order of 175 mg./100 ml. of blood with an individual variation of approximately 15 mg. above and below that figure.

If sugar and ketones are found in a dog's urine and the urine has been examined because the clinical examination has suggested the possibility of diabetes mellitus there is little need to carry out a blood sugar estimation for diagnostic purposes. It is, however, of interest to know the blood sugar level in these cases and even after fasting for twenty-four hours the blood sugar still remains phenomenally high, levels of upwards of 200 mg. being quite common and figures of over 400 mg. are not rare.

If sugar alone is found in a dog's urine and a second sample confirms the presence of sugar without ketones it will be necessary to eliminate the possibility of the case being one of renal glycosuria resulting from a low renal threshold for sugar.

Hypoglycæmia appears to be an exceedingly rare condition in dogs. It is a waste of time to carry out a blood sugar estimation on a dog to determine the existence of hyperglycæmia unless its possible presence has been established by the demonstration of glycosuria.

In cattle and sheep the blood sugar level normally shows wide variations generally falling within the range 40-80 mg./100 ml.

Blood sugar estimation on a single isolated sample of blood from cattle or sheep is of no value in diagnosis.

In very young baby pigs hypoglycæmia develops very rapidly if the pigs are not receiving sufficient milk, the condition being aggravated by an unduly cold environment. As a general rule the circumstances involving the litter of piglets suggest the nature of the condition and a blood analysis is not necessary.

UREA.—Blood urea estimations are usually restricted to dogs and much less frequently cats. As the blood urea level is an accurate yard-stick of renal function, blood urea estimations are employed to confirm or refute a tentative clinical diagnosis of nephritis. The blood urea figure is also of value in formulating a prognosis in cases of nephritis.

The normal blood urea in dogs falls within the range of 15-40 mg./100 ml. In nephritis there is usually a marked increase in the blood urea to a figure in excess of 120-150 mg./100 ml. In more severe cases the figure may be within the range of 200-300 mg./100 ml. or even more.

Prognosis must be in part at least assessed on the dog's general condition, but as a guide to prognosis it may be said that between 200 and 300 mg./100 ml. the prognosis is doubtful and if substantially above 300 mg./100 ml. the prognosis is quite hopeless.

It must be appreciated that factors other than renal disease may cause alterations in the blood urea levels. Thus intestinal obstruction, dehydration due to vomiting and dehydration due to profuse diarrhœa may cause an increase in the blood urea level. As a rule in these cases the blood urea does not exceed 100 mg./100 ml. but exceptional cases have been encountered where the blood urea was as high as 150 mg./100 ml. Only a limited study of blood urea levels has so far been made in the other species of domesticated animals. These suggest that with the exception of ruminants the normal blood urea levels fall within a range comparable to that in dogs.

CALCIUM.—In the domesticated animals the blood calcium level normally falls within the range of 9-11 mg./100ml. Milk fever in cows and lambing sickness in ewes are associated with a precipitate fall in blood calcium to a figure as low as 3·5 mg./100 ml.

When the response to normal therapy for these diseases by the injection of soluble calcium salts proves unsatisfactory it will be found useful to have a blood analysis done to determine the levels of calcium, magnesium and inorganic phosphate. Such an investigation becomes of greater value if it can be carried out on a series of cases in the herd or flock concerned. The results may serve as a guide to the clinician in his choice of therapy.

In bitches suckling a litter of puppies, there may develop an acute hypocalcæmia manifested by signs of intense nervous excitement. The condition can usually be identified by the circumstances of onset and the clinical picture, but if desired can be confirmed by the demonstration of a very low blood calcium figure.

MAGNESIUM.—It is principally in cattle and sheep that reductions in blood magnesium are responsible for acute and frequently rapidly fatal illness.

In ruminants the blood magnesium normally falls within the range of 2·5±0·5 mg./100 ml. In acute magnesium deficiency the figure may drop to as low as 0·5 mg./100 ml. As a rule it is found that all the animals at risk are showing a greater or lesser reduction in blood magnesium. It is then useful to determine the blood magnesium status of the herd or flock and this can be done by taking blood from a representative sample of the animals.

A condition of low blood magnesium occurs in calves, the clinically affected animals showing signs of acute nervous excitement, convulsions and death. In this instance, too, the position can be assessed by taking blood samples from those animals exposed to a regime identical with that experienced by the animals that have died.

INORGANIC PHOSPHATES.—In association with disturbances of blood calcium and blood magnesium depression of the inorganic blood phosphate levels have been demonstrated. When circumstances have suggested the need for an enquiry as to the calcium and magnesium status of the animals involved, it is probably wise to extend the enquiry to include the inorganic phosphate level.

In cattle the normal blood level for inorganic phosphate is 2·5-9 mg./100 ml.

BILIRUBIN.—Conjugated bilirubin (cholebilirubin) is normally excreted from the healthy liver cells. If the passage of bile is obstructed conjugated bilirubin cannot pass on to the duodenum. It then appears in the plasma and is subsequently excreted in the urine. An immediate direct Van den Bergh test then indicates the presence of conjugated bilirubin in the blood, suggesting the existence of obstructive jaundice, which the clinician may already suspect from the clinical evidence presented.

Bilirubin formed from the breakdown of hæmoglobin (*i.e.* hæmobilirubin) does not give a direct reaction to the Van den Bergh test. If the serum proteins are precipitated with alcohol, bilirubin dissolves in the supernatent fluid, and the addition of the diazo reagent produces a colour reaction known as the indirect reaction. A positive indirect Van den Bergh test does not distinguish between bilirubin (hæmobilirubin) and conjugated bilirubin (cholebilirubin) if both should be present in the serum. As bilirubin is always present in serum albeit in small amounts the indirect test is of limited value and if both bilirubin and conjugated bilirubin are present a positive result may be quite confusing. For these reasons the Van den Bergh test has been found to be of no value in attempting to differentiate the various forms of toxic and infective jaundice but the direct test may be of help in confirming the presence of obstructive jaundice.

QUANTITATIVE VAN DEN BERGH TEST.—The serum of normal dogs has been found to contain 0·1 mg. of bilirubin per 100 ml. A mild degree of jaundice just recognisable by inspection of the sclera gives a bilirubin figure of 0·5 mg./100 ml. Severe jaundice with intense pigmentation of the visible membranes may give a figure as high as 7·0 mg./100 ml.

This method of expressing the results in terms of mg./100 ml. is more satisfactory than that of arbitrary figures quoted as an icteric index.

The quantitative Van den Bergh test is of little value in differential diagnosis of the cause of jaundice, but it does provide a measurement of the progress of a case of jaundice.

TRANSAMINASE.—Normally there is present in the blood demonstrable quantities of the two forms of transaminase, glutamic-pyruvic transaminase (G.P.T.) and glutamic-oxalo-acetic transaminase (G.O.T.). When tissue cells rich in these two substances are damaged there is an increased liberation of them into the blood stream and this can be measured by estimating the transaminase levels. The two tissues in which this reaction is most marked are liver and heart muscle.

When liver cells are damaged both glutamic-pyruvic transaminase (G.P.T.) and glutamic-oxalo-acetic transaminase (G.O.T.) blood levels increase; the increase in level of G.P.T. is much greater than that of G.O.T. When heart muscle is damaged the increase in G.O.T. level is greater than that of G.P.T.

Studies of transaminase levels has shown that their estimation is of some value in the differential diagnosis of liver disease. There are, however, limitations. The most marked rises occur in cases where the liver damage is recent and severe, as, for instance, in acute toxic or infective jaundice. When the liver damage is old standing but not progressive the blood transaminase levels may drop to within the normal range. If the liver damage is only slowly progressive the increase in blood transaminase level may not be of an order that is significant.

The normal transaminase levels in a limited number of normal dogs have been found to be of the following order : Glutamic-pyruvic transaminase (G.P.T.) 53±13 units per 100 ml. and Glutamic-oxalo-acetic transaminase (G.O.T.) 49±17 units per 100 ml.

In cases of proven acute liver damage figures obtained were : Glutamic-pyruvic transaminase up to 800 units per 100 ml. and Glutamic-oxalo-acetic transaminase up to 520 units per 100 ml. In a limited series of estimations in other species of domesticated animals the transaminase levels have been found to lie within a much wider range than those given for dogs.

The value of transaminase estimations as an aid to diagnosis of myocardial damage in the domesticated animals has not yet been established.

COPPER.—Studies of the copper status for the purposes of diagnosis may be required in cattle and sheep. It is extremely doubtful if blood copper estimation on a sample from one animal is of any validity in differential diagnosis as blood copper values in normal animals are subject to very wide variations. If there are a number of animals of the same age and type exposed to the same environmental conditions, samples taken from all the animals or a representative sample of the whole group may give an indication of the copper status of the group. In assessing the significance of blood copper estimations from such a group sample it is necessary to consider the extent to which the individual samples show scatter over the normal range. It is only if the samples show a consistently low figure that the results can be assessed as being significant.

Liver biopsy samples give a more accurate indication of the copper status of a group of animals. In assessing the significance of copper estimations on liver biopsy specimens it is as important as with blood samples to consider the range of the results.

Blood copper values in normal cattle fall within the range of 0·08 to 0·12 mg./100 ml. and in sheep 0·07 to 0·12 mg./100 ml.

Liver copper values in normal cattle are upwards of 100 p.p.m. D.M. and in sheep upwards of 200 p.p.m. D.M. In cattle in copper deficiency the liver values may be as low as 5 p.p.m. D.M., and in sheep 25 p.p.m. D.M. or even lower.

COBALT.—Since blood cobalt estimations are of doubtful value in the clinical diagnosis of cobalt deficiency other methods must be used. These fall into two categories soil and herbage analysis and test therapy.

Samples of soil can be taken at any time of the year. Each sample should consist of two pounds of soil. If the soil appears to be very variable it is wise to take several samples to provide a representative cross section of the area. The analysis should consist not only of an estimate of the cobalt content of the soil but also of a general soil analysis that will indicate any factor preventing the cobalt being available to the plants, such as a high calcium carbonate content with a high pH value.

Herbage samples should be taken at the period of maximum growth. In Great Britain that is usually in the months of May, June and July. Autumn and winter samples do not give an accurate picture of the cobalt status of the herbage. The herbage sample must be fully representative since plants vary considerably in their ability to take up cobalt from the soil. If necessary separate samples of different types of herbage may be taken for analysis.

Soil and herbage analyses for cobalt content are carried out in laboratories specialising in this class of work.

If resort is made to test therapy it should be carried out by administering a massive dose such as 0·5-1 g. of a soluble cobalt salt in aqueous solution by mouth. If at all possible some animals should be left undosed as controls. These can be dosed at a later date if those dosed first show a clear cut response to cobalt therapy. If at the end of a month the results are equivocal, those dosed should receive a second dose while the control animals are still left undosed.

FÆCES

PANCREATIC DEFICIENCY IN DOGS.—The existence of pancreatic deficiency as distinct from deficiency of the secretion of the cell islets of Langerhans leading to diabetes mellitus, will have been suggested by a clinical history of a dog that in spite of a voracious appetite is in poor bodily condition and is passing very bulky, soft but formed, evil-smelling fæces. In some cases it will be possible by naked eye examination to detect the presence of globules of unemulsified fat. If necessary an examination for fat globules may be made microscopically when examining a smear of fæces under the microscope to see whether the muscle fibres in the diet have been digested.

In the majority of normal dogs the fæcal emulsion will digest the photographic emulsion in dilutions of 1 in 500 to 1 in 1000. It is, however, found that the trypsin content of the fæces varies very considerably. If there is no evidence of undigested fat in the fæces and the muscle fibres in the fæces appear to have been digested, a low trypsin content, as shown by digestion of a dilution not higher than 1 in 100, should be regarded as indicating the need to examine further samples of fæces for their trypsin content.

TOXICOLOGICAL INVESTIGATIONS

LEAD.—In the living animal suspected of suffering from lead poisoning, blood and fæces may be examined for their lead content. For this purpose a sample of unclotted blood is required and it is desirable to furnish the laboratory with at least 30 ml. of blood, and 1 to 2 ounces of fæces.

Blood levels of lead in normal animals are found to be less than 0·25 p.p.m. and fæcal levels less than 35 p.p.m. The relationship between blood levels and fæcal levels is dependent on whether a single large dose of lead has been ingested or whether ingestion has continued over a period of time. If a single does has been ingested the blood level will rise and remain elevated, while the fæcal level at first high may drop as the lead is excreted from the alimentary canal. If successive doses have been ingested the blood level is elevated and the fæcal level remains high until ingestion ceases and the lead is excreted.

If the blood level of lead is substantially above 0·25 p.p.m. this can be taken as indicating the possibility of lead poisoning. If the fæcal levels are high, such as 100 p.p.m. or even much more this adds force to the chemical diagnosis, but low fæcal figures do not refute the evidence of an increased blood level of lead.

In the case of dead animals, kidney is the best tissue for analysis and if the lead content exceeds 25 p.p.m. this is indicative of lead poisoning, and in regard to liver 20 p.p.m. of lead.

At all times endeavours should be made to find the source of lead and confirm its existence by chemical analysis.

FLUORINE.—The clinical manifestations of fluorosis are (i) the dental lesions and (ii) bone and joint fluorosis causing lameness.

The lesions of dental fluorosis develop in those permanent teeth formed and erupted during a period when excess of fluorine compounds have been ingested. Bone and joint fluorosis develops in animals ingesting a fairly high concentration of fluorine compounds, frequently developing within four weeks of the animals going into a contaminated pasture.

In normal ruminants the fluorine content of urine does not exceed 5 p.p.m. ; a figure of over 10 p.p.m. indicates that the animal has ingested a greater quantity of fluorine than is normal and is in consequence excreting fluorine in the urine. There is an indeterminate zone between 5 and 10 p.p.m. of fluorine in urine.

In regard to dental fluorosis the ingestion of the fluorine compounds causing them occurred months before they became manifest, so the urinary flourine may have no relevance to dental lesions.

In regard to bone and joint fluorosis if the animals are still going on the contaminated pasture that caused the lesions it is to be expected that the urinary fluorine would be high, possibly 20-40 p.p.m.

It must be emphasised that adult cattle with a urinary fluorine content greatly in excess of 10 p.p.m. have been found to be and to remain in perfect health.

While the lesions of a dental fluorosis are sufficiently characteristic to suggest a tentative diagnosis, those of bone and joint fluorosis are not ; indeed the lameness closely resembles that associated with aphosphorosis.

It is therefore necessary to seek confirmation of the absorption and storage of fluorine compounds.   In the living animal this can be done by removing the last segment of the tail for the purpose of fluorine analysis. The value of this method was investigated in twenty cattle known to be suffering from fluorosis.   In these animals teeth and other bones were analysed for fluorine content and it was shown that the last segment of the tail gave an adequate indication of the fluorine status.

In the case of possible litigation it may be necessary to sacrifice one of the affected animals in order to obtain teeth bone and other tissues for fluorine analysis.

In normal animals the fluorine content of teeth and bone is of the order of several hundred parts per million, usually below 500 p.p.m.   In affected animals the fluorine content is upwards of 1000 p.p.m. frequently within the range of 2000-3000 p.p.m. or higher.

Herbage analyses are useful as a means of establishing the source of fluorine.   The degree of contamination varies very considerably and so undue significance should not be placed on the fluorine content of an isolated sample of herbage.   Continued ingestion for many weeks of herbage containing more than 25 p.p.m. of fluorine compounds will cause bone and joint fluorosis, the length of time reducing as the concentration rises.

Continued ingestion of less contaminated herbage will cause dental fluorosis in adolescent animals during the period their permanent teeth are being formed.

ORGANO-PHOSPHORUS COMPOUNDS.—The laboratory carrying out the cholinesterase estimation will usually advise on the significance of their findings.   The findings are expressed in terms of the extent to which acetyl choline is converted to acetic acid stated as a percentage.   In normal animals the percentage conversion rate is 75.   In organo-phosphorus poisoning the percentage conversion is reduced to as little as 30.

It may well be that this estimate of cholinesterase activity is not a specific test for organo-phosphorus poisoning, but if taken in conjunction with history and clinical evidence it is a useful piece of confirmatory evidence.   The degree to which cholinesterase activity is depressed forms some guide to prognosis and the need for urgent antidotal therapy.

BRACKEN.—In bracken poisoning in horses the blood thiamine level is depressed from a normal level of about 8·5 μg/100 ml. to 3·5 μg/100 ml. (Evans 1951).

REFERENCE

EVANS, E. T. R., EVANS, W. G., and ROBERTS, H. E. (1951).   Brit. vet. J., vol. cvii, pp. 364, 399.

In bracken poisoning in cattle there is a marked reduction in the total leucocyte count, in the red cell count and in the thrombocyte count. The blood picture is not specific of bracken poisoning. If, however, the history of grazing on bracken pastures is available and the animals are showing the high temperatures and general picture of hæmorrhage from mucous membranes, such a blood picture assists the establishment of a diagnosis.

PART II

CLINICAL BACTERIOLOGY

Since the purpose of clinical bacteriology in differential diagnosis is essentially to demonstrate the presence or absence of a causal organism, the results obtained tend to be capable of straight forward interpretation. The nature of the material and its source will in the majority of cases indicate the type of organisms for which an examination should be made. In some cases it may be necessary for the clinician to indicate whether any special examinations are required. For instance, in the case of pleuritic fluid from the pleural cavity of a dog exclusion of tuberculosis may be an important part of the bacteriological investigation. A concise clinical history of the case from which the material has been obtained will be of great assistance to the bacteriologist in deciding the scope of investigation to be made. It is essential for the bacteriologist to know the species of animal from which the material was derived.

PART III

CLINICAL HELMINTHOLOGY

In the living animal there are forms of helminthiasis in which the causal parasite can be directly identified, if not in species at least in genus ; for instance tapeworm infestations in dogs, or the identification of larvæ as in parasitic bronchitis in cattle and filaroides infestation of the respiratory mucous membrane in dogs. There are, however, many instances when the evidence is less direct as for instance worm egg counts.

In interpreting worm egg counts the clinician must take into account the history and clinical evidence and he must also consider the possibility of other intercurrent disease. It is always important to remember that worm egg counts may have been markedly influenced by administration of anthelmintics, e.g. the depression of egg-laying following phenothiazine dosage. The possibility of some other intestinal disease being present concurrently with helminthiasis must be borne in mind when considering the significance of a worm egg count. An example of this was the case of a four year old Shorthorn bull with persistent profuse diarrhœa. A worm egg count showed 900 strongyle eggs per gram, but the fæces were found to contain large numbers of the bacilli of Johne's disease.

In the case of a dead animal a total and differential worm burden estimation may be made, but in the course of the post-mortem examination any significant lesions will have been noted.

PART IV

CLINICAL HÆMATOLOGY

The assistance in clinical diagnosis that can be derived from hæmatological investigations fall into two main parts. The first concerns the investigation of the red cell picture in relation particularly to anæmia ; the second is the investigation of the white cell picture with a view to deriving information as to the general nature of a disease process, the nature of which is clinically obscure. It may well be that the cause of anæmia is revealed by changes in the white cell picture, and on that account in obscure cases of anæmia a complete blood examination should be carried out.

RED BLOOD CELL PICTURE

All the requisite information for a complete study of the red cell picture can be obtained from a combination of the following investigations : (i) hæmoglobin estimate, (ii) red cell count, (iii) Hæmatocrit (Packed Cell Volume) and (iv) a stained blood film. If for any reason the source of material is limited or the facilities for examination are restricted quite useful information can be derived from a hæmoglobin estimation by the Tallqvist Method and the microscopic examination of a stained blood film.

HÆMOGLOBIN.—The hæmoglobin content provides a direct index of the " quality " of a sample of blood. The mean and standard deviation for the various species of animals are given in Table V. When the hæmoglobin content is below the normal range the animal is anæmic. It is, however, necessary to consider the environment of the animals or group of animals. Thus in the case of hill sheep, especially ewes in lamb, there is quite frequently a progressive loss of condition throughout the winter. This loss in condition is accompanied by a degree of anæmia that falls into a particular category because it is a clinical feature of all the animals in the group. If they survive what the hill sheep farmer terms the " hungry gap " their condition will improve with the spring growth of herbage and coincidentally the blood picture will return to normal. On the other

TABLE V

Means and Distribution

Species	White Count 10³ per c.mm.	Percentage Neutrophils	Percentage Lymphocytes	Percentage Monocytes	Percentage Eosinophils	Haemoglobin g./100 ml.	Red Count 10⁶ per c.mm.	Hæmatocrit	M.C.V. cµ.	M.C.H.C. Percentage
Horse	9·0±1·6	58±12	29±11	5±2·5	7±3·5	10·0±1·5	7·0±0·7	28±3·5	40±4	35·5±3·0
Mule (Neser, 1923)	12·9±2·1	46·2±8·5	43·6±7·9	2·8±1·1	6·9±2·9	11·8±1·2	8·1±1·2	35±2·9	45·7±9·4	33·8±5·6
Donkey (Neser, 1923)	13·4±1·8	34·6±6·6	51±6·1	4·7±2·8	9·2±2·6	10·6±1·6	6·2±1·0	36·5±3·8	50·7±2·2	31·4±2·0
Cow	7·0±2·0	30·0±9·8	52·0±11·8	7·0±2·7	11·0±11·9	11·0±1·5	6·0±0·8	35·0±4·1	57·0±7·3	33·0±2·8
Sheep	9·2±3·1	24±9	68±10	3±2·7	4·4±4·5	12·4±1·4	11·5±1·8	29±4·0	27±4	41·1±4·0
Goat	7·7±2·7	50·3±10·7	43·7±10·9	3·6±3·2	2·3±2·5	11·5±1·8	12·6±2·6	27·7±5·0	22·4±3·6	42·0±5·3
Pig (Fraser, 1938)	14·7±4·5	53±11	38±13	4±2·0	4±2·0	12·1±1·3*	5·6±0·7*	37±4·3*	71±5*	30·3±1·8
Dog (Mayerson, 1930)	11·3±3·3	74±7	20±5·4	4±3·0	2±2·0	13·0±1·8	6·1±1·0	39±5·8	59±8	34·3±4·5
Cat (Landsbergh from Wintrobe, 1942)	17·2±6·6	59	33	1	7	10·5±2·1	7·2±1·0	40±6·1	57±6	27·0±4·1

Venn, 1946

With acknowledgement to H. H. Holman.

hand the clinical picture of such sheep may be complicated by helmin-thiasis, either gastro-intestinal parasitism or liver fluke infestation when this anæmia of late winter is a clinical manifestation of helminthiasis complicated by a low plane of nutrition.

RED CELL COUNT.—It is widely recognised that red cell counts are only accurate to within approximately 10 per cent. In many animals the effect is that allowing for the possible error a red cell count falls within the range of one standard deviation of the mean (see Table V). As the day to day variation in the red cell count may exceed this error it can be neglected. In any case there is no clinical significance in such minor deviation. If the mean red cell count is 6·0 million, the clinician becomes actively interested when the figure has fallen to a figure of 3·0 million or a little lower.

When the red cell count is low and the hæmoglobin has also been found to be low, it is most important that a stained blood film be examined. This will reveal whether there is any sign of regeneration. (See page 357). In this way it is possible to distinguish between anæmia due to blood loss and anæmia due to failure of production, if that has not already been possible from the findings of the clinical examination. (See Chapter V, p. 150)

HÆMATOCRIT.—The hæmatocrit or packed cell volume provides an indication of the red cell picture that is of itself of immediate value for the blood of a markedly anæmic animal must obviously have a reduced hæmatocrit reading.

In many cases of anæmia it is found that reductions in hæmoglobin, red cell count and hæmatocrit are comparable in degree, the exceptions are when there is some marked change in the hæmoglobin concentration in the red cell or in the size of the red cells.

The hæmatocrit estimation is necessary if the mean corpuscular hæmoglobin concentration is to be calculated.

STAINED BLOOD FILM.—The microscopic examination of a stained blood film is obviously an essential part of investigating the red cell picture for without it no information is available as to the morphology and staining characteristics of the red blood cells.

If the bone marrow is capable of responding to a stimulus to produce more blood cells to make good blood loss there will appear in the blood immature erythrocytes and their appearance is described as evidence of regeneration (or regenerative changes). The earliest regenerative changes are the appearance of cells with unusual staining characteristics, either staining with a bluish tinge (Polychromasia) or stippling with purple granules (Punctate basophilia). When the stimulus to regeneration has been pro-longed or has been repeated both very large and very small erythrocytes may be seen (Anisocytosis) and there may also be seen variations in the shape of the red cells (Poikilocytosis).

Further evidence of regeneration can be obtained if necessary by making a special preparation by the technique of supra-vital staining to demonstrate the presence of reticulocytes (see p. 360). In aplastic anæmia due to gross bone marrow damage reticulocytes may be absent from such a preparation.

ERYTHROCYTIC INDICES.—From the information obtained from the hæmoglobin estimation, red cell count and hæmatocrit, it is possible to calculate the mean corpuscular hæmoglobin concentration and the mean corpuscular volume. From these indices it is possible to state whether the anæmia is normochromic or hypochromic and whether it is macrocytic, normocytic or microcytic.

It must be admitted that these erythrocytic indices are not of very great material value in assisting in determining the cause of anæmia in the domesticated animals. Thus a low mean corpuscular hæmoglobin concentration may be demonstrated in heavily parasitised sheep, but it is of more clinical importance to recognise the presence of the parasitic gastroenteritis which is the cause of anæmia. There are certain terms used to describe various changes in the red cell picture.

OLIGOCYTHEMIA simply means reduction in the number of red blood cells.

POLYCYTHEMIA means an abnormally high number of red blood cells. It appears to be a normal state in racing greyhounds.

HYPOPLASTIC AND APLASTIC ANÆMIA.—These terms are used to describe anæmia due to reduced bone marrow activity or to a suspension of bone marrow activity. This is seen in bracken poisoning in cattle and in lympho-sarcoma of the bone marrow in the dog.

MACROCYTIC ANÆMIA is one in which there is an increase in corpuscular size. This may be due to regenerative changes and its recognition is therefore of value in prognosis.

MICROCYTIC ANÆMIA is one in which there is a decrease in the corpuscular size. This too may be evidence of regeneration or attempts at regeneration. Microcytic anæmia may be associated with widespread tumour metastases.

HYPOCHROMIC ANÆMIA is one in which the mean corpuscular hæmoglobin concentration is low and is a feature of anæmia due to iron deficiency or copper deficiency.

BONE MARROW STUDIES.—The true criterion of hypoplastic or aplastic anæmia is a microscopic examination of the bone marrow.

Bone marrow studies in the domesticated animals have not yet reached a stage where their regular use in differential diagnosis can be advocated. It is therefore necessary to base a tentative diagnosis of hypoplastic or aplastic anæmia on the relative or complete absence of signs of regeneration.

CLOTTING TIME.—Some attention has been focussed on the value of estimating the clotting time as an aid to diagnosis in suspected cases of poisoning with the anticoagulant type of rat poison usually referred to as Warfarin. In a severe case of warfarin poisoning the clotting time of dog's blood may be delayed for as much as half-an-hour when compared with a normal clotting time of less than five minutes. Prolongation of clotting time is not specific for warfarin poisoning, but if taken in conjunction with other clinical evidence adds force to a tentative diagnosis.

It is generally considered that there is an increase in the clotting time in cases of liver damage and in leukæmia, but it has not been found that this is sufficiently marked to be significant.

In all animals there are substantial variations in the normal clotting time. Holman (1956) gave normal clotting times as follows : Horse 3·5-11 minutes, cows and goats 2·5-11·5 minutes, and sheep 1·5-6 minutes. Watt (1961) estimated the clotting time in dogs to vary from 3-10 minutes.

REFERENCES

HOLMAN, H. H. (1956). *Diagnostic Methods in Veterinary Medicine.* 4th Edition, p. 375.
WATT, J. G. (1961). Personal Communication.

BLOOD SEDIMENTATION RATE.—The blood sedimentation is increased in many diseases but there is no specific significance in the increase. The rate is markedly increased in severe cases of anæmia. It is decreased in cases of hæmoconcentration. An increase in the sedimentation rate was observed in a proportion of a small number of dogs known to be affected with tuberculosis but when studied further the results were not consistent.

WHITE BLOOD CELL PICTURE

The combination of a total white cell count and a differential white cell count make it possible to determine the percentage proportion and the absolute figures for the different types of white blood cells. While an increase in the total white cell count is an indication of abnormality, it is of little or no help in differential diagnosis unless the differential white count is also available. If there are any restrictions in the facilities available for investigating the white cell count the wisest course is to concentrate on a stained blood smear from which a differential count can be made and at least some general estimate made as to whether the proportion of white cells is greater than normal.

The means and distribution of the white blood in the various species of domesticated animals are given in Table V (page 378).

The term leucocytosis implies an increase in the total white blood cell count while the term leucopœnia implies a decrease in the total white blood cell count. The term panleucopœnia is used when the reduction in white cells involves all types of cell. Thus in the virus disease feline enteritis a feature is the presence of a marked panleucopœnia.

NEUTROPHILS.—Since inflammation is the normal response to trauma or bacterial infection and since the polymorphonuclear neutrophil cells are actively involved in the defensive mechanisms of the body the most common change in the white cell picture is an increase both in the proportion and in the absolute numbers of the leucocytes. The immediate effect of a stimulus causing an increase in neutrophils is that the proportion of immature neutrophils increases, that is to say, the proportion of non-lobulated cells increases in relation to the lobulated. This shift in proportion as between lobulated and non-lobulated neutrophils has been spoken of as Schilling's Shift to the Left. The more intense and the more recent the stimulus the more marked is the increase in proportion of immature neutrophils. In old-standing cases of infection, though there may be a high neutrophil count, the proportion of immature cells is not so marked. As a general rule the neutrophil response to bacterial infection is more marked than to non-infected tissue damage.

It must be appreciated that a neutrophilia with a marked increase in the proportion of immature cells is merely an indication of a defensive reaction. It is not specific for any particular system of the body or for any individual organ. On the other hand the establishment of a neutrophilia does point to the nature of the disease process and does assist the clinician in differential diagnosis.

Day to day studies of the white cell count show that the percentage of neutrophils and their distribution between mature and immature cells can vary very rapidly and a complete reversal of the position can occur within five days.

NEUTROPŒNIA.—A marked neutropœnic reaction is a feature of uncomplicated virus infection and is seen in the mucosal disease complex in cattle, in swine fever in pigs, in distemper in dogs and in feline enteritis. If, however, the disease becomes complicated by secondary infection the picture will change as the defences against bacterial infection are mobilised and the neutropœnia changes to a neutrophilia.

EOSINOPHILS.—Normally the percentage of eosinophils is relatively low; indeed they may be absent in differential counts made from apparently healthy animals.

A degree of eosinophilia is associated with parasitic helminthiasis, in which the parasites penetrate the tissues, e.g. these helminths burrowing in the mucous membrane of the alimentary tract. In animals recovering from infections, including helminth infections, there develops a phase of eosinophilia which is referred to as the eosinophilia of recovery.

As the proportion of eosinophils in normal animals may be so low as to be practically non-existent it is obviously impossible to describe an eosinopœnia.

BASOPHILS.—The proportion of basophils is normally very low. Marked changes in the basophils are not observed. In the course of eosinophilia of recovery a small increase in basophils may be seen.

Neutrophils, eosinophils and basophils are produced in the bone marrow, and are sometimes referred to as the granular cells. Depression of the bone marrow from any cause will lead to a reduction in these granular cells, a state referred to as agranulocytosis.

Depression of the bone marrow may be the result of a disease process invading it as in the rather rare case of lympho-sarcoma involving that tissue. External influences such as X-rays and other forms of irradiation can damage the bone marrow. The toxic action of some drugs is exerted on the bone marrow. When this side action of a drug is known it is usually avoided in therapeutics. Part of the toxic action in cattle of bracken poisoning is that of a bone marrow poison.

Excessive production of granular cells is a feature of myeloid leukæmia —a disease that appears to be very rare in the domesticated animals.

LYMPHOCYTES.—The lymphoid tissue from which the lymphocytes are derived though involved in the defensive mechanisms of the body does not usually respond to infection by the production of greater numbers of lymphocytes.

In the case of lympho-sarcoma a lymphocytosis may be observed and when the number of the lymphocytes becomes very high a proportion is seen to be abnormal in shape with distorted nuclei. Unfortunately a marked increase in the lymphocytes and the appearance of abnormal forms may only be found in the later stages of the disease when it is clinically obvious that the animal cannot survive long. The blood picture in these cases may be a complex one. Thus a three year old male white miniature poodle with a history of listlessness, lack of appetite and loss of condition for about six weeks was found to be markedly anæmic. No evidence of blood loss could be found. The red cell count was below three million and there was no sign of regeneration. The total white cell count was over 20,000 and the lymphocytes represented 30 per cent. of the total count. In three days, by which time it was obvious the dog could not survive much longer, the total white count was over 40,000 and the proportion of lymphocytes nearly 50 per cent. Many of the lymphocytes were abnormal in shape with distorted nuclei. A diagnosis of aplastic anæmia associated with the development of lympho-sarcoma probably involving the bone marrow was advanced. Post-mortem examination confirmed the diagnosis. Similarly the changes in the lymphatic picture only became well established in the later stages of a case of lympho-sarcoma involving the wall of the small intestine.

MONOCYTES.—In chronic defensive reactions the proportion of monocytes may increase. The significance of this is not clearly understood.

In cases of lympho-sarcoma there is also a monocytosis but as both what appear to be normal lymphocytes and abnormal monocytes are seen the distinction between the two may really be impossible. In such circumstances the two types of white cell should be classed as one group. It appears that the monocytes play a part in the defence mechanism. Their precise role is not understood.

CHAPTER XX

POST-MORTEM TECHNIQUE

IT is not necessary to give here the full details of post-mortem technique ; such details can be found in standard works on the subject. The following points should be observed when making a post-mortem examination in the field for the purpose of establishing a diagnosis, particularly in epizootic disease.

Before commencing the post-mortem examination all equipment that is likely to be required in the course of the examination should be got ready at the site where the operation is to be performed. Rubber boots and a rubber apron are necessary to protect the clothing of the operator and any assistant. The use of rubber gloves is at all times desirable, but if there is any reason to suspect that the cause of death is a disease that may affect man the use of rubber gloves is absolutely essential. The use of rubber gloves minimises contamination of the hands during the making of a post-mortem examination and, therefore, reduces the time required for cleansing the hands at the end of the operation. If rubber gloves have not been worn, the hands must be thoroughly cleansed before proceeding to other tasks. It should be appreciated that complete disinfection of the hands after handling tuberculosis material is extremely difficult and so, if possible, rubber gloves should always be worn when handling such material. An adequate supply of reliable disinfectant solution must be available, but the merits of thorough washing of the hands with soap and water should not be discounted. The instruments required are large knives, scalpels, tissue forceps, bone forceps and saw. Glass slides, a platinum loop and a spirit-lamp are needed if smears from organs or tissue fluids are to be made ; if these are to be examined on the spot, stains and a microscope must also be provided, but this examination is necessarily restricted to places where adequate light is available. Separate containers must be available for the reception of organs and parts of organs, tissue fluids and visceral contents. If material is to be submitted to a bacteriological examination the containers must have been sterilised by boiling. Glass jars of the type used for bottling fruit are ideal for use as containers.

Provision must be made for taking notes at the time of the post-mortem examination ; if there is any reason to expect that an enquiry concerning liability, or that litigation may follow, the notes taken must be full and complete.

2 B

These notes must indicate :

(1) The place, date and time of the post-mortem examination, and the name and address of the person who authorised the post-mortem examination.

(2) A description of the dead animal, dealing with such points as species, breed, sex, age and any means of identification.

(3) Time of death, if known.

(4) The state of the body : (a) rigor mortis, (b) body heat, (c) tympany and protrusion of rectum, (d) signs of putrefaction.

(5) External abnormalities, including evidence of skin parasitism.

(6) Abnormalities found during the post-mortem examination.

(7) Description of material removed for further examination and the nature of the examination intended.

(8) The results of such examinations if made by the person making post-mortem examination, or the nature of any report received subsequently.

(9) Opinion as to the cause of death.

Other relevant details of the case will be available from the case record.

Unless the cause of death is fully obvious, steps must always be taken to eliminate anthrax in the case of cattle, sheep and pigs. If there are any external signs of swelling in the region of the throat in the case of pigs, horses and dogs, similar steps must be taken. In the case of the carcase of a fur-bearing animal presented for post-mortem examination, the possibility of anthrax should be borne in mind and excluded before proceeding with the post-mortem examination.

Except when there are very good reasons for making a partial post-mortem examination, the practice of doing so is to be discouraged, as not only may relevant details of the case concerned be missed, but an opportunity of studying the tissue changes resulting from disease has been neglected. It is only by systematic study of all tissue changes caused by disease that progress in the science of diagnosis can be achieved.

In some cases, the clinician may decide only to perform a partial post-mortem examination as the course of the animal's illness may have already indicated the probable nature of the malady that caused death. Thus, a fatal case of colic may have been tentatively diagnosed as volvulus and all that may be thought necessary is that the abdomen should be opened and the existence of an intestinal twist confirmed.

TECHNIQUE.—A thorough inspection of the animal's body must first be carried out. If possible the immediate surroundings of the place where the animal died should also be inspected. Signs of struggling prior to death may be significant. The proximity of any danger such as high-power electric cables or poisonous plants should be observed. The position of the body and its general state in relation to the time that has elapsed since death should be noted.

In many cases it is found convenient to secure the carcase firmly on its back; but in the case of cattle it may be more convenient to lay the carcase on its left side so that the mass of the rumen is below the intestines; in horses the depth of the abdomen makes removal of the intestinal mass difficult, and this is facilitated if the animal is laid on its side. In both cattle and horses severing of the upper fore and upper hind limbs facilitates access to the body cavities.

Incise the skin from the symphysis of the mandible to the brim of the pelvis; in the case of cows the incision must be continued on both sides of the udder so as to free that organ from the skin. Reflect the skin on either side of this incision. Note the state of the subcutaneous tissue. Remove the mammary glands in the female and examine the inguinal region on both sides. The mammary glands are examined by incising their substance. If the associated lymph glands have been removed with the mammary glands they should also be incised. Examine the umbilicus. Incise the abdominal wall from the xiphoid cartilage to the pelvis, make a transverse incision in one flank from the longitudinal incision to the lumbar region, remove the two flaps of the abdominal wall thus formed. Note the presence and nature of fluid or other abnormality in the abdominal cavity. If required take specimens. Inspect the contents of the abdominal cavity without disturbing them.

Remove the sternum intact by cutting through the costochondral junctions and separate the two sides to expose the thoracic cavity. In the case of a carcase lying on its side, if the ribs are severed near the vertebral column and at the costochondral junctions, the entire side of the chest wall can be removed in one piece. Inspect the thoracic cavity and its contents before displacing them. Take specimens of fluid if required.

If septicæmic changes indicate the need for a bacteriological examination, the best material to despatch to the laboratory is an intact long bone from which the bulk of the flesh has been removed. For this purpose, in the larger animals, a metacarpal or a metatarsal bone may be sent, while, in the smaller animals, the radius or the tibia are suitable.

The abdominal organs can now be methodically removed. Ligature the rectum in two places and deal similarly with the duodenum; incise each organ between the ligatures. Remove the intestines with their contents. Note the state of the blood vessels, especially the portal vein. Ligature the œsophagus and remove the stomach and its contents. Inspect the peritoneum for signs of inflammation, subserous hæmorrhages, etc.

Remove the liver, cut open the bile ducts and make multiple incisions into the substance of the liver, noting its appearance, colour and consistency. Take any specimens required. Examine the diaphragm. Remove the kidneys and adrenal glands, detach any fat and, especially in pigs, examine for subcapsular hæmorrhages. Section each kidney by a longitudinal incision ; examine the cut surfaces. Strip the capsule from each ; note any adherence of the capsule to the underlying tissue. Section each adrenal gland. Take specimens. Cut through the pelvic symphysis and examine the pelvic organs ; while doing so examine the external genitalia. Remove the bladder and associated organs. In the female remove the ovaries, uterus and vagina with the bladder. Examine the bladder, associated glands and genitalia.

Separate the tongue from the mandible and remove the tongue, larynx, trachea, lungs and heart. Examine these organs and also examine the regional lymphatic glands.

In ruminants incise the rumen, examine its contents, take a specimen if necessary, and then empty the rumen. Examine the reticulum and omasum. Incise the greater curvature of the stomach and empty its contents into a container. Open the stomach, wash the mucosa and inspect the mucous membrane ; in ruminants examine for parasitic helminths, and if necessary make a smear from the mucous membrane and examine the smear microscopically for the smaller helminths.

Inspect the intestinal mass for any gross abnormality, e.g. volvulus or intussusception. Detach the intestine from its mesentery and while doing so examine the mesenteric lymphatic system. Open the intestine throughout its length, examining the contents and taking specimens at intervals. In the case of suspected enterotoxæmia of sheep, in which a specific diagnosis is required, samples of intestinal contents should be taken in order that the specific clostridial toxin can be identified. In order that destruction of the toxin may be prevented a small quantity of chloroform should be added. Wash the mucosa and inspect it. Examine the carcase lymph glands.

If the nervous system is to be examined turn the carcase over. By means of a syringe armed with a long needle—both previously sterilised—withdraw a specimen of the cerebrospinal fluid. This is done by passing the needle through the atlanto-occipital space into the cisterna magna. The cranium must next be opened ; this is best done by sawing through the bones forming the vault of the skull and then raising the cut portions with a lever, completing the operation of separating the detached portions of bone with bone-forceps.

In order to expose the spinal cord the laminæ on either side are severed and the spinous processes removed ; it will be found more convenient to do this commencing with the last lumbar vertebra and working forward. When the brain and cord have thus been exposed they can be removed for examination. If macroscopic examination fails to reveal any lesion in the brain or cord it must not be concluded that no lesion exists, since degenerative process may only be visible in the nervous tissue after microscopic examination of the tissue.

PACKING AND DESPATCH OF MATERIAL FOR LABORATORY EXAMINATION

The Post Office regulations make it an offence to despatch through the post matter that can damage other matter in transit in the mails. Organs, viscera and their contents should be despatched by rail or carrier. The choice of material to be sent for laboratory examination is dependent on the findings of the post-mortem examination. In general, it may be said that, if the findings of the post-mortem examination suggest the existence of an ante-mortem bacteræmia or septicæmia, an intact long bone from a limb may be forwarded to a laboratory for bacteriological examination. If poisoning is suspected, the material forwarded for analysis should be the stomach contents and portions of liver and kidney. In the case of ruminants, it is well to send contents from both the rumen and the abomasum. Separate containers should be used for parenchymatous organs, viscera with their contents and any other tissues selected. Whatever the material, it must be enclosed in an impervious container. For this purpose, glass jars with tops that can be closed efficiently are ideal but a tin with a closely fitting lid does very well. The container or containers are then placed in a packing case or box sufficiently large to permit the container being surrounded by some material such as sawdust so that any leakage will be absorbed. The package must be clearly labelled so as to indicate the sender's name, the nature of the material enclosed and the type of examination required. A covering letter should be despatched to the laboratory by post repeating and, if necessary, elaborating the details given with the package.

Preservative must not be added to material that is to be chemically analysed. Tissues that are to be sectioned for histological examination are best preserved by wrapping in a piece of clean cloth thoroughly moistened in 5 per cent. solution of formalin. No preservation must be added to material that is to be examined bacteriologically, as doing so renders cultivation or biological tests impossible.

It is essential that material intended for bacteriological or pathological examination should reach the laboratory while still fresh. Where there is likely to be delay in transit or when the weather is very warm, ice may be used to preserve the material in transit.

For this purpose, a large watertight container is required. The jars or tins are packed in this with a mixture of ice chips and sawdust. Such an arrangement has only a temporary action in preventing decomposition.

CHAPTER XXI

DIAGNOSIS OF POULTRY DISEASES

J. G. CAMPBELL, D.Sc., PH.D., F.R.C.V.S.

Introduction—Structure—Diagnosis of Disease on the Farm—Destruction of Fowls—Post-mortem Technique—Packing of Material for Laboratory Examination—Special Diagnostic Methods in the Field

THE poultry industry now occupies a position of major importance in the agricultural economy of this country, and as a result considerable attention is being directed to the husbandry of poultry, and to their diseases and dietary deficiencies. Although a great deal of this work is being carried out by specialised centres, there are still numerous occasions when the general practitioner may be asked to diagnose disease and to advise the poultry farmer what measures to take in order to prevent the disease spreading, and eventually to eradicate it completely from his stock. Treatment of the individual is admittedly uneconomic in the case of poultry, unless the bird is a valuable specimen, but this fact in itself is advantageous as one can sacrifice a fowl with little financial loss in order to ascertain by post-mortem examination the condition affecting the flock. It is thus desirable for the veterinary practitioner to have at least a basic knowledge of the disease problems facing the poultry farmer engaged in the various specialised branches of the industry, whether egg or meat production, and including the rapidly expanding production of broilers.

STRUCTURE

Only the salient differences from mammalian anatomy will be mentioned here. For further details the reader is advised to consult Bradley's *The Structure of the Fowl*.

Birds are hot-blooded oviparous vertebrates, adapted with few exceptions for flying. They have a high metabolic rate; for example, the temperature of the domesticated fowl is about 106° F. ; its heart rate is 250-300 per minute, and its respiration rate varies from 18-30 per minute under resting conditions.

The long bones of the skeleton contain air cavities which communicate with air-sacs in the thorax and abdomen, and so with the lungs. These latter are fixed to the sides of the thorax, and are incompletely separated from the abdomen by a rudimentary diaphragm.

The digestive system differs considerably from that of mammals. Fowls have no teeth, the tongue is hard and pointed, and the beak is very sensitive. The pharynx leads into the œsophagus, which is character-ised by a dilatation about two-thirds of the way down its length, called the crop. This organ is a storage place for food, and contains no glands except in the regions near the œsophagus proper. The food here under-goes a preliminary softening before it is passed on to the glandular stomach or proventriculus, which is a small fusiform organ situated between the two lobes of the liver and adjacent to the small rounded spleen.

The muscular gizzard is situated immediately after the proventriculus, and its function is to grind up grain, etc., previously softened by storage in the crop and the digestive juices in the proventriculus. Grit and small stones within the gizzard facilitate this process.

The intestinal tract in the fowl is about five times the length of the body. It consists of the duodenum, in the form of an elongated loop surrounding the pancreas, the ileum, two blind diverticulæ or cæca branching off at the junction of the ileum and the very short large intestine, and a cloaca or common cavity into which the urinary, repro-ductive and digestive tracts open.

In the hen, the reproductive organs consist of an ovary (represented by the left organ, the right having practically disappeared during develop-ment) and a single oviduct terminating in the cloaca. Occasionally the vestige of the right oviduct may be seen, and sometimes it becomes cystic. The reproductive organs of the cockerel call for no special attention from the clinical aspect.

Diagnosis of Disease on the Farm

In adult fowls the following are the main points to look for in the flock. The mortality rate : is it high or low, and do the birds die suddenly or sicken and die slowly ? A high mortality with sudden deaths suggests an acute infection such as fowl pest (" Newcastle disease ", or more strictly, avian pneumoencephalitis), fowl cholera or fowl typhoid. Poisoning must also be borne in mind, although here the death rate, though high, is usually confined to a definite area on the farm.

Most infectious diseases of poultry produce characteristic symptoms. For example, fowl pest, which is a notifiable disease, should be suspected if there occurs a sudden fall in egg production together with an outbreak of coughing and gasping and decline in food consumption, especially if a number of birds develop nervous symptoms, such as torticollis and chronic spasms involving the legs or wings.

In typhoid, a disease which is a septicæmia accompanied by a well-marked toxæmia, the injury to the intestine allows entrance into the system of non-specific intestinal toxins, and liver injury causes an excessive destruction of the red blood cells. Anæmia and a greenish diarrhœa are common, together with intense thirst and depression. An elevated temperature is not unusual and may be 110-112° F. A more chronic form of the disease also occurs, characterised by occasional deaths, and may be more difficult to diagnose, but post-mortem and laboratory examination quickly establish a diagnosis.

With fowl cholera the facial appendages appear cyanotic instead of anæmic as in typhoid. The droppings are watery and often grey or yellow in colour. Such birds as may linger for a few days appear stupid and will not eat or drink. They become emaciated, may be lame from localisation of the disease in the joints, and may exhibit difficult respiration owing to excessive mucous in the respiratory tract.

A slowly progressive emaciation of individual fowls in a flock, lameness, anæmia and a scurfy appearance of the facial appendages, diarrhœa and occasional sudden deaths ; all these symptoms, when taken together, suggest tuberculosis, and immediate steps should be taken to confirm the diagnosis and apply control measures.

Blood in the droppings, unthriftiness and a hunched-up appearance of the affected birds are symptomatic of coccidiosis, and microscopical examination of the droppings may reveal the oöcysts, or a post-mortem examination of a typical case will quickly establish a diagnosis.

There are two main forms of fowl pox, and in the past these were considered as separate diseases. Firstly there is a skin form, in which warty growths appear on the comb, wattles and at the commissures of the mouth and eyes. These tend to coalesce to form large, brown, scabby growths. Secondly, in the mouth form, yellowish necrotic material is found attached to the tongue or to the larynx. This form is often known as the diphtheritic type, a name which is useful to remember, as, in diphtheria, the false membranes are difficult to remove from the underlying mucosa, and forcible removal leaves a raw bleeding surface below, which is quickly covered again by membranes. The chronic form of infectious coryza closely resembles this type of fowl pox, but the caseous material in the palatine cleft, on the tongue or larynx is easily removed in catarrh, leaving an intact mucosa beneath. However, in such cases if sufficient affected birds are examined, some will usually be found to have the typical epithelial form first mentioned. Definite diagnosis of pox can only be made in the laboratory, where sections of lesions may be examined, and transmission experiments carried out. Fowl pox in all its forms is a very debilitating disease, and egg production may practically cease.

Severe attacks of coughing in a number of birds, with the ejection of blood-stained mucous, difficult bubbling respiration and cyanosis of the mucous membranes, suggest an outbreak of infectious laryngo-tracheitis, and a few typical cases should be sent alive if possible to a laboratory for examination, whilst all other birds should be isolated and the worst affected destroyed. The breathing in laryngo-tracheitis is very characteristic. The neck is extended in a straight line, and with the eyes closed, the bird breathes in through the open beak with a loud wheezing or bubbling sound. The neck is then withdrawn to a normal position, the eyes open, and the bird exhales. Affected birds usually prefer to remain in a sitting position.

Fowl paralysis is not now generally regarded as being a part of the leucotic complex of disease in fowls. In its typical form, *i.e.* neuro-lymphomatosis, the symptoms are usually sufficiently characteristic to establish a confident diagnosis. Outbreaks of paralysis are not uncommon in flocks, affecting mainly young birds between the ages of 10-20 weeks. The etiology is not definitely established, and its infectivity in the stage when usually seen—the nervous form, is debated. It has been suggested that this is a chronic manifestation exhibited by the survivors of an acute infectious disease primarily affecting young chicks, and that the " chronic " stage is not commonly infectious.

The symptoms for which to look in neuro-lymphomatosis are commonly lameness, varying from a slight disability to complete flaccid paralysis of the affected leg, drooping wings, spasmodic twisting of the head and neck into unusual positions, together with less specific symptoms such as impacted crop, indigestion, diarrhœa, etc., all of which may be due to an impairment of the nerve supply to the digestive tract. In a fairly early case of leg paralysis the leg can still be used to a certain extent. The toes are frequently bunched together in a clutching position, and the " clutch " or " perching reflex " is impaired. This reflex may be easily tested by holding the bird at the base of its wings with one hand and lowering it suddenly so that the foot to be tested comes into contact with the extended fore-finger of the other hand. Normally the toes will clutch the finger as in perching, but a case of leg paralysis is unable to do this, and the bird fails to grasp the finger. Apart from actual mechanical injury, lameness may also be due to staphylococcol infection of the " hock " joint, characterised by heat and swelling, or to articular gout, with deposits of urates in and around the toe joints. If the wing is affected the bird is unable to retain it in the normal folded position, and so it droops, sometimes to the extent of trailing the primary feathers along the ground.

Ocular lymphomatosis is characterised by distorted or paralysed pupils, frequently with a notched border, together with a loss of pigmentation, so that the normal orange-red iris becomes greyish, resulting in the so-called " pearly-eye." This form of paralysis is usually taken to indicate that the bird is infected, but the virus is latent. Such birds should be culled from the flock, and certainly never used for breeding purposes.

The third form of fowl paralysis—the visceral type—is difficult to diagnose in life, and is often confused with lymphoid leucosis at post-mortem examination, of which more will be said in the section dealing with post-mortem findings. Visceral fowl paralysis frequently involves the ovary which is inactive, pale and granular in appearance. In this condition it is often spoken of as " tumorous," but in fact it is more correctly called an ovarian lympho-granuloma.

THE DESTRUCTION OF FOWLS

It may occasionally happen that the veterinary surgeon wishes to kill an ailing fowl and proceed immediately to a preliminary post-mortem examination, in order to obtain some idea of the nature of the disease, so that suitable preventive measures for the rest of the flock can be instituted without further delay. Such an examination may lead to a reasonably definite diagnosis, as, for example, in the case of tuberculosis or fowl paralysis. However, the value of a post-mortem examination in the field is usually not so much the establishment of a quick diagnosis, but the elimination of certain conditions. Any practitioner who proposes to perform careful autopsies on poultry should do so where facilities ensuring a more reliable diagnosis exist.

Fowls are commonly destroyed by dislocation of the neck. The legs and tips of the wings are grasped in one hand, and the other hand holds the head so that it rests between the hollow of the thumb and index finger. Bend the head back at right angles to the neck and push downwards firmly until the bones in the neck separate. Cease traction as soon as the bones are separated, otherwise the head may be pulled off. Birds frequently struggle for a short time after destruction, this being purely a reflex action.

In the case of large birds such as geese and turkeys, destruction is best done by means of a Burdizzo emasculator. With this instrument, the vertebræ can be separated and the spinal cord and jugular veins severed without breaking the skin.

POST-MORTEM TECHNIQUE

An adequate post-mortem examination of the fowl can be performed with a minimum of instruments, all that is required being a stout pair of curved scissors, a knife, a pair of dissection forceps and a pair of bone forceps. Some enamel trays and a spring balance weighing up to 15 lb. will complete the equipment. If chicks are to be examined it is useful to have a small tray filled with hard wax to which the chicks can be pinned, but nailing the wings and legs of the spread-eagled chick to a board is also quite satisfactory.

Adult fowls for post mortem should be examined to ascertain the breed, sex, weight and condition, signs of external disease or injury and whether the neck is broken or not. Externally, the comb and wattles should be examined for signs of fowl pox, typified by brown warty, often coalescing growths, the eyes should be examined, noting the colour of the iris—whether normal orange-red or pearly grey in hue—and whether the pupil is distorted or has a ragged or contracted appearance (ocular form of fowl paralysis).

The nostrils may be plugged with caseous material, and similar signs of an exudate may be found in the mouth, in the palatine cleft or attached to the tongue and entrance to the larynx. If these can be removed easily, leaving an intact mucous membrane below, the chronic form of infectious coryza is suggested, but if they strip with difficulty, leaving an ulcerated surface beneath, fowl pox is probable. Signs of ecto-parasitism are provided by dull rough plumage and lice eggs may be found attached to the base of the feathers, especially in the cloacal region. Scaly leg is characterised by crusts and hypertrophied scales on the unfeathered parts of the legs. Inflammation of the vent, with necrosis, encrustation and a foul odour is indicative of " vent gleet " or infectious cloacitis. Finally, external tumours may be found growing on almost any part of the body.

The feathers should now be damped by holding the bird under a running tap, preferably with warm water. The bird is laid on its back on the tray, and with the scissors a transverse incision is made in the loose skin just caudal to the termination of the sternal keel. The skin may now be torn away, leaving the abdominal and pectoral muscles exposed. Care should be taken not to rupture the crop at this stage. With the knife, or by manual blunt dissection, separate the fascia joining the inner aspects of the thighs to the lateral aspect of the abdominal wall and disarticulate the hip joints by pressing down on the femoro-tibial joint with the flat of the hands so that the body lies flat on the tray.

Lay open the abdomen, either by using scissors and forceps or the knife, and make two deep incisions each side in the breast muscles so that the ribs are exposed. These must now be severed with the scissors, working towards the head, and if possible by cutting through the costo-chondral junctions. The coracoids and clavicles will need to be cut with the aid of the bone forceps. The entire breast may now be lifted upward and forward, exposing the thoracic contents and the remainder of the abdominal organs.

At this stage fluid, exudate or egg material may be noticed in the abdominal cavity. Ascites in fowls is usually characterised by a straw-yellow fluid, and is commonly associated with ovarian cancer, with multiple transcœlomic implantations of tumour tissue on to the serosa of the abdominal contents.

Occasionally a cyst-like structure of variable size and containing a clear colourless fluid will be found near the posterior part of the abdominal cavity and attached by a slender cord to the cloaca. This is a persistent cystic right oviduct and is a developmental abnormality.

A yellowish exudate covering the intestine and mesentery is an indication of peritonitis, frequently a sequel to rupture of an ovarian yolk sac, with consequent liberation of yolk material into the cavity. It may also be found associated with a specific infectious disease such as typhoid. A dirty, dark, foul-smelling exudate is usually found to be due to perforation of the bowel, either by a foreign body or by rupture of an ulcerated portion.

The oviduct may be impacted with inspissated egg material, forming a large firm mass, and again, peritonitis is a frequent sequel to this condition.

Petechial hæmorrhages may be present on the visceral pericardium and in the heart muscle, and the pericardial sac may contain a small quantity of fibrinous exudate. This suggests fowl cholera, and the lungs and intestines together with the abdominal fat should be inspected to see if similar petechiæ are present in these sites. A film made from the heart blood and stained with Leishman or methylene blue will show numerous bipolar organisms (*Pasteurella aviseptica*) in a positive case, when examined with the oil immersion objective. If no organisms can be detected microscopically, consideration should be given to the possibility of poisoning by Sulpha drugs, especially Sulphaquinoxaline.

The surface of the heart and liver may be covered with a white crystalline or chalky deposit, indicating visceral gout, a sequel to nephritis, and commonly brought about by feeding an unbalanced diet containing an excess of protein. In such cases the kidneys are usually swollen, pink and the tubules are visibly engorged with creamy urates.

An enlarged mottled liver suggests leucosis, especially if the spleen and kidneys are similarly involved. The average weight of the normal liver is in the region of 50 grams, but in leucosis weights of 300 or even 500 grams are not uncommon. Discrete white tumours in the liver are indicative of lymphocytoma (lymphoid leucosis) and similar growths may be found in other viscera, although if the lungs are involved a diffuse cellular infiltration is the rule. Solid, discrete, white or yellowish growths in the lungs and in the kidney, etc. are typical of fibro-sarcoma. Such tumours are often mucinous. Erythroleucosis is characterised by a swollen bright red friable liver, spleen and kidneys, and a bright red semi-liquid bone marrow; while a blood film will show many immature red blood cells (hæmocytoblasts, etc.).

If the liver is enlarged and has a greenish or bronze sheen, and shows small necrotic foci, fowl typhoid should be suspected, especially if peritonitis is also present. Yellowish caseous nodules of varying size in the liver and spleen suggest tuberculosis and the intestines should be examined for similar lesions in the wall. A smear stained by the Ziehl-Neelsen technique and examined with the oil-immersion lens, usually shows numerous acid-fast bacilli.

Heavy mortality in turkeys, especially in the first three months, associated with weakness and a persistent yellow diarrhœa, is probably due to "blackhead" or infectious entero-hepatitis (*Hæmophilus meleagridis*). In such cases post-mortem examination reveals roughly circular, flat, dryish necrotic lesions, yellowish in appearance and somewhat depressed below the level of the liver surface. The cæca show mucosal inflammation, necrosis and occasionally caseous casts in the lumen.

Next, the alimentary tract should be removed. With forceps seize the large intestine at its termination and sever the intestine from the cloaca with scissors, pull it up and cut the mesenteric attachments. In this way the length of the intestine may be pulled out up to the duodenum. Next, reflect the liver to the left and cut through the œsophageal-proventriculus junction. Sever the attachments with the liver, taking care not to puncture the gall bladder, cut the gizzard attachments and remove the alimentary tract. Slit open the intestines with scissors and examine the mucosa for any inflammatory changes. Large round worms (*Ascaridia galli*) will be easily detected, and are often found associated with pale, flaccid intestines. Small punctate hæmorrhages may indicate an infestation with "thread worms" (*Capillaria sp.*), not easily detectable by naked eye examination, but if some of the mucoid contents of the bowel are mixed with a little water in a dish, and examined over a dark background, they may be seen as very thin threads. Small (*circa* 1-2 mm.) oblong bodies are usually tape-worm segments (*Davainea sp.*). In each of these cases microscopical examination of a smear of bowel contents diluted with a drop of water on a slide will provide immediate confirmation. *Capillaria* eggs are elongated ovals, with a polar plug at each end, and tapeworm eggs exhibit the typical hexacanth embryo. Round, pale spots are occasionally seen to be shining through the wall of the unopened gut, and a microscopical examination of a scraping from such a case usually demonstrates the oöcysts of *Eimeria necatrix*. Severe cases of coccidiosis are characterised by an intense hæmorrhagic enteritis affecting the duodenal loop and the rest of the small intestine, and in such cases oöcysts may be difficult to demonstrate, but a dried smear stained with Leishman's stain and examined with the oil-immersion lens will show many minute spindle-shaped merozoites.

Cæcal coccidiosis, due to *E. tenella*, is usually found in young chickens up to 8-10 weeks of age and only rarely in older birds. The cæca are inflamed, often dark red in colour, and in an acute case the lumen contains much free blood. Chronic cases are characterised by the presence of caseous plugs in the cæca.

The cæca may be grossly enlarged, with multiple projecting caseous abscesses in the walls, and this condition is known as chronic typhlitis. It is frequently bilateral in distribution and its etiology is uncertain. In some instances it appears to be infectious.

The gizzard should now be opened with the knife and the proventriculus slit open with scissors. Hæmorrhages in the sub-mucosa of the proventriculus are often associated with similar petechiæ in the rest of the intestinal tract and, especially if found in conjunction with pneumonia, may indicate fowl pest. In all cases where this disease is suspected, blood samples or portions of lung should be sent to the Ministry laboratories for hæmagglutination inhibition tests (see Chapter on Clinical Bacteriology, p. 333). In geese the horny gizzard lining may be found to be ulcerated and to strip easily from the underlying tissue. If the whole organ is immersed in water, the white threads of *Amidostomum sp.*, the gizzard worm, will be seen floating up with the head end embedded in the gizzard wall.

Next, slit open the upper alimentary tract, commencing at the angle of the mouth, and using scissors, continue the cut down through the pharynx and œsophagus to the crop. White pustules scattered down the length of the œsophagus indicate a vitamin A deficiency.

The crop may be found impacted with vegetable material, such as tangled grass stems or cabbage stalks, etc., and the impaction may continue down to the proventriculus and gizzard.

The trachea should now be slit open along its length and examined for caseous exudate, or hæmorrhagic mucus. In the first case infectious bronchitis is suggested, especially if broilers are involved, and the air sacs should be examined for cloudiness ; and in the second case infectious laryngo-tracheitis should be suspected.

Adult pullorum disease (*Salmonella pullorum* infection) is characterised by discoloured angular pedunculated ova in the ovary. The contents of such mis-shapen ova are frequently pasty in consistency.

If fowl paralysis is suspected, the peripheral nerves should now be examined, and indeed this should always be done as a routine measure in post-mortem examinations of young fowls up to a year of age. The vagi lie on each side of the neck, associated with the carotid artery and jugular veins, and on the right side, medial to the œsophagus. They should be of the thickness of a piece of stout thread. In paralysis cases they may show fusiform enlargements, or a general enlargement involving the whole length of the nerve. There is a normal fusiform enlargement at the base of the neck, due to a large ganglion, and this should not be confused with a fowl paralysis lesion. The brachial plexus will have been exposed already and should now be examined. The nerves are normally white and exhibit faint transverse striations. If swollen, translucent and with an absence of striation, fowl paralysis is probable. Similarly the sciatic nerve may be exposed by cutting longitudinally into the ribbon-like adductor muscle about a half-inch posterior to the femur, and what has been said regarding the appearance of the brachial nerves also applies here. The roots of the sciatic nerves should always be examined, as well as the main nerve trunk in the leg. They may be exposed by dissecting away the surrounding kidney tissue, since they pass through this organ as a lumbar plexus. Other nerves may be found to be obviously enlarged, such as the splanchnic and the intercostals, but if fowl paralysis is present in its neural form (neurolymphomatosis) then it is fairly safe to confine one's examination to the vagus, brachial plexus and sciatic nerves, as these are the most commonly affected.

Fowl paralysis lympho-granulomata occur most commonly in the ovary as a firm lobulated somewhat translucent growth, often containing many white spots about the size of a pin's head. Other organs which may be involved are the bursa of Fabricius, heart, kidney, lungs and intestines. In all such apparent tumour cases the nerves should be examined, since, when enlargements are present, an important differential diagnostic aid is afforded between lymphocytoma and the lympho-granulomata of fowl paralysis.

The kidneys may be swollen and grey in colour, due to a diffuse infiltration with lymphoid cells (lymphoid leucosis). If the convoluted tubules are very prominent and shine through the capsule, and minute white crystals are abundant, then nephritis (frequently associated with visceral gout) is present. The abdominal and thoracic air-sacs may contain a grey velvety material, indicative of pneumomycosis, caused by a mould *Aspergillus sp.*

The foregoing list of common post-mortem findings must not be assumed to be specific for the diseases mentioned. Disease is rarely constant in its manifestation, and so all pathological changes must be carefully correlated with the history, age, sex and species before a diagnosis is made, and frequently recourse to the laboratory is essential for a final diagnosis. No mention has been made of the post-mortem examination of very young chicks as in all cases it is much more satisfactory to send them straight to the laboratory.

THE PACKING OF MATERIAL FOR LABORATORY EXAMINATION

If possible, a typically affected live bird should be submitted to the laboratory. Failing this an unopened freshly dead or killed bird, securely packed in a strong cardboard box after wrapping in paper, should be sent, together with a full history of symptoms, etc. The submission of organs alone for bacteriological examination is not satisfactory, but if, *e.g.* intestines suspected of containing worms, or tumorous organs are sent, they should be placed in a 10 per cent. solution of formalin in a water-tight container and carefully packed to prevent breakage.

SPECIAL DIAGNOSTIC METHODS IN THE FIELD

Under this heading comes (a) tuberculin testing, and (b) the rapid (stained antigen) test for pullorum disease. Tuberculin testing has been dealt with in Chapter XII, which the reader should consult.

The technique of the stained antigen test is essentially very simple, and if only a few birds are to be tested occasionally, very little equipment is required. If, however, frequent large-scale testing is contemplated, it would be advisable to get special equipment such as is used by the veterinary staff of the Ministry of Agriculture and Fisheries.

All that is required for a few tests is a bottle of stained antigen, a rubber teated pipette, a spirit lamp, cotton wool, a bottle of alcohol, a stout triangular Hagedorn needle, a porcelain plate or enamel tray, a grease pencil, and a wire loop such as is used in bacteriology for inoculating cultures. The loop should be enlarged so that it can hold a fair-sized drop of blood (about 5-6 mm. diameter is sufficient).

With an attendant holding the bird to be tested, a few feathers are plucked from the inner aspect of the " elbow " joint, and the part wiped with cotton wool damped with alcohol. Sterilise the wire loop, prick the brachial vein with the needle and take up a loopful of blood and mix with a drop of antigen about the size of a shilling, previously placed on the plate or tray by means of the pipette. Mix antigen and blood thoroughly with the loop and then gently rock the plate for about half a minute.

A rapid agglutination, characterised by a granular clumping in the mixture, indicates a carrier fowl. The speed of the agglutination varies with the external temperature, and therefore testing should be done inside a building. Generally speaking, a deposit not appearing until after one minute should be disregarded or labelled " doubtful " for subsequent retest. The loop must be sterilised by flaming after every individual test. It must be remembered that carriers of fowl typhoid also react to this test as there is a cross-agglutination, and only a bacteriological examination will distinguish between the two diseases.

APPENDIX I

SYNOPSIS OF CASE RECORDING

DESCRIPTION OF PATIENT.—Species, breed, sex, age.

OWNER'S COMPLAINT.

HISTORY OF CASE.—Past history. Immediate history.

SYMPTOMS AND PRELIMINARY GENERAL EXAMINATION OF PATIENT.—General appearance. Behaviour. Expression. Bodily condition. Condition of skin and coat. Rate and character of respirations. Appearance of abdomen. Posture. Gait. Abnormal acts. Visible mucous membranes. Eye. External surfaces of the body. Pulse. Temperature.

CLINICAL SIGNS ARISING FROM SYSTEMS OF THE BODY.—Digestive system and abdomen. Respiratory system. Circulatory system. Urinary system. Nervous system. Skin. Lymphatic system. Sense organs. Genitalia. Locomotor system.

SPECIAL DIAGNOSTIC PROCEDURES.

DIAGNOSIS, DIFFERENTIAL DIAGNOSIS AND ETIOLOGY.

PROGNOSIS.

TREATMENT.

PROGRESS OF CASE.

TERMINATION.

POST-MORTEM EXAMINATION.

DISCUSSION.

REFERENCES.

APPENDIX II

SCHEDULED DISEASES IN GREAT BRITAIN

Under the Diseases of Animals Act 1950 orders are made in respect of certain contagious and infectious diseases of animals, the diseases in respect of which these orders are made being known as the diseases scheduled under the Act. The term notifiable disease is sometimes applied to the diseases so scheduled because of the obligation imposed on any veterinary surgeon who encounters a case or suspected case of such diseases to notify the existence of it to the police when the order in respect of the diseases requires notifying.

Some of the scheduled diseases have not occurred in Great Britain for some time and the purpose of maintaining an order in force is to provide legal sanction for the methods required to prevent their re-introduction.

The diseases still occurring in Great Britain in respect of which notification is required are :—

Anthrax
Foot and Mouth Disease
Swine Fever
Atrophic Rhinitis of Swine
Certain forms of Bovine Tuberculosis

(The forms of bovine tuberculosis that must be notified are tuberculosis of the udder, tuberculous emaciation, chronic cough with definite clinical signs of tuberculosis and animals excreting or discharging tuberculous material. As a result of the successful campaign to eradicate bovine tuberculosis from Great Britain the notification of cases of bovine tuberculosis will soon be a thing of the past).

Fowl pest is notifiable but not to the police ; the owner or veterinary surgeon is required to notify the suspected presence of disease to the Veterinary Laboratory of the Ministry of Agriculture, and the owner is also required to send the carcase of the bird to the laboratory. Fowl pest includes fowl plague and Newcastle disease.

The diseases no longer occurring in Great Britain but of which notification of cases or suspected cases is still required should the disease be re-introduced are :—

Cattle Plague (Rinderpest)
Glanders or Farcy
Epizootic Lymphangitis

402

Parasitic Mange (Sarcoptic and Psoroptic only) of Horses, Asses
  and Mules
Contagious Bovine Pleuro-Pneumonia
Rabies
Sheep Scab
Sheep Pox

For further information in regard to the control of diseases of animals
in Great Britain the reader should refer to the Handbook of Orders
Relating to Diseases of Animals published by H.M. Stationery Office,
London.

APPENDIX III

INCUBATION PERIODS

The accurate estimation of the incubation periods of infective and contagious diseases is, under field conditions, somewhat difficult. The exact time of infection cannot always be determined, and the onset of the symptoms may be so gradual that the precise time when the incubation period ended cannot be stated accurately.

In diseases which are acute and show a sudden onset of characteristic symptoms, the incubation period can be stated with some precision, but even in such diseases the infecting agent may vary in its virulence. An animal may have a natural or acquired resistance to a particular infection, and where the immunity is not sufficient to prevent establishment of disease it may suffice to prolong the period before the onset of symptoms. In the more insidious diseases, the disease process may be established long before the symptoms of disease occur ; as, for instance, in tuberculosis, where a lesion may be demonstrated at about three weeks after infection although the particular animal may never exhibit symptoms of disease. Again, the time of onset of symptoms may be conditioned by the route or site through which infection gained access to the body. In certain diseases, the causal agent, though present, does not become active without the intervention of some activating agent. In diseases carried by an insect the occurrence of infection is dependent on the activity of the vector ; if the disease can be transmitted artificially the incubation period so determined may be used to assess the probable time of natural infection.

In most diseases some assistance in determining the incubation period may be obtained by a study of the events following experimental infection. It must, however, be realised that the conditions prevailing for natural infection are not entirely comparable to those associated with the artificial production of a disease. Under experimental conditions a lethal or definitely infective dose of the causal agent is directly introduced into the body, whereas under field conditions much smaller doses may be acquired, and the variety of other factors already mentioned have to be considered. It is necessary that the incubation period quoted for any disease should extend sufficiently to cover all reasonable, contingencies, but in some diseases, while a wide range must be given, it can often be claimed that the commonly experienced incubation period falls within much narrower time limits.

ACUTE CONTAGIOUS AND INFECTIVE DISEASES

Disease	Range	Average	Remarks
Anthrax . . .	Not more than 10 days	...	Usually very short
Distemper canine . .	3-7 days	4 days	...
Foot and mouth disease .	2-10 days	48-72 hours	Shorter period more usual
Influenza equine . .	3-10 days	4 days	...
Influenza piglet . .	10-14 days	...	...
Pleuropneumonia, contagious bovine	1-3 weeks	2 weeks	Onset very insidious
Pustular dermatitis, contagious . . .	4-7 days	...	...
Rabies canine . .	9 days-15 months	1-2 months	...
Rabies equine and bovine	9 days-15 months	1-3 months	...
Rinderpest . .	3-9 days	...	...
Strangles . . .	3-8 days	...	...
Swine erysipelas . .	1-5 days	3-5 days	...
Swine fever . . .	5-10 days	...	...
Tetanus . . .	1 day-3 weeks	4-15 days	...
Variola ovina . .	Virulent 2-7 days Benign 10-20 days	...	...
Variola vaccinia . .	3-6 days	...	...

CHRONIC DISEASES WITH AN INDEFINITE SUBCLINICAL STAGE

The presence of an established infection in the body is probable after the period stated, during which period the capacity to react to an allergic test will have developed.

Disease	Range	Average	Remarks
Glanders . . .	1-3 months	1 month	...
Johne's disease . .	1-3 months	1 month	Clinical signs seldom seen in less than 18 months
Tuberculosis . .	1-3 months	1 month	The appearance of clinical signs may be indefinitely delayed.

DISEASES WITH AN UNDEFINABLE INCUBATION PERIOD

Blackquarter and braxy are diseases which are dependent for their development on the action of some exciting factor, consequently it is impossible to state an incubation period for these diseases.

The disease of sheep, louping-ill, is transmitted by an insect vector *Ixodes ricinus* ; the incubation period following subcutaneous injection of virus is from seven to fourteen days, following experimental tick infestation from eight to eighteen days. (Data supplied by Dr D. R. Wilson, Moredun Institute, Gilmerton, Midlothian.)

In the disease of sheep known as scrapie, and thought to be due to a virus, the incubation period is known from clinical experience to be at least eighteen months.

In parasitic mange the incubation period is very variable as the disease may remain dormant for a very long time. Following massive infections in susceptible animals, lesions may be demonstrable in fourteen days.

INDEX

PRINTED IN GREAT BRITAIN BY OLIVER AND BOYD LTD., EDINBURGH